LITTLE, BROWN'S PAPERBACK BOOK SERIES

Basic Medical Sciences

Boyd & Hoerl	Basic Medical Microbiology
Colton	Statistics in Medicine
Hine & Pfeiffer	Behavioral Science
Kent	General Pathology: A Programmed Text
Levine	Pharmacology
Peery & Miller	Pathology
Richardson	Basic Circulatory Physiology
Roland et al.	Atlas of Cell Biology
Selkurt	Physiology
Sidman & Sidman	Neuroanatomy: A Programmed Text
Siegel, Albers, et al.	Basic Neurochemistry
Snell	Clinical Anatomy for Medical Students
Snell	Clinical Embryology for Medical Students
Streilein & Hughes	Immunology: A Programmed Text
Valtin	Renal Function
Watson	Basic Human Neuroanatomy

Clinical Medical Sciences

Clark & MacMahon	Preventive Medicine
Daube et al.	Medical Neurosciences
Eckert	Emergency-Room Care
Grabb & Smith	Plastic Surgery
Green	Gynecology
Gregory & Smeltzer	Psychiatry
Judge & Zuidema	Methods of Clinical Examination
MacAusland & Mayo	Orthopedics
Nardi & Zuidema	Surgery
Niswander	Obstetrics
Thompson	Primer of Clinical Radiology
Wilkins & Levinsky	Medicine
Ziai	Pediatrics

Manuals and Handbooks

Alpert & Francis	Manual of Coronary Care
Arndt	Manual of Dermatologic Therapeutics
Berk et al.	Handbook of Critical Care
Bochner et al.	Handbook of Clinical Pharmacology
Children's Hospital Medical Center, Boston	Manual of Pediatric Therapeutics
Condon & Nyhus	Manual of Surgical Therapeutics
Friedman & Papper	Problem-Oriented Medical Diagnosis
Gardner & Provine	Manual of Acute Bacterial Infections
Iversen & Clawson	Manual of Orthopaedic Therapeutics
Massachusetts General Hospital	Clinical Anesthesia Procedures
Massachusetts General Hospital	Diet Manual
Massachusetts General Hospital	Manual of Nursing Procedures
Neelon & Ellis	A Syllabus of Problem-Oriented Patient Care
Papper	Manual of Medical Care of the Surgical Patient
Shader	Manual of Psychiatric Therapeutics
Snow	Manual of Anesthesia
Spivak & Barnes	Manual of Clinical Problems in Internal Medicine: Annotated with Key References
Wallach	Interpretation of Diagnostic Tests
Washington University Department of Medicine	Manual of Medical Therapeutics
Zimmerman	Techniques of Patient Care

Little, Brown and Company
34 Beacon Street
Boston, Massachusetts 02106

*Handbook
of
Clinical
Pharmacology*

Felix Bochner, M.D., F.R.A.C.P.

Senior Lecturer in Medicine,
University of Queensland, Brisbane, Australia

George Carruthers, M.D., M.R.C.P. (U.K.),
F.R.C.P. (C.)

Assistant Professor of Medicine and
Honorary Lecturer in Pharmacology,
University of Western Ontario,
London, Ontario, Canada

Jens Kampmann, M.D.

Research Associate,
Clinical Pharmacology Research Unit,
University of Copenhagen, Copenhagen, Denmark

Janice Steiner, M.B., B.S., F.R.A.C.P.

Lecturer in Clinical Pharmacology,
Medical Research Council Clinical Pharmacology Unit,
Radcliffe Infirmary, Oxford, England

With an introductory chapter by

Daniel L. Azarnoff, M.D.

Distinguished Professor of Medicine and of Pharmacology,
and Director, Division of Clinical Pharmacology,
University of Kansas College of Health Sciences and
Hospital School of Medicine, Kansas City, Kansas

Little, Brown and Company, Boston

Handbook
of
Clinical
Pharmacology

Contents

11. *Drug Profiles* 87

In the following list the terms given in capital letters are subtitles within this chapter.

*Not presently available in the United States.

*Not presently available in the United States.

Preface

*P*roliferation of drug information represents only one aspect of the rapid growth of medical knowledge. Numerous studies of therapeutic indications, pharmacokinetics, and pharmacodynamics appear in the scientific literature and ultimately in textbooks, advertising literature, and circulars from drug information services and regulating agencies. However, this wealth of information often loses value by reason of its inaccessibility in circumstances of greatest relevance, such as in the assessment or treatment of a sick patient at the bedside or in the office.

Acutely aware of this difficulty and frustrated by the lack of a convenient source of "hard" data, we began to collect, evaluate, and tabulate the available data on commonly used drugs. The concept of this book was that it would be a readily available, informative source that would help solve many frequently posed problems, such as the adjustments of drug dosage in patients with renal and hepatic disease and the potential adverse effects and possible interactions of these drugs with other medications. Since we were then involved in research and were concerned with teaching clinical pharmacology and therapeutics to the medical and allied professions at the University of Kansas School of Medicine and at our home institutions, we believed it was also important to provide some relevant referencing of the primary literature for those seriously interested in gaining an in-depth knowledge of a particular drug. We trust that the description of each drug will answer most of the questions that are asked and that the references will permit the interested reader to evaluate related literature more easily. The chapters on the use of drugs in specific clinical conditions and age groups and on the definition of many of the terms commonly used in the clinical pharmacology literature should provide general background information and encourage more meaningful reading of the literature.

The fundamental goal of the book is the development of a critical and rational approach to the prescribing of drugs. It is commonly accepted that modern therapeutic efforts fall somewhat short of diagnostic accuracy, a failure that unfortunately may negate diagnostic excellence. We hope that this handbook will promote improved use of drugs through a better appreciation of their activity, and that the format of this text will lead to frequent, convenient consultation.

F. B.
G. C.
J. K.
J. S.

Acknowledgments

*W*e thank the sponsoring agencies that made it possible for us to undertake fellowships in clinical pharmacology at the University of Kansas School of Medicine. Felix Bochner was a Clinical Sciences Fellow of the National Health and Medical Research Council of Australia. George Carruthers was a Fogarty International Fellow of the United States National Institutes of Health from the Queen's University and Belfast City Hospital, Northern Ireland. Jens Kampmann was the recipient of a Merck Sharp & Dohme International Fellowship in Clinical Pharmacology from The Merck Company Foundation, Rahway, New Jersey. Janice Steiner received a traveling fellowship of the Postgraduate Medical Committee of the University of Sydney, Camperdown, New South Wales, Australia.

We are grateful to all our colleagues for their encouragement. In particular we thank Isami Shudo, M.D., for help in the early stages of preparation and Danny Shen, Ph.D., John Straughan, M.D., and Jim Hosler, M.D., for their valuable comments. Harry Shirkey, M.D., Visiting Professor of Pediatrics from Tulane University, New Orleans, Louisiana, provided helpful remarks on dosage adjustments for children.

The assistance of Roxanne Hackler and Debbie Waring, who typed the manuscript, and the additional secretarial help of Mary Witthaus, Patti Wolters, and Dorothy Howard are acknowledged with deep gratitude.

Our special thanks go to Daniel L. Azarnoff, M.D., Distinguished Professor of Medicine and of Pharmacology at the University of Kansas, for all his help and guidance. In addition, Dr. Azarnoff has written a chapter on rational drug therapy that provides a stimulating introduction to the text.

Finally, we thank Lin Richter and the staff of Little, Brown and Company for their expert advice and assistance at all stages of manuscript preparation.

*Handbook
of
Clinical
Pharmacology*

Notice

The indications and dosages of all drugs in this **Handbook** have been recommended in the medical literature and conform to standards generally acceptable in medical practice. The medications described do not necessarily have specific approval by the Food and Drug Administration for use in the diseases and dosages for which they are recommended. The package insert for each drug should be consulted for use and dosage as approved by the FDA. Because standards for usage change, it is advisable to keep abreast of revised recommendations, particularly those concerning new drugs.

Do We Achieve Rational Drug Therapy?

Daniel L. Azarnoff

I

It has been estimated that the cost of drugs was 9.3% of the $104.2 billion spent on health care in the United States in 1974 [8]. However, the percentage is greater, since unwarranted adverse reactions to drugs contribute to the cost included in the remaining 90%. Economic losses estimated in the billions of dollars due to illness and even death brought about by today's potent drugs add further to the expense.

Stedman's Medical Dictionary [21] defines rational therapy as a plan of treatment of disease based on the correct interpretation of the symptoms and a knowledge of the physiological action of the remedy. In other words, the physician must make the correct diagnosis and understand the pathophysiology of the disorder before deciding whether or not to treat a patient with a drug. If the answer is affirmative (and it definitely should not always be), the physician should know enough about drugs to select the right one and to administer it by the right route in the right amount at the right intervals for the right length of time. In addition, the physician must be aware of the potential for interactions with environmental, genetic, and disease-related factors. In general, physicians make the correct diagnosis with a reasonable degree of accuracy, but I am less sure that we are familiar with the pathophysiology of the disorder or the pharmacology of the drugs.

Irrational Drug Prescribing

Evidence of irrational prescribing by physicians is not difficult to find. Based on pharmaceutic production data, the consumption of prescription drugs in the United States has been estimated to have doubled over the past 10 years [20]. The average practitioner now writes about 8000 prescriptions per year. In 1975, greater than five prescriptions per capita were written in Australia, whereas from 1961 to 1971 approximately three per capita were written [24]. One must wonder if this 60% increase is the result of a more sickly population in 1975 or if the population is 60% or even 10% healthier as a result of increased drug usage. I doubt that either is true. In patients matched for age, sex, and illness, American physicians used almost 4 times as many drugs for the specific and nonspecific treatment of a variety of illnesses as did their Scottish counterparts [13]. As might be expected, the incidence of adverse effects was significantly higher in the American patients. Although it was not possible to obtain outcome results, there is no evidence that the Scottish patients were getting poorer care or were in poorer health. A review of prescribing

behavior revealed that two-thirds of all outpatient physician en-
counters resulted in the writing of at least one prescription [14].
We must ask ourselves whether these prescriptions were warranted or were used only to get rid of the patient. The ten most
common indications for a prescription drug were insomnia, pain,
constipation, anxiety, congestive heart failure, blood clotting,
preoperative medication, bronchospasm, infection, and nausea.
Described even in generous terms, we appear to be a nation of
constipated, infected, wheezing, nauseated, anxious, throm-
bophlebitic insomniacs with failing hearts.

In an evaluation of physicians' prescribing habits, it was found
that for more than 40% of prescriptions issued, the prescriber
expected only a "hopeful" or "possible" value in patients with
trivial conditions [15]. Greater than 90% of physicians in one
community wrote one or more prescriptions for the common
cold; 60% were for antibiotics or sulfonamides despite their
known ineffectivness for this condition. Unwarranted and irrational use by physicians of dangerous drugs, such as chloramphenicol, has also been documented [18]. Even though safety
may not be a factor, irrational prescribing has been documented
in a study in which it was estimated that in Great Britain vitamin
B_{12} usage was at least 4 times greater than the actual need [3].
Such irrational prescribing, if nothing else, adds to the cost of
medical care.

Even after making the proper diagnosis and properly selecting
and prescribing a drug, inadequate attention to the patient may
still preclude satisfactory drug utilization. A significant number of
patients never have their prescriptions filled and, even if they do,
do not take the medication as directed by the physician [1]. At least
in part, inadequate communication between the physician and
patient is also responsible for this lack of compliance and breakdown in rational therapy.

Can physicians be utilizing drugs rationally when they continue
to prescribe drugs in a manner that contradicts the current evidence? Why do the sales of sulfonylureas continue to rise when
the University Group Diabetes Program (UGDP) study indicates
they are of no benefit in the maturity onset diabetic and may
hasten the onset of cardiovascular mortality [22]? Why are hormones still prescribed for the prevention of miscarriages or as a
test for pregnancy despite the lack of evidence that they are
effective for these indications and may produce birth defects [5,
9]? Why do we continue to prescribe clofibrate for the hyper-
lipidemic male patient with a previous myocardial infarction
when this drug was demonstrated to be ineffective in preventing
further cardiovascular morbidity and mortality in the Coronary
Drug Project [4]? In fact, a significant increase in the incidence of
thrombophlebitis, pulmonary embolus, and gallstones in patients
receiving clofibrate was well documented in this study.

I believe we must conclude from these observations that drug
therapy is not optimum. Rational drug therapy can no longer be
based on a memorized schedule of dosage and contraindications.
Drugs no longer are the herbals of yesteryear with questionable
pharmacological activity; rather, they are potent chemicals with a
potential for extensive harm as well as good. The practicing

physician is certainly not ignorant, negligent, nor unconcerned; he is busy and harried, working many hours per week. Importantly, however, he spends, on an average, less than 20 minutes a day reading the drug-related medical literature, which, unfortunately, is all too frequently inaccurate, irrelevant, unavailable, or misleading.

In considering the reasons for the lack of optimal drug therapy, we can classify drug-prescribing abuses [19] and perhaps identify the causes.

Overprescribing

Overprescribing exists when the drug is not needed or is given in a dose that is too large, for a period that is too long, or in a quantity that is too great for the patient's immediate needs. One cause of overprescribing is the use of drugs, such as sedatives, as a means of alleviating the patient's complaints when actually more complex solutions are required. The physician frequently uses the prescription as a means of terminating the visit. In a comparison of physicians and nurse practitioners it was found that after 1 year there was an increase in the use of vitamins and tonics (self-administered to some extent) in the physician-treated group of patients, whereas the use of tranquilizers and sedatives significantly decreased in the group followed by the nurses [2]. Could the difference be that the nurse practitioners took the time to talk to the patients?

Another cause of overprescribing is the desire to guarantee that everything possible that can be done has been done. This approach has been called by Kunin [11] the use of "drugs of fear," i.e., agents that help the physician resolve his own fear of failing to give the patient what he believes is the very best drug. Patients may also be responsible for the physician's overprescribing when they imply they have not received adequate attention unless they receive a prescription, or when they apply pressure to obtain a prescription that the physician would not ordinarily give. The prescribing of an antibiotic for a viral upper respiratory infection is a good example of this type of pressure. The physician assumes that, if he does not prescribe the antibiotic, the patient will go to another doctor who will prescribe it, so he may as well.

Underprescribing

Underprescribing is the failure to prescribe a required medication, such as a drug to lower blood pressure in a hypertensive patient. Inadequate dosage or administration for too brief a period also falls in this category. The reasons for this type of abuse include overemphasis on the risk of a useful drug, a skepticism about the efficacy of a drug for a particular indication, or a bad experience with a few patients in one's own practice.

Incorrect Prescribing

Incorrect prescribing occurs when the drug is given for the incorrect diagnosis, when the wrong drug is selected for the indication, or when the prescription is prepared improperly. Physicians' illegible handwriting is legendary.

Incorrect prescribing also occurs when a physician is not aware of or forgets that genetic and environmental factors or the disease per se may alter the patient's response to a drug. For example, cigarette-smoking may markedly accelerate the rate of elimination of a variety of drugs [17, 23]; low plasma albumin concentrations, as found in patients with the nephrotic syndrome, are associated with an increased fraction of unbound clofibrate and phenytoin, but the steady-state concentration of the unbound drug is not altered because of compensatory changes [7]; and downward dosage adjustments are necessary in patients with portacaval shunts who receive drugs with a significant first-pass effect [6].

An adverse response, such as a skin rash, is obvious to the physician and the patient, but the prevention of a satisfactory response, which is common, is much less readily discernible. Both may be the result of incorrect prescribing. For example, the "usual" dose of theophylline may not control bronchospasm in the patient who smokes due to induction of theophylline metabolism [10], whereas inhibition of phenytoin metabolism by isoniazid may result in ataxia in patients previously showing no signs of toxicity from the same dose. The latter is most likely to occur in patients who are slow acetylators of isoniazid [12]. In this instance, the drug interaction becomes clinically significant only in individuals with certain genetic determinants.

Multiple Prescribing

Abuses caused by multiple prescribing may occur when the patient visits and receives prescriptions from more than one physician, when the patient uses nonprescription drugs along with prescription drugs, or when the physician does not withdraw one drug before starting another or prescribes a brand-name product that contains several different drugs. In such instances the physician often forgets or is not aware that he is prescribing more than one active drug. The latter, as well as other examples, provides a cogent reason for prescribing only by generic name. If it is preferred or is necessary to prescribe a specific manufacturer's product, the generic name can be written first on the prescription, followed by that of the manufacturer.

Achieving Rational Drug Therapy

Today, healthy individuals as well as those who are chronically ill may receive drugs for long periods of time. Therefore, it behooves us to eliminate unwarranted drug utilization. What is required to accomplish this goal? I believe we need several approaches:

1 Improve and extend education about the rational use of drugs, starting in medical school and continuing throughout the practitioner's career. An educational program on rational uses of digitalis was undertaken for the house staff at a Montreal hospital. Simply emphasizing the importance of body weight and renal function when prescribing loading and maintenance doses of digoxin reduced the incidence of toxicity in this hospital from 21.4% to 12.3% over a 2-year period [16].

2 Reduce both the blatant and insidious pressures from patients and commercial sources that coerce the practitioner to increase drug utilization.

3 Provide sources of unbiased information about drugs.

4 Inculcate in the physician the realization that the selection and rational use of drugs is certainly as, and possibly even more, intellectually stimulating and rewarding than making the correct diagnosis.

Once the correct diagnosis is established, we must decide whether or not drug therapy is warranted. Frequently it is not. We must remember that the designation of a drug as safe and effective by a regulatory agency means only that the drug is statistically better than a placebo. *Statistically better* may mean better by only a few percentage points and be of little, if any, clinical consequence. Would you use a drug for a minor symptom if you knew the chance of producing a desirable effect was only 1 in 20? Some of us probably do.

Next we should set realistic goals by asking ourselves, "What am I trying to accomplish by administering this drug?" The goals should be both short- and long-term. For example, a short-term goal in treating diabetes mellitus would be control of the patient's blood sugar and a long-term goal would be prevention of retinopathy and nephropathy. End points should be defined to monitor both efficacy and toxicity. To do this, the relevant physiological, biochemical, behavioral, and physical characteristics should be measured at appropriate intervals. The patient's condition is not static. Therefore, we must continually review our treatment regimen and make any changes that are necessary by alterations in the patient's disease or response. All too often we prescribe a drug, such as digitalis for congestive heart failure, and years later the patient is still taking the drug at the same dosage originally prescribed. In the interim we have given little if any consideration to whether or not the use or initial dosage of this drug is still appropriate.

I have briefly set forth my views on the current status of drug therapy and made several broad suggestions for improvement. A major need is for nonbiased drug information. You may imagine my pleasure when the authors of this book informed me that they were gathering and critically reviewing the pharmacokinetic data available for many of the most commonly used drugs. As well-trained internists as well as clinical pharmacologists, Drs. Bochner, Carruthers, Kampmann, and Steiner are well qualified for this undertaking. For months I watched them put the information they gathered to use at the bedside of many patients. Soon it became obvious that their colleagues could also use the information profitably and, so, this book.

We should all strive to maximize the rational use of drugs, not rationalize the maximal use of drugs. This book will be a great help.

References

1 Blackwell, B.   The drug defaulter. *Clin. Pharmacol. Ther.* 13:841–848, 1972.
2 Chaiton, A., Spitzer, W. O., et al.   Patterns of drug use. A community focus. *Can. Med. Assoc. J.* 114:33–37, 1976.
3 Cochrane, A. L., and Moore, F.   Expected and observed values for the prescription of vitamin B_{12} in England and Wales. *Br. J. Prev. Soc. Med.* 25:147–151, 1971.
4 Coronary Drug Project Research Group. Clofibrate and niacin in coronary heart disease. *J.A.M.A.* 231:360–381, 1975.
5 Dieckmann, W. J., Davis, M. E., et al.   Does the administration of diethylstilbestrol during pregnancy have therapeutic value? *Am. J. Obstet. Gynecol.* 66:1062–1075, 1953.
6 Gugler, R., Lain, P., et al.   Effect of portacaval shunt on the disposition of drugs with and without first pass effect. *J. Pharmacol. Exp. Ther.* 195:416–423, 1975.
7 Gugler, R., Shoeman, D. W., et al.   Pharmacokinetics of drugs in patients with the nephrotic syndrome. *J. Clin. Invest.* 55:1182–1189, 1975.
8 *Health in the United States (1975).* (A chartbook: Department of Health, Education and Welfare publication [HRA] 76-1233.) Washington, D.C.: U.S. Government Printing Office, 1976.
9 Herbst, A. L., Poskanzer, D. C., et al.   Prenatal exposure to stilbestrol. A prospective comparison of exposed female offspring with unexposed controls. *N. Engl. J. Med.* 231:360–381, 1975.
10 Hunt, S. N., Jusko, W. J., et al.   Effect of smoking on theophylline disposition. *Clin. Pharmacol. Ther.* 19:546–551, 1976.
11 Kunin, C. M.   Use of antibiotics. A brief exposition of the problem and some tentative solutions. *Ann. Intern. Med.* 79:555–560, 1973.
12 Kutt, H., Brennan, R., et al.   Diphenylhydantoin intoxication. A complication of isoniazid therapy. *Am. Rev. Resp. Dis.* 101:377–384, 1970.
13 Lawson, D. H., and Jick, H.   Drug prescribing in hospitals. An international comparison. *Am. J. Public Health* 66:644–648, 1976.
14 *National Disease and Therapeutic Index.* (Reference File, Diagnosis, July 1967–June 1968.) Ambler, Pa.: Lea Assoc. 1968.
15 *National Disease and Therapeutic Index.* (Reference File, Diagnosis, The common cold, October 1967–September 1968.) Ambler, Pa.: Lea Assoc., 1968.
16 Ogilvie, R. I., and Ruedy, J.   An educational program in digitalis therapy. *J.A.M.A.* 222:50–55, 1972.

17 Pantuck, E. J., Kuntzman, R., et al. Decreased concentration of phenacetin in plasma of cigarette smokers. *Science* 175:1248–1250, 1972.

18 Ray, W. A., Federspiel, C.F., et al. Prescribing of chloramphenicol in ambulatory practice. *Ann. Intern. Med.* 84:266–270, 1976.

19 Report by Working Party 1975, Council of Europe, European Public Health Community. Abuses of medicines. II. Prescription medicines. *Drug Intel. Clin. Pharm.* 10:94–110, 1976.

20 Rucker, D. T. Drug use. Data, sources and limitations. *J.A.M.A.* 230:880–890, 1974.

21 *Stedman's Medical Dictionary* (23rd ed). Baltimore: Williams & Wilkins, 1976.

22 The University Group Diabetes Program. A study of hypoglycemic agents on vascular complications in patients with adult-onset diabetes. II. Mortality results. *Diabetes* 19 (Suppl. 2):789–830, 1970.

23 Vaughn, D. P., and Beckett, A. H. The influence of smoking on the intersubject variation in pentazocine elimination. *Br. J. Clin. Pharmacol.* 3:279–283, 1976.

24 Wade, D. N. The background pattern of drug usage in Australia. *Clin. Pharmacol. Ther.* 19:651–656, 1976.

Drug Information: A Means to Improve Prescribing

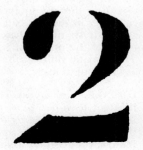

Appropriate therapy is the logical extension of a correct diagnosis. Treatment with medicines forms a unique bond for most efforts to relieve suffering and eradicate disease. In modern clinical practice an extensive array of drugs is prescribed and vast quantities of medicine are consumed. There is little doubt that many patients experience improvement in health as a result of this effort, but many derive little or no benefit, while others suffer the additional problems of drug-induced side-effects and diseases.

The bizarre drug interaction, like the unusual physical sign or clinical syndrome, excites enormous interest. The majority of problems with drugs are, unfortunately, not associated with the dramatic or unusual but with common medications used in the treatment of common diseases.

Prescribing difficulties are of two main types: (1) *qualitative,* in which the therapeutic agent is inappropriate in terms of its efficacy or the benefit-risk ratio is insufficient to merit its use, and (2) *quantitative,* in which an appropriate drug is applied in inadequate or potentially toxic doses.

The factor of cost should also be considered. The patient may be put to the discomfort and expense of an unnecessarily extensive or complicated regimen, a treatment schedule that is inadequate for his disease, or a schedule that further aggravates his disordered health. There is the additional expense of increased consultation, prolonged hospitalization, and lost working time while his original disease is treated inappropriately or inadequately and his drug-induced disorders are evaluated.

In summary, the patient's life may be impoverished in quality and diminished in duration by inappropriate, inadequate, or excessive use of medications.

Clinical pharmacology is a discipline that seeks to improve the art of drug therapy by increasing our knowledge of drugs and their value in disease. Such knowledge cannot be applied in a vacuum. It should be based on a sound diagnosis and a clear concept of the underlying physiological derangement.

Therapeutic skill can be developed by repeatedly posing the following questions:

What is the basic diagnosis?
What are the defects in normal physiology?
What is the rational drug (or nondrug) *therapy?*
What can reasonably be expected from drugs, considering the natural progression, remission, and variation of the disease?

How will improvement be assessed? Subjectively by the patient, subjectively by the clinician, or by some objective measurements?
How long will treatment be pursued (an acute crisis, a chronic disorder, lifetime maintenance)?

These are the conscious or unconscious decisions that formulate a prescription. Failure to pose the questions, even if they cannot be adequately answered, leads at best to vagueness and at worst to negligence in therapeutic decision-making.

Two further specific questions remain:

What is the appropriate dose, considering the nature and severity of disease, intercurrent illness, age, and weight?
What are the potential problems (side-effects, toxicity, interactions with concurrent medications, including nonprescription medicines and social drugs, especially alcohol)?

The last questions have been posed separately, since they represent the major contribution in recent years of advances in clinical pharmacology. The concept that all patients with the same disease do not require equal doses of medicine has long been recognized. It is hoped that the reasons for this variation are gradually being appreciated and will lead to improved standards of therapeutics.

The aim of this book is the improved use of medicines through a rational appreciation of the action of drugs on disease and of the diseased body on drugs.

To encourage familiarity with these aspects of drugs and illness, the text has been kept brief, the style didactic, and the outlines of individual drugs consistent. The definition of terms (Chapter 10) should assist the reader to comprehend the complexities behind the apparently simple act of swallowing a tablet or receiving an injection. Chapter 10 and the chapters on specific prescribing problems in childhood, old age, pregnancy, lactation, renal disease, and liver disease are designed to help clarify and elaborate specific statements in the descriptions of individual agents and to increase the reader's awareness of drug dynamics and kinetics.

In considering more than 100 common medications, an attempt was made to be as comprehensive as possible. Nevertheless, there must necessarily be omissions. Some drugs have been excluded because their use is restricted to small specialized units (this is not to detract from their clinical importance). Certain drugs are excluded or are categorized within a group because they are "me-too" agents that all too often produce little advantage over their predecessors. Other drugs have been excluded either because their therapeutic effects are marginal or because their benefit-risk ratios are disproportionate to other available agents. For the reader who is disappointed at the absence of his favorite medication, the development of a profile for that drug could be a valuable exercise.

Trade names have been omitted; when patents exist there is usually only one trade name anyway. When there is more than one trade name the clinician should evaluate cost-effectiveness, dosage forms, and bioavailability, if relevant, and he or she may choose to make a note of this information beside the generic name for ease of reference.

The profile of each drug adheres to a consistent, logical pattern composed of the following information (listed in the order in which it is discussed):

1 Introduction
2 Absorption
3 Distribution
4 Elimination
5 Dosage schedule
6 Special dosage situations
7 Therapeutic concentrations
8 Adverse reactions
9 Interactions
10 Reviews and references

Introduction

The introductory paragraph provides a general outline of the chemical, pharmacological, or therapeutic group to which the drug belongs, a brief description of its pharmacological activity, and its major clinical indications. This information should provide some sense of the scope of activity of the drug, including potential limits of usefulness and the nature of possible toxicity.

Absorption

It is an essential feature of an oral drug which is expected to act systemically that it is absorbed from the gastrointestinal tract and that it reaches the systemic circulation in a form which is therapeutically active. Certain simple corollaries follow: if a drug is not absorbed it cannot act systemically; if absorption is poor, oral doses must greatly exceed parenteral doses; if absorption is slow, the effect may be delayed; if absorption is unduly fast, side-effects associated with high levels may occur soon after dosage; if absorption is erratic, clinical effects may be unpredictable. Oral absorption depends on disintegration of the preparation, dissolution of the active drug, transfer across the gastrointestinal tract wall, and passage through the portal vein to the liver. The drug must then pass in the hepatic veins to the systemic circulation.

It is increasingly appreciated that some drugs do not easily pass the gut wall because of their polarity, solubility, or formulation. This is a problem of drug absorption. Other drugs may undergo extensive metabolism on their first exposure to enzymes in the gut wall or the liver, so that little, if any, active drug remains for systemic activity—the so-called first-pass effect. These are factors that affect the systemic bioavailability of a drug or specific preparation, that is, the fraction of the swallowed dose that eventually appears in the systemic circulation. It has become clear that differences in absorption may be caused by the variation in formulation among different manufacturers and occasionally between batches of the same manufacturer. These points are mentioned under specific drugs, if relevant.

Distribution

Drugs bind to plasma proteins and pass to extracellular fluids and body tissues to a variable extent. The volume of distribution (V_d) is a hypothetical volume, but its magnitude gives some concept of the extent to which a drug is taken up by tissues other than plasma. When the apparent volume of distribution of a drug is very large, e.g., digoxin (5–7 L/kg), it should be appreciated that some tissues have a great avidity for digoxin and that plasma concentrations will be very small. Indeed, it is known that skeletal muscle, which accounts for 30–50% of total body weight, has digoxin levels 10–20 times greater than plasma, while cardiac muscle levels may be 30–60 times greater than plasma. Plasma concentrations of digoxin are of the order of 1 nanogram (ng = 10^{-9} g) per milliliter. When the volume of distribution is small, e.g., gentamicin (0.25 L/kg), most of the drug remains in plasma, although there is clearly sufficient permeation of infected tissues to exert a bactericidal effect. Concentrations of gentamicin in plasma are therefore relatively higher than those of digoxin, even allowing for dosage differences, i.e., several micrograms (μg = 10^{-6} g) per milliliter.

Specific physiological distribution of drugs in man has not been extensively studied for obvious reasons, although some autopsy and biopsy data have been assessed. When data concerning the distribution of drugs into milk, psychotropic agents into brain or cerebrospinal fluid, cardiovascular drugs into the heart or blood vessels, and antibiotics into cerebrospinal fluid, bile, urine, or joint spaces are known, the information is given under the specific drug.

Protein binding is a measure of the affinity of drug in plasma for the plasma proteins, albumin in particular. This fraction of drug in plasma is considered pharmacologically inert. It is generally accepted that only unbound or "free" drug is available for pharmacological activity, toxic effects, metabolism, and renal excretion, although probable exceptions exist.

Drugs that are extensively protein bound (greater than 90% of total plasma drug) demand special attention. Because the fraction of unbound drug in plasma is small, changes in binding may produce substantial changes in effect. Knowledge of total plasma protein concentration is important with this group of drugs, since a reduction in albumin will produce a relatively higher concentration of unbound drug. The fraction of unbound drug in plasma may be increased in uremia because of qualitative changes in plasma proteins or interference by some unknown endogenous waste products.

The result of diminished protein binding because of hypoalbuminemia, uremia, or displacement by another drug depends on three factors: (1) the extent of displacement, (2) the enhanced clearance of increased unbound drug, and (3) the redistribution of unbound drug. The sum of these effects is often difficult to predict. Information on specific drugs is given when it is available.

Elimination

The metabolic and excretory pathways of the liver and kidneys, which are responsible for the removal of endogenous wastes, are also used to eliminate drugs and other exogenous substances. Many drugs follow a pattern of conversion or biotransformation to more polar, less lipid-soluble, less active metabolites by hepatic oxidation followed by conjugation with sulfate or glucuronide. The polar metabolites are generally excreted in bile or urine.

This broad outline of elimination has many exceptions. Some drugs undergo extensive or completed metabolism in this manner, while others are excreted almost or totally unchanged. Specific metabolic processes include acetylation, which is partly genetically determined by an autosomal dominant gene. Dealkylation and other processes occasionally lead to the formation of active metabolites. Urine flow and pH may occasionally influence the urinary clearance of drugs and their metabolites, e.g., salicylate, quinidine, and phenobarbital.

The rate at which the total process of metabolism and excretion progresses is described by the elimination rate constant (K or k_{el}). The elimination rate constant is the negative slope of the curve of the natural logarithm of the plasma concentration versus time. When the curve of the more common logarithm (base 10) of the plasma concentration versus time is plotted on appropriate coordinates, the elimination rate constant is the slope multiplied by 2.303. The rate of elimination is more conveniently expressed as the half-life ($t_{\frac{1}{2}}$), sometimes referred to as the $t_{\frac{1}{2}}$ beta, since it is calculated from the terminal or beta phase of the drug elimination curve (see Half-life: Alpha and Beta Phases, p. 76). (Nomenclature may vary in multicompartmental models.) During this time, half the drug present at the beginning is eliminated. The half-life is easily determined from the terminal phase of the log concentration versus time graph or may be calculated from the elimination rate constant:

$$t_{\frac{1}{2}} = \frac{\ln 2}{k_{el}} = \frac{0.693}{k_{el}}$$

Half-life is a simple expression of the duration of survival of a drug in plasma or other tissues and has important implications for the dosage frequency of most drugs. The half-life and elimination rate constant are dependent on two important factors: the volume of distribution (V) and the total clearance (Q_B) of the drug from the body.

$$Q_B = V_d \cdot k_{el}$$

$$Q_B = V_d \frac{0.693}{t_{\frac{1}{2}}}$$

or $$t_{\frac{1}{2}} = 0.693 \frac{V_d}{Q_B}$$

It is clear from the last equation that $t_{\frac{1}{2}}$ may be shortened by reduction in the volume of distribution, by enhanced clearance, or by a combination of these changes. Conversely, $t_{\frac{1}{2}}$ may be prolonged when the volume of distribution is increased, the clearance diminished, or both. The $t_{\frac{1}{2}}$ may remain the same when changes in clearance and volume of distribution exactly balance each other. In summary, the half-life depends on both the amount of plasma or tissue cleared from a drug in a given time and the distribution of the drug throughout the tissues.

Dosage Schedule

The dosage schedule represents the clinician's appraisal of the patient's therapeutic requirements. There are two important aspects of any dosage schedule. The total daily dose of drug should reflect the nature and severity of the illness to be treated and the patient's age, weight, and concurrent disease status. The dosage frequency ideally represents an attempt to produce continuous safe and effective concentrations of the drug in the patient's tissues in a manner that is convenient for the patient and that will encourage his compliance. A poor dosage schedule is one that fails in one or more of these respects.

The dosage interval depends on the half-life of the drug, the safety or therapeutic index of the drug, the character of the concentration-response curve, and the minimum effective plasma concentration. If a drug has a very short half-life, it would seem reasonable to give it frequently. However, if it is possible to produce high plasma concentrations of such a drug in a safe manner, clearly it may be administered less frequently. Benzyl penicillin is a good example of this situation; it has a half-life in plasma of only 30 minutes, but a large dose once or twice daily is quite satisfactory. When half-life is short and safety is limited, the rational mode of treatment is a carefully monitored intravenous infusion, e.g., oxytocin, with a $t_{\frac{1}{2}}$ of about 5 minutes. When the dose response or concentration response is "flat," the dosage interval may be prolonged, for example, with beta blockers.

The rate of decline of effect (R) is related to the elimination rate constant (k_{el}) and the slope of the log concentration-effect graph (m) by the equation

$$R = \frac{k_{el}m}{2.303} = 0.3 \ \frac{m}{t_{\frac{1}{2}}} \ \text{(expressed in appropriate units)}$$

The duration of effect (t_d) depends on the initial amount of drug in the body (X_0), the minimum amount necessary to produce the desired effect (X_{min}), and the rate at which drug is removed (k_{el}).

$$t_d = \frac{2.303}{k_{el}} \log X_0 - \frac{2.303}{k_{el}} \log X_{min}$$

It is not always possible to give drugs with longer half-lives as infrequently as one might expect. Gastrointestinal disturbance associated with a large single dose or toxicity associated with the rapid development of high peak levels may necessitate a divided-dose regimen.

When a metabolite is active it is, of course, relevant to consider its half-life in the overall dosage plan. Although the $t_{\frac{1}{2}}$ for allopurinol is 2 or 3 hours, the active metabolite oxypurinol or alloxanthine has a $t_{\frac{1}{2}}$ of 18–30 hours, so that a single daily dose of allopurinol is perfectly rational and has been shown to work in practice.

Many standard dosage schedules are based on an attitude that medicines should be taken with meals or at least 3 times daily. Increased awareness that a divided-dose regimen increases the likelihood of poor compliance and that a dose once or, at most, twice daily is adequate for many drugs, should lead to a reevaluation of what has become almost a reflex—the writing of t.i.d. or q.i.d. on a prescription.

Once-or-twice-daily dosage, when suitable, offers additional practical and psychological advantages over more frequent dosage schedules. The school child and the elderly can more readily be supervised in taking their medications and the worker is permitted to take the drug in the privacy of his home. It has been argued that it is better to miss only one of four divided doses than half or all of the day's total intake. But the object of the exercise is to create a situation where no doses will be omitted!

The importance of clearly explaining to the patient the drugs, their effects, the doses to be taken and the frequency of dosage, the aims of therapy, and the possible duration of treatment cannot be overemphasized. A comment on the cost of the drug may be salutary. It is unfortunate that patients often have no concept of the properties or activity of their medications, the basis for their use, or the aims and limitations of their effects. It is hardly surprising that many patients are bewildered about the indications for their medicines and careless about their use of drugs. A few moments of explanation by the clinician may draw attention to problems previously not considered and may even provide a chance to reevaluate a regimen that is becoming complex, unwieldy, or potentially hazardous.

The nurse and pharmacist may play a valuable role in reinforcing the information transmitted to the patient by the physician.

Special Dosage Situations

The clinician must develop a system of warnings about particular groups of high-risk patients, that is, patients in whom drugs must be given with more than the usual degree of caution. The newborn, the child, the elderly, the pregnant woman near term, and the lactating woman are easily identified. However, the newly pregnant or "potentially" pregnant female, the patient with moderate derangement of hepatic or renal function, and the alcoholic or other drug abuser are more difficult to identify. Yet for all of these patients a simple determination of dosage by body weight will fail to produce a rational regimen for many drugs.

A number of clichés are worth remembering. A child is not a small adult. A serum creatinine of 1 mg/dl in a 20-year-old male who weighs 70 kg reflects a totally different renal function than the same serum concentration in a 75-year-old female who weighs 50 kg. An "extremely safe" drug may become mutagenic in the early weeks of pregnancy. A total serum bilirubin of 0.8 mg/dl may conceal a well-compensated case of gross cirrhosis. An obese person who weighs 150 kg may have the skeletal muscle mass of a person half that weight.

The urgency for making value judgments carefully is modified by the known toxicity of the drug, the necessity for early treatment, and the proximity of laboratory facilities.

Further information on this important aspect of drug utilization is given in the descriptions of individual drugs and in the chapters dealing with specific problems.

Therapeutic Concentrations

For many drugs there is a range of plasma concentrations that is associated with a clinical improvement in the majority of patients. Additional plasma concentrations, below which effect is generally not apparent and above which an intolerable incidence of toxicity develops, have also been defined. Plasma concentrations of drugs in these groups are described as *subtherapeutic* and *toxic*, respectively. Plasma concentrations in the high therapeutic range may be considered potentially toxic.

The therapeutic plasma concentration is not a magical range that guarantees successful treatment without adverse effect. Some patients require only a low plasma concentration, presumably because of differences in disease severity, tissue sensitivity, or pathophysiology. A low therapeutic or even subtherapeutic concentration may be adequate for their management. This level usually cannot be predicted in advance. A *cautious, supervised* trial of drug withdrawal from such patients and others in whom disease is reversible may demonstrate their ability to manage without medications as a result of natural improvement in their disease state or, conversely, it may demonstrate their continued requirement of the medicines. Many patients remain on medicines that, although once relevant to their care, are no longer necessary and have become essentially a habit that the patient or his clinician may be reluctant to break. Some patients, by nature of overwhelming disease or a different pathophysiology, may fail to respond to high therapeutic concentrations of drug.

Adverse reactions may occur within the so-called therapeutic concentration range. They may represent normal biological variation, enhanced sensitivity, idiosyncrasy, altered protein binding, or variations in the "milieu intérieure," which may be superficially characterized by electrolyte disturbances. There may be summation or synergy with other medications.

The measurement of drug concentration may be inaccurate, or the sample may be taken at an inappropriate time (see Chapter 3). The methodology may be disturbed, for example, by hemolysis, bile pigmentation, and the presence of other drugs or interfering metabolites. Laboratory errors, both human and mechanical, may also occur.

When dosage or plasma concentration and response are not compatible by normal standards, pharmacodynamic, pharmacokinetic, or analytical interference should be considered. Many important interactions between drugs and disease have been exposed in this way.

Adverse Reactions

Any drug effect that is not desired is an adverse reaction. Many drugs have clearly predictable side-effects that are directly related to the known pharmacological properties of the drug. A simple example is the dryness in the mouth and blurring of vision associated with the use of atropine in the treatment of bradycardia. The anticholinergic action of atropine is desirable to increase heart rate but is a nuisance when the atropine influences other tissues. The bradycardia associated with the use of digoxin and the postural syncope experienced by hypertensives after the administration of guanethidine are other examples of unwanted effects (side-effects) that often accompany the therapeutic effect of a drug.

Other adverse effects include dose-related toxicity on systems or receptors other than those that the drug is meant to influence. Deafness with gentamicin, fluid retention with phenylbutazone, and cholestasis with methyltestosterone are directly dosage-related and will predictably occur in a high percentage of people if the amount of drug given exceeds a certain level.

Idiosyncratic effects are effects that occur sporadically and suggest a specific genetic defect. In general, such side-effects are uncommon, occasionally very serious, and usually incompletely understood. Examples of this type of adverse reaction are malignant hyperpyrexia and apnea with suxamethonium, hemolytic anemia with quinine in G6-PD deficiency, and crises in porphyria with barbiturates.

Allergic effects are related to disturbances of the immunological system. Such adverse effects include the hemolytic anemia of methyldopa, the anaphylactic shock of penicillin, and many skin reactions.

The manifestations of overdosage are generally a combination of the exaggerated pharmacological effects of the drugs and the nonspecific acute toxic signs and symptoms related to poisoning of the vital respiratory, cardiovascular, and central nervous systems. Usually, treatment is nonspecific and supportive but is directed at these two major types of symptoms and signs. Pharmacological antagonism is often considered but is generally not possible. Symptomatic management is concerned with the support of the cardiovascular and respiratory systems and with fluid, electrolyte, and acid-base balance until the body eliminates a sufficient quantity of the drug for the patient to recover spontaneously. Specific aspects of poisoning are described in the individual drug profiles in Chapter 11.

Interactions

Many reports of drug interactions in man are anecdotal and bear little scientific weight. There are other reports of animal and test-tube studies that are not reproducible in man. Some interactions have little clinical significance because the drugs involved do not have major effects alone or in combination, or the increase or decrease in effect is relatively insignificant on a flat dose-response curve.

There are so many possibilities for drug interaction that it is perhaps surprising and fortunate that relatively few have major clinical significance. The major clinical interactions probably involve alterations in the rate of metabolism of one drug by another and the additive effect of a number of drugs with similar properties. A drug may interfere with the renal clearance of another drug or may compete with another drug at receptor sites. Specific examples that appear relevant because of their frequency or because they are potentially hazardous are described under the individual drugs. Special attention should be given to drugs that are taken for long periods of time, to preparations sold over the counter, and to medicines with potentially dangerous therapeutic effects, e.g., the anticoagulants and hypoglycemic agents.

Conclusion

Prescribing a drug involves little mental or physical effort—to do it badly! A little more effort may produce considerable benefits for individual patients and for society. It is hoped that the contents of this short book will alert the reader to the possible problems associated with many common drugs that are used daily and will assist the clinician to use those drugs in a more rational and effective manner.

Measurement of
Drugs in
Plasma

3

It is generally assumed that the biological effect of a drug is related to its concentration and duration at the receptor site. It is also assumed that the majority of drugs in plasma achieve equilibrium with the drug at the receptor site. Thus, indirectly, drug levels in plasma reflect pharmacological effect, if other factors such as pH and electrolytes remain constant.

Recent technological advances have made it possible to measure the plasma concentrations of many drugs. The purpose of this chapter is to outline the circumstances in which it is useful to make these measurements and to indicate the limitations in the interpretation of the values obtained. Therapeutic plasma concentration ranges, when available, are given in the text on the individual drugs and will not be discussed further here.

Figure 1 provides in schematic form the reasoning that may be used to decide whether or not a plasma drug level measurement will help in evaluating treatment of the patient.

Under most circumstances, it is useful to measure plasma drug levels only if these relate directly to pharmacological or toxic effects. Even when this relationship exists, the pharmacological effect may be easy to measure, making a knowledge of plasma drug levels unnecessary. This especially applies to the following drugs: diuretics, hypoglycemic agents, antihypertensives, anticoagulants, analgesics, sedatives and hypnotics, uricosuric agents, hypolipidemics, and most antimicrobial agents.

Indications for Plasma Level Monitoring

The following indications are generally accepted for plasma level monitoring.

1 The drug is used as a prophylactic, e.g., anticonvulsant drug, antiarrhythmic drug.
2 There is a narrow therapeutic range, with serious toxicity occurring at levels close to the therapeutic range, e.g., digitalis, gentamicin.
3 Toxic drug effects are easily confused with the disease process itself, e.g., nausea, vomiting, and arrhythmias due to digitalis, arrhythmias due to theophylline.
4 Oral dosage is erratically related to plasma levels because of poor gastrointestinal absorption, zero-order kinetics or first-pass metabolism, e.g., salicylates, tricyclic antidepressants, propranolol.
5 Tolerance is suspected, e.g., narcotic analgesics, barbiturates.
6 Prognosis and management are related to blood level after

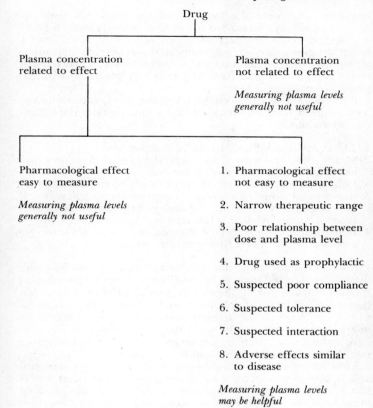

Figure 1 *Schematic model for determining the potential value of measuring the plasma level of a drug.*

acute overdose, e.g., acetaminophen, barbiturates, ethanol.
Under certain circumstances, plasma levels may be indicated whether or not a direct plasma concentration-response relationship exists.

7 Noncompliance with the regimen is suspected.
8 The possibility of malabsorption of the drug exists.
9 The patient is suspected of drug overdosage or abuse, but it cannot be confirmed by the history.
10 A drug interaction is suspected.

The indiscriminate measurement of drugs in plasma is usually of little value and may be misleading. The measurement must be made in conjunction with a proper clinical assessment of the patient and a thorough knowledge of the disease state, its severity, and its expected response to therapy. In addition, the presence of hepatic and renal insufficiency must be assessed. Considerations should include the duration of treatment, the dose, the form, frequency, and route of administration, the time of the last dose, and the plasma concentration required to produce a given pharmacological effect (if different effects require different levels). Other drugs that are being administered concurrently may interact with the drug in question and should be noted. Finally, much of the drug history may have very little relationship to reality if patient compliance is poor.

When blood is drawn to establish that the therapeutic range has been reached, samples should ideally be taken under the following conditions:

1 The distribution phase should be complete.
2 Steady state should have been achieved. This will occur 4 or 5 half-lives after initiation of treatment.
3 If the drug has a short half-life, peak (1 or 2 hours after administration) and trough (predose) measurements are advisable. If the drug has a long half-life, the timing of the blood collection in relation to the last dose is less critical.
4 If plasma levels are to be estimated during an infusion, remember to take blood from the opposite limb!

It is easy to understand that if these basic rules are not followed, the results obtained may not be readily interpreted. For instance, if blood is taken during the distribution phase, the plasma concentration will be spuriously high. Such a level is not representative of the level at the receptor site but may erroneously be interpreted as being in the toxic range. Digoxin and digitoxin have prolonged distribution phases of 6–10 hours, and therefore estimations during this time will be misleading.

After the initiation or adjustment of therapy, drug concentration in plasma will increase or decrease over a period of 4 or 5 half-lives until a new steady state is reached. Although drug measurements may be helpful during this time, they may not accurately reflect the final steady-state level. This is particularly important in those drugs that have dose-dependent kinetics, e.g., phenytoin.

Plasma concentrations of drugs with short half-lives may fluctuate widely during a single dosage interval. To characterize the plasma concentration profile, it is essential that blood be drawn when concentrations are likely to be at their maximum and minimum. In this way, it is possible to determine whether the drug levels at any stage are in the toxic or subtherapeutic ranges. Armed with this knowledge, one may then adjust dosage intervals and the individual dose on a rational basis.

Summary

Estimations of plasma concentrations of certain drugs may be clinically useful when made in conjunction with a thorough evaluation of the patient. The timing of blood sampling in relation to dosage is often of critical importance in interpreting the result. Knowledge of the therapeutic plasma concentration and other aspects of the pharmacokinetics of the drug are essential to the proper evaluation of any drug level.

Reviews

Azarnoff, D. L. (Ed.). Report of the second Deer Lodge conference. *Clin. Pharmacol. Ther.* 16:129–288, 1974.

Koch-Weser, J. Drug therapy: Serum drug concentrations as therapeutic guides. *N. Engl. J. Med.* 287:227–231, 1972.

Reidenberg, M. (Ed.). Individualization of drug therapy. *Med. Clin. North Am.* 58:905–1161, 1974.

Drugs and
Renal Disease

4

Altered Therapeutic Response

Patients with impaired renal function have a higher incidence of adverse drug reactions than patients with normal kidney function. Possible reasons for increased toxicity and altered therapeutic response in patients with poor renal function are summarized below.

Absorption

There is no information concerning drug absorption in uremia, although increased gastrointestinal motility associated with diarrhea might reduce the bioavailability of drugs with limited solubility.

Volume of Distribution

Changes in muscle mass, plasma proteins, and fluid disposition may alter drug distribution in the body.

Protein Binding

Decreased concentration of albumin and qualitative changes in the ability of albumin to bind drugs may increase unbound fraction of drug.

Excretion

Diminished glomerular filtration and tubular secretion may impair renal elimination of unchanged drug and active metabolite(s).

Metabolism

Acetylation is often inhibited in uremia. Mixed function oxidation may be enhanced.

Tissue Sensitivity

Changes in electrolytes and altered tissue responsiveness may account for an increased sensitivity to some drugs in uremia.

Excretion

With normal renal function the fraction of drug or active metabolite undergoing renal excretion varies from drug to drug but is relatively constant for each individual drug. For drugs that are excreted unchanged by the kidneys, the rate of elimination is diminished and the half-life is prolonged when renal function is impaired. In general, changes in endogenous creatinine clearance relate extremely well to changes in the clearance of the drug. It appears less important to know if the drug is excreted by glomerular filtration or tubular secretion, since the renal clearance of most drugs parallels the glomerular filtration rate even when tubular secretion is the main route of excretion. Therefore, knowledge of the endogenous creatinine clearance and the fraction of the drug or its metabolite(s) excreted by the kidneys enables one to predict with some measure of confidence the dosage adjustments necessary in the various degrees of renal impairment. It must always be remembered, however, that such adjustments are merely a compromise for lack of exact knowledge.

Serum creatinine can be used as a substitute for endogenous creatinine clearance only if the age-dependent reduction in renal function and the sex and body weight of the patient are considered. A nomogram may be of assistance in estimating creatinine clearance (Figure 2).

The overall objective for dosage adjustment in renal disease is to reduce the rate of drug administration to equal the decrease in drug elimination, thereby achieving the same average amounts of drug in the body.

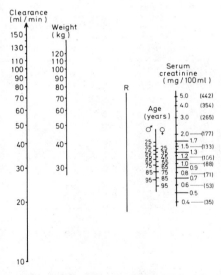

Figure 2 *Nomogram for evaluation of endogenous creatinine clearance. Use of the nomogram: connect with a ruler the patient's weight and the patient's age. Note the point of intersection on R and keep the ruler there. Turn the right side of the ruler to the appropriate serum creatinine value and the left side will indicate the creatinine clearance in milliliters per minute (ml/min). Serum creatinine values in $\mu mol/l$ are given within parentheses. (From J. Kampmann, K. Siersbaek-Nielsen, et al., as reprinted from* Lancet *1:1132–1133, 1971. By kind permission of the authors and publishers.)*

Rules for Changing Drug Dosage in Renal Impairment

1 Decide the appropriate dosage regimen for the patient as if renal function were normal.
2 Determine the fraction of drug and any active metabolite that is excreted unchanged by the kidneys (see individual drugs).
3 Determine the renal function by measurement of endogenous creatinine clearance. If this is not available, a reasonable estimate may be obtained (Figure 2).
4 Calculate the dosage-adjustment factor from Table 1. This factor is the ratio of the half-life of the drug in the uremic patient and the half-life of the drug in the normal person.
5 Use the dosage-adjustment factor in one of the following ways, after considering which is most appropriate for the appropriate drug.
  a Divide the dose you determined for normal renal function by the dosage-adjustment factor and continue with the same dosage interval.
  b Continue with the same dose but multiply the dosage interval you determined for normal renal function by the dosage-adjustment factor.
  c Reduce the dose and prolong the dosage interval appropriately.

Table 1 *Dosage-Adjustment Factors*

% Excreted Unchanged in Urine	Creatinine Clearance (ml/min)						
	0	10	20	40	60	80	120
10	1.1	1.1	1.1	1.1	1.1	1.0	1.0
20	1.3	1.2	1.2	1.1	1.1	1.1	1.0
30	1.4	1.3	1.3	1.2	1.2	1.1	1.0
40	1.7	1.6	1.5	1.4	1.3	1.1	1.0
50	2.0	1.8	1.7	1.5	1.3	1.2	1.0
60	2.5	2.2	2.0	1.7	1.4	1.3	1.0
70	3.3	2.8	2.3	1.9	1.5	1.3	1.0
80	5.0	3.7	3.0	2.1	1.7	1.4	1.0
90	10.0	5.7	4.0	2.5	1.8	1.4	1.0
100	∞	12.0	6.0	3.0	2.0	1.5	1.0

The values in Table 1 have been derived from the following formula:

$$\text{Dosage-adjustment factor} = \frac{1}{F (kf - 1) + 1}$$

where

F = fraction of drug excreted unchanged

kf = relative kidney function, calculated by dividing the actual or derived creatinine clearance by 120 ml/min

Examples

Digoxin: F = 0.75 (about 75% excreted unchanged in the urine). If you would have given a patient 0.25 mg digoxin orally daily had renal function been normal, the dose for this patient with a creatinine clearance of 60 ml/min is 0.25/1.6 = 0.16 mg orally daily, since the dosage-adjustment factor is

$$\frac{1}{0.75 \ (60/120 - 1) + 1} = 1.6$$

Similarly, if you would have given another patient 0.375 mg daily had renal function been normal, the dose for this patient with a creatinine clearance of 20 ml/min is 0.375/2.7 = 0.139 mg daily, since the dosage-adjustment factor for digoxin in a patient with creatinine clearance of 20 ml/min is

$$\frac{1}{0.75 \ (20/120 - 1) + 1} = 2.7$$

Gentamicin: F = 0.9 (about 90–100% excreted unchanged in the urine). If you would have given a patient 80 mg at 8-hour intervals had renal function been normal, the dosage interval for this patient with a clearance of 60 ml/min is 80/1.8 = 44 mg every 8 hours, or 80 mg every 8 × 1.8 = 14.4 hours, or, adjusting dose and dosage interval, 40 mg every 7.2 hours, since the dosage-adjustment factor is

$$\frac{1}{0.9 \ (60/120 - 1) + 1} = 1.8$$

Similarly, if the creatinine clearance had been 20 ml/min, the dosage regimen for this patient would have been 80/4 = 20 mg every 8 hours, or 80 mg every 4 × 8 = 32 hours, or, adjusting dose and interval, 30 mg every 12 hours, since the dosage adjustment factor is

$$\frac{1}{0.9 \ (20/120 - 1) + 1} = 4.0$$

It is important to realize that the dosage-adjustment factor gives the drug regimen for the uremic patient relative to the regimen for the *same* patient if that particular patient's kidney function had been normal. This enables the physician to change the dosage regimen according to the needs of each individual patient. Of course, the calculated dosage regimen has to be modified by common sense and practical considerations. For instance, in the digoxin examples, the practical dosage regimen would have been 0.125 mg daily and in the first gentamicin example a suitable regimen would be 40 mg every 8 hours.

The decision to reduce dose, increase the dosage interval, or modify both depends on several considerations. Lowering the dose reduces the peak plasma concentration of drug. Prolonging the dosage interval reduces the trough concentration of drug in plasma. A regimen of combined-dose reduction and dosage-interval prolongation may maintain a more uniform serum concentration. For digoxin and most antiarrhythmic agents a dosage reduction is most suitable to avoid the high potentially toxic peaks. For bactericidal antibiotics, prolonging the dosage interval is the most usual method. When either of these methods is likely to produce toxic peaks or subtherapeutic troughs, a combination of dose reduction and interval prolongation offers the best modification of the dosage schedule (see previous examples).

The rules previously discussed apply primarily to modifications of maintenance dose therapy. In most cases the usual loading dose can be given. It is obvious from Table 1 and the dosage-adjustment formula that alterations in dosage are most important for drugs with renal excretion of unchanged drug above 50% or active metabolites that are extensively eliminated in urine and that dosing considerations are seldom of clinical importance unless renal function deteriorates below 50% of normal. In addition, only drugs with a low therapeutic index need to be considered seriously. Therefore, in clinical practice only a relatively small group of drugs poses any significant problem in renal disease. These drugs are:

Aminoglycosides, e.g., gentamicin, kanamycin, streptomycin, tobramycin
Cephaloridine
Colistin
Digoxin
Ethambutol
Lithium
Methotrexate
Procainamide
Sulfonamides

Conditions for the Validity of the Dosage-Adjustment Factor

1 First-order kinetics in the therapeutic concentration range.
2 Metabolites of the drug are assumed to be inactive and non-toxic. If metabolites are active the dosage-adjustment factor may be calculated separately for the metabolites (active metabolites with renal excretion include N-acetyl procainamide [NAPA] from procainamide, hydroxyacetohexamide from acetohexamide, oxypurinol from allopurinol, and glycinxylidide [GX] and monoethylglycinxylidide [MEGX] from lidocaine).
3 No differences in the absorption, distribution, and metabolism of the drug between normal and uremic patients.
4 No alterations in drug sensitivity in uremic patients (unchanged concentration-effect relationship).
5 A direct relationship is assumed between creatinine clearance and the renal elimination of the drug.
6 Stable kidney function.

These conditions are essential for the exact application of the dosage-adjustment factor. However, in reality they often cannot be fulfilled because of changes in metabolism, distribution, and sensitivity, which sometimes result from renal insufficiency. Nevertheless, in the practical clinical setting, the dosage-adjustment factor will allow reasonably accurate modifications of regimens. When available, specific information is included with the description of each drug.

Protein Binding and Volume of Distribution

The unbound fraction of several acidic drugs (phenytoin, salicylate, diazoxide, clofibrate, several sulfonamides) may be increased in uremia, even when the concentration of the serum albumin is normal. The reduction in binding of phenytoin is related to the decrease in renal function (20% unbound drug at a serum creatinine level of 10–12 mg/dl compared to about 10% unbound with normal renal function). One practical implication of this information is that the uremic patient whose total plasma phenytoin level is below the therapeutic range may still have adequate seizure control because the unbound concentration is in the desired therapeutic range (1–2 μg/ml). For the same reason toxicity may result if the total plasma phenytoin concentration is in the middle or high usual therapeutic range. If necessary, total and unbound plasma concentrations should be measured.

In contrast to acidic drugs, the protein binding of basic drugs seems to be normal in uremic patients, with triamterene being the one known exception. Little is known about neutral drugs, but available information shows that the unbound fraction of digitoxin is increased in uremia.

It has been shown for some highly bound drugs, such as phenytoin and clofibrate, that in patients with nephrotic syndrome and essentially normal creatinine clearance the decreased serum albumin is associated with a proportional increase in the fraction of unbound drug. However, because of an increase in clearance (V_d · k_{el}) the total levels decrease and unbound concentration does not change significantly.

Little is known about alteration in volume of distribution in renal diseases, but it has recently been shown that the volume of distribution for phenytoin is increased in nephrotic patients.

Metabolism

The metabolism of 25-hydroxy-cholecalciferol, procaine, insulin, and cortisol is reduced in uremia. Reduced metabolism with prolongation of half-life has also been demonstrated for several drugs that are acetylated—sulfisoxazole, p-aminosalicylic acid, procainamide, and hydralazine—but not for isoniazid. The clinical relevance of this phenomenon is uncertain, but a decrease in dose would appear reasonable. In uremic patients with normal concentrations of serum albumin, increased metabolism has been demonstrated for phenytoin. In nephrotic patients with low serum albumin, increased metabolism has been demonstrated for phenytoin and clofibrate.

Tissue Sensitivity

Uremic patients may have an increased sensitivity to the anticholinergic side-effects of chlorpromazine and to the CNS-depressing action of narcotic analgesics and sedatives.

Measurement of Plasma Concentrations of Drugs

The uremic patient may benefit from the measurement of drugs such as digoxin and the aminoglycosides, which may be essential to his recovery but which may further threaten his health if used inappropriately. Further measurements of drug in plasma may be necessary with changing renal function or the intervention of dialysis procedures.

Additional Drugs That Require Specific Attention in Uremia

Anticoagulants	Increased bleeding tendency
Ulcerogenic drugs (phenylbutazone, indomethacin, ibuprofen, salicylates, baclofen)	Possibly increased tendency to ulceration
Potassium sparing drugs (spirolactone, triamterene, amiloride)	Increased risk of hyperkalemia
Potassium supplements	Increased risk of hyperkalemia
Aminoglycosides⎫ Gold ⎪ Tetracyclines ⎪ Cephaloridine ⎪ Sulfonamides ⎬ Mercurials ⎪ Phenylbutazone ⎪ Amphotericin B ⎪ Phenacetin ⎪ Methicillin ⎭	Potentially nephrotoxic
Probenecid and sulfinpyrazone	No uricosuric effect in uremia
Thiazides	Not effective as diuretics but useful as antihypertensives
Phenformin	Contraindicated because of enhanced risk of lactic acidosis

Reviews

Bennett, W. M., Singer, I., et al.   Guide to drug therapy in renal failure. *J.A.M.A.* 230:1544–1553, 1974.

Dettli, L.   Individualization of drug dosage in patients with renal disease. *Med. Clin. North Am.* 58:977–985, 1974.

Dettli, L.   Drug dosage in renal disease. *Clin. Pharmacokin.* 1:126–134, 1976.

Fabre, J., and Balant, L.   Renal failure, drug pharmacokinetics, and drug action. *Clin. Pharmacokin.* 1:99–120, 1976.

Kampmann, J., Siersbaek-Nielsen, K., et al.   Rapid evaluation of creatinine clearance. *Acta Med. Scand.* 196:517–520, 1974.

Reidenberg, M.   *Renal Function and Drug Action.* Philadelphia: Saunders, 1971.

Reidenberg, M. Effect of disease states on the plasma protein binding of drugs. *Med. Clin. North Am.* 58:1103–1109, 1974.

Reidenberg, M. Drug metabolism in uremia. *Clin. Nephrol.* 4:83–85, 1975.

Reidenberg, M. The binding of drugs to plasma proteins from patients with poor renal function. *Clin. Pharmacokin.* 1:121–125, 1976.

Tozer, T. N. Nomogram for modification of dosage regimens in patients with chronic renal impairment. *J. Pharmacokin. Biopharm.* 2:13–28, 1974.

Drugs and
Hepatic Disease

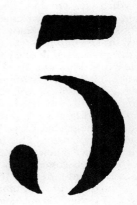

The Influence of Liver Disease on Drug Metabolism

The effect of liver disease on the disposition of drugs may be considered in two parts: (1) the effect of hepatocellular loss itself, with an absolute decrease in the quantity of metabolizing enzymes, and (2) the effect of altered hepatic perfusion, such as that which often occurs in cirrhosis.

Parenchymal liver disease has been shown to affect the half-lives of some drugs but not others (Table 2), even though all are eliminated primarily by hepatic metabolism. The extent of hepatic destruction and the reserve capacity of the remaining liver to metabolize an individual drug (including enzyme induction) must be of some importance. However, it has become evident that other factors, such as alterations in protein binding, may lead to changes in the concentration of unbound drug and the volume of distribution, which may be of greater significance than altered metabolism in influencing the half-life and clearance of the drug.

Alterations in hepatic blood-flow patterns have proved equally difficult to quantitate, although elegant pharmacokinetic models now exist to explain the relationship of blood flow to hepatic uptake of drugs. In these models, it has been shown that certain drugs, such as propranolol, meperidine, propoxyphene, and lidocaine, have a very high clearance by the liver, to the extent that the liver may remove more than the unbound fraction of the drug in the blood. Thus, in one passage through the liver essentially all the drug is removed from plasma and from the erythrocytes. On the other hand, drugs such as antipyrine, warfarin, tolbutamide, diazepam, phenylbutazone, and phenytoin are not so extensively removed from the circulating blood, and their removal is confined to the unbound fraction. The extent to which a drug is cleared in one passage through the liver is referred to as the extraction ratio. For a drug like lidocaine the extraction ratio is about 0.9, whereas for antipyrine it is 0.1. For drugs with a high extraction ratio, extraction by the liver is dependent on the amount of blood flowing past functioning cells. Alterations in liver blood flow, such as those produced by cardiac failure or the portasystemic shunting of cirrhosis, cause large changes in the clearance of drug. This has been well shown for lidocaine and meperidine. When the extraction ratio is low, alterations in liver blood flow become much less critical. Drugs with a high hepatic clearance ratio are said to be liver blood-flow dependent.

Changes in protein binding have variable effects on the half-lives of drugs. Propranolol is highly cleared but when the un-

Table 2 *Effect of Parenchymal Liver Disease in Man on the Elimination Half-life of Various Drugs*[a]

Prolonged $t_{\frac{1}{2}}$	Unchanged $t_{\frac{1}{2}}$
Amobarbital	Chlorpromazine
Carbenicillin	Dicumarol
Chloramphenicol	Pentobarbital[a]
Diazepam	Phenylbutazone[a]
Hexobarbital	Phenytoin
Isoniazid	Salicylic acid
Lidocaine	Tolbutamide[a]
Meperidine	
Meprobamate	
Pentobarbital[a]	
Phenobarbital	
Phenylbutazone[a]	
Prednisone	
Rifampin	
Tolbutamide[a]	

[a]Half-life has been reported to be both prolonged and unchanged in different studies.

bound fraction increases, the unbound propranolol distributes to other tissues. The increased distribution produces an increase in the apparent volume of distribution and prolongation of the half-life, since there is less drug available to the liver. When only unbound drug is cleared during passage through the liver, e.g., phenytoin and warfarin, an increase in the unbound fraction, such as that which may occur in the nephrotic syndrome, leads to increased hepatic extraction with a reduction of half-life.

The degree of portasystemic shunting may also have important effects on the first-pass metabolism of drugs. An increase in the oral systemic bioavailability of highly cleared drugs may occur in patients with advanced cirrhosis and in patients who have undergone surgical portacaval shunting.

The difficulties to date in defining and predicting the degree to which drugs are affected by individual liver disease processes lie in obtaining quantitative liver function tests in man, in the wide variability of the normal half-life and clearance of a given drug (so that only gross changes become apparent), and in the mixed picture of hepatocellular and vascular disorganization, which occurs in cirrhosis and other liver disorders. Drugs that have been demonstrated to produce adverse clinical effects when their pharmacokinetics are altered by liver disease include meperidine, diazepam, and barbiturates. The clinical effects are seen in both hepatitis and cirrhosis. The half-life is prolonged in patients with hepatic parenchymal disease, and therefore steady-state plasma levels for a given dose are higher than in normal subjects. However, it must also be remembered that for drugs with a high therapeutic index, even large increases in half-life may not produce clinical difficulties.

The Hepatoxicity of Drugs

Drugs may damage the liver as a dose-related phenomenon (Table 3) or as an allergic reaction in which the response occurs irregularly and infrequently in the population, usually at low dosage and often in association with other hypersensitivity phenomena (Table 4). In either case, the basic mechanism appears to be the metabolic activation of chemically stable drugs to alkylating, arylating, or acylating agents within the body.

Table 3   *Drugs That Are Toxic to the Liver*

Liver Disorder	Drugs
Acute hepatitis	Acetaminophen (paracetamol)
	Tetracyclines
	Isoniazid
	Salicylates
	6-Mercaptopurine
	5-Fluorodeoxyuridine
	Mithramicin
	Mitomycin
	Actinomycin D
	Ferrous sulfate (large doses)
	Ethanol
Cirrhosis	Methotrexate
	Arsenic (presinusoidal intrahepatic portal hypertension)
	Ethanol
Cholestasis	17 α-Methyltestosterone
	Estrogens
	Azathioprine
Neoplasm	Chlorambucil
	Oral contraceptives

Dose-related hepatotoxicity may be expressed as cell necrosis such as that which occurs with acetaminophen (paracetamol), phenacetin, and isoniazid as well as with the more classic hepatotoxins such as carbon tetrachloride. In acetaminophen poisoning, cellular damage occurs when a toxic metabolite is produced in excess of the available glutathione. Thus, instead of forming an inactive conjugate with glutathione, the metabolite forms covalent linkages with macromolecules in the hepatocyte and necrosis ensues. Drugs that accelerate the formation of the active metabolite by enzyme induction, e.g., phenobarbital, ethanol, and phenytoin, may potentiate the hepatotoxic effect of acetaminophen. Unfortunately, it is not possible to raise hepatic

Table 4 *Drugs That Cause Hypersensitivity Reactions in the Liver*

Liver Disorder	Drugs
Acute hepatitis	Halothane
	Para-aminosalicylic acid
	Rifampin
	Isoniazid
	Iproniazid
	Phenelzine
	Pheniprazine
	Isocarboxazid
	Ethionamide
	Pyrazinamide
	Methimazole
	Long-acting sulfonamides
	Nitrofurantoin
	Pyridium
	Phenytoin
	Phenylbutazone
	Propylthiouracil
Chronic active hepatitis	Oxyphenisatin
	Methyldopa
Cholestasis	Chlorpromazine
	Promazine
	Prochlorperazine
	Mepazine
	Trifluoperazine
	Chlorpropamide
	Acetohexamide
	Carbutamide
	Erythromycin estolate
	Methylthiouracil
	Imipramine
	Organic arsenicals
	Gold

glutathione levels by systemic administration, since it does not penetrate the hepatocyte. However, other sulfhydryl (—SH) containing substances, such as cysteamine and methionine, may prove valuable and have been suggested as an antidote for acetaminophen poisoning. Direct toxicity of drugs may also be manifested by cirrhosis (the classic example is ethanol), by dose-related cholestasis (e.g., methyltestosterone), and by neoplastic change (e.g., chronic chlorambucil therapy).

Allergic hepatic reactions have been ascribed to a large number of drugs, which are listed in Table 4. Histologically and clinically, the reactions may be manifested as hepatocellular disease, chole-stasis, or a combination of both. The hepatocellular process may, furthermore, be manifested as acute or chronic active hepatitis. The mechanism is unknown, although it has been postulated that an activated drug metabolite linked to a macromolecule in the liver might serve as a hapten for antibody production or, alterna-tively, that intracellular proteins, liberated by the initial damage caused by the metabolite, might serve as antigens.

Measurement of Plasma Concentration of Drugs

When liver disease is advanced or when marked fluctuation in liver function is assessed by conventional biochemical tests, the measurement of drugs known to be extensively metabolized in the liver may be helpful in regulating dosage. Ideally the concentration of unbound drug should be known, especially if there is marked reduction of the albumin concentration in plasma. This is often technically difficult, and therefore careful observation of clinical effect is the usual means of adjusting dos-age.

Additional Drugs That Require Specific Attention in Liver Disease

A small group of drugs has the potential to worsen the clinical status of a patient with liver disease by mechanisms other than those already discussed. Furosemide and the thiazide diuretics, by promoting potassium loss and metabolic alkalosis, may provoke the development of hepatic encephalopathy. Morphine and other analgesics, sedatives, and tranquilizers may also precipitate he-patic encephalopathy, possibly as a result of increased brain "sen-sitivity" to centrally acting drugs, although reduction of the rate of metabolism of these drugs, modification of their distribution, and changes in their protein binding may also play a part in this adverse reaction. If possible, hypoglycemic agents should be avoided in patients with advanced liver disease, since these pa-tients have reduced hepatic glycogen stores and are particularly susceptible to hypoglycemic coma. Anticoagulants may also pro-duce an exaggerated response in patients with liver disease as a result of diminished ability to form the clotting factors. Patients with cholestasis may also fail to absorb the fat-soluble vitamin K necessary for hepatic formation of Factors II, VII, IX, and X, with resulting prolongation of the prothrombin time.

Conclusion

Current research of the absolute measurement of hepatocellular function, liver blood flow, and the mechanisms of hepatic injury by drugs may help answer two important questions: What dosage adjustments are necessary for specific drugs metabolized by the liver? How can hepatotoxicity of drugs be predicted or avoided? At present, while this exact information is lacking, clinical judg-ment is essential when drugs belonging to either of these categories must be used.

Reviews

Black, M. Liver disease and drug therapy. *Med. Clin. North Am.* 58:1051–1057, 1974.

Mitchell, J. R., and Potter, W. Z. Drug metabolism in the production of liver injury. *Med. Clin. North Am.* 59:877–885, 1975.

Schenker, S., Hoyumpa, A. M., Jr., et al. The effect of parenchymal liver disease on the disposition and elimination of sedatives and analgesics. *Med. Clin. North Am.* 59:887–896, 1975.

Wilkinson, G. R., and Shand, D. G. Commentary: A physiological approach to hepatic drug clearance. *Clin. Pharmacol. Ther.* 18:377–390, 1975.

Medication During Pregnancy

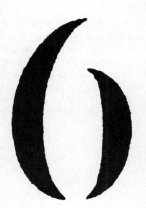

Influence of Pregnancy on Drug Metabolism

There is little information on the effect of human pregnancy on drug metabolism. One might expect altered pharmacokinetics in pregnancy for a number of reasons:

1 Serum albumin concentration is decreased.
2 Blood volume and body water are increased.
3 Creatinine clearance is increased.
4 The placenta is a potential site of drug metabolism.

These changes might be thought likely to produce important alterations in protein binding, distribution, and elimination of many drugs. However, information on maternal drug metabolism is available for only a few drugs:

1 The protein binding of sulfisoxazole is reduced.
2 Salicylamide conjugation is reduced.
3 Meperidine demethylation is decreased.
4 Phenytoin clearance is increased.

No general recommendations can be made until further information is available concerning other drugs.

Effect of Maternally Administered Drugs on the Fetus and Neonate

Factors Affecting Drug Transfer from Mother to Fetus

Most drugs cross the placenta by passive diffusion. The molecular weight of the drug influences its transfer across the placenta. Most substances with molecular weights of less than 500 (which includes the majority of drugs and their unconjugated metabolites) cross the placenta easily, especially if they are nonionized and lipid-soluble.

The effect of protein binding on the placental transfer rate of a drug depends on whether the drug is lipophilic and nonpolar or hydrophilic and polar. Lipophilic drugs do not appear to be greatly influenced by protein binding, and their transfer rate is governed by placental blood flow. Hydrophilic drugs are much more affected by protein binding and diffuse across the placenta at slower rates.

It must be remembered that the unbound *concentration* of a drug is pharmacologically active. It has been shown that the unbound *fraction* of sulfonamides, barbiturates, and phenytoin is substantially higher in the fetus than in the mother. Thus a low ratio of fetal-to-maternal *total* drug concentration may still result in the fetus being exposed to a concentration of the unbound drug that is similar to the unbound concentration in maternal plasma.

The Fetus

All drugs entering the fetal circulation go first to the liver, where some passes to the portal vein and the remainder to the ductus venosus, which bypasses the liver parenchyma. Thus, theoretically, the first-pass metabolism of drugs may be diminished in the unborn.

As a rule, the capacity for drug metabolism in the fetus is less than in later stages of postnatal development. Although substantial amounts of drug-metabolizing enzymes have been detected in human fetal liver, the fetus appears to depend largely on maternal metabolism for drug elimination. It is possible that there is recirculation of drugs and metabolites in the fetus by the fetus swallowing amniotic fluid into which urine has passed. This interesting possibility has yet to be explored.

Teratogenesis

Teratogenesis may be defined as any birth defect—morphological, biochemical, or behavioral—that may be induced at any stage of gestation and may be detected at birth or later. It has been estimated that the average pregnant woman takes about eight drugs during her pregnancy. Of these, only 20% have been prescribed by her physician. Because of the high incidence of

Table 5 *Drugs Associated with Teratogenesis*

Drug	Clinical State
Aminoglycosides	Deafness
Anti–folic acid drugs	Aminopterin during first trimester produces fetus with multiple defects: growth retardation, cranial dysostosis, cleft palate, mandibular hypoplasia, ear anomalies Methotrexate given during first trimester produces abnormal cranial bones, absent digits
Chloroquine	Deafness; neurological deficit
Diethylstilbestrol	Clear cell carcinoma of genital tract in adolescent girls
Lithium	Possible cardiovascular abnormalities
Phenytoin	Malformation of fingers; cleft palate (incidence may be similar in epileptic patients not on phenytoin)
Tetracycline	Stained teeth; depressed skeletal growth
Thalidomide	Phocomelia; hearing loss
Warfarin	Given in first 10 weeks, hypoplastic nasal structures

drugs taken during pregnancy, teratogenesis has become an increasingly important issue.

The occurrence of a congenital malformation is dependent on the interplay of the following factors, which are known to influence teratogenicity:

1 Nature of the responsible agent
2 Accessibility of the agent to the fetus
3 Duration of exposure to the agent
4 Stage of fetal gestation

Prior to implantation (the first 2 weeks following conception) the embryo is generally considered to be resistant to environmental agents other than radiation, possibly because there is no direct circulatory link between the mother and embryo. This interval is

Table 6 *Drugs Affecting the Neonate*

Drug	Clinical State
Alcohol	Acute withdrawal and delirium tremens–like state
Antithyroid drugs	Neonatal goiter; hypothyroidism
Aspirin	Factor XII deficiency; reduced platelet function
Chloramphenicol	Gray syndrome; cardiovascular collapse
Coumarin anticoagulants	Intrauterine death; postnatal hemorrhage
Heroin (maternal addiction)	Low birth weight; withdrawal syndrome
Lithium	Cyanosis; flaccidity; lethargy; possible goiter
Magnesium sulfate (intravenous)	Respiratory difficulty; flaccidity
Methadone (mother on methadone program)	Withdrawal syndrome
Norethisterone	Masculinization of female
Phenobarbital	Hemorrhagic disease of newborn;[a] withdrawal syndrome; hyperexcitability
Phenytoin	Hemorrhagic disease of newborn[a]
Primidone	Hemorrhagic disease of newborn[a]
Reserpine	Nasal discharge; sternal retraction; lethargy; poor feeding
Sulfonamides	Kernicterus
Thiazide diuretics	Thrombocytopenia with hemorrhage
Vitamin K (synthetic water-soluble analogues)	Hyperbilirubinemia with increased risk of kernicterus

[a]Responds to vitamin K.

from conception to the time of the mother's first missed menstrual period. The time of organ formation in humans is approximately from 13 to 56 days of gestation; from days 15 to 25 for the nervous system, from days 20 to 40 for the heart, and from days 24 to 48 for the limbs. After the first trimester most organs are formed, although the genital apparatus, teeth, and central nervous system continue to mature. Any malformation will be closely related to the stage of development at the time of exposure to the teratogenic drug or other external agent.

Tables 5 and 6 contain, in alphabetical order, what are considered to be documented instances of drugs causing either neonatal injury or teratogenesis. Only the reports considered to be fairly free from controversy have been included.

Conclusion

Ideally the pregnant woman should not receive any drugs throughout her pregnancy, except for the hematinics, iron, and folic acid if they are considered necessary. This statement, however, ignores the very real situation of pregnancy complicated by disease or discomfort requiring some therapeutic intervention. The physician must then decide, after careful evaluation of the benefit-risk ratio, whether or not medication is justified. If the situation demands that treatment be given and if a choice exists, a well-established agent not implicated in teratogenesis or neonatal disease should be selected and administered in the smallest dose for the shortest possible duration compatible with effective therapy.

Reviews

Eriksson, M., Catz, C. S., et al. Drugs and pregnancy. *Clin. Obstet. Gynecol.* 16:199–224, 1973.

Krauer, B., and Krauer, F. Drug kinetics in pregnancy. *Clin. Pharmacokin.* 2:167–181, 1977.

Mirkin, B. L. Prenatal pharmacology: Placental transfer, fetal localization, and neonatal disposition of drugs. *Anesthesiology* 43:156–170, 1975.

Mofenson, H. C., Greensher, J., et al. Hazards of maternally administered drugs. *Clin. Toxicol.* 7:59–68, 1974.

Sutherland, J. M., and Light, I. J. The effect of drugs upon the developing fetus. *Pediatr. Clin. North Am.* 12:781–806, 1965.

Medication During Lactation

7

Breast-feeding provides a situation in which the suckling infant may become the unintentional recipient of medications taken by the nursing mother. At first glance the problem might appear to be of some importance, since most drugs pass into breast milk to a varying extent. In addition, the young baby has several attributes that make him unduly susceptible to the effects of drugs. He has a low body weight. His kidneys and liver are immature, and thus his ability to eliminate drugs is generally less than that of his mother and accumulation may easily occur. Evidence of early toxicity may be masked by the obvious lack of symptomatology and the difficulty in interpreting nonspecific complaining behavior. There may also be difficulty in attributing nonspecific signs to drug effect, especially if the signs are not representative of the same overdose state in the older child or adult. On rare occasions the child's genetic makeup may produce a deficiency in his ability to metabolize some drugs in the same manner as the mother.

On the other hand, certain factors mitigate the adverse effects on the baby of drugs taken by the mother. He may already have been exposed to the drug in utero and therefore may have developed some capacity to deal with it, probably by enzyme induction. Some agents, such as insulin and epinephrine, are destroyed in the gastrointestinal tract and thus their presence in milk poses no problem. Casual exposure of the mother to drugs may produce only occasional intermittent challenges that do not disturb the child, since the opportunity for the drug to accumulate is diminished.

As with any drug effect, the overwhelmingly important aspects are the amount of drug consumed and the sensitivity of the individual. The amount of drug received by the baby is clearly dependent on the concentration of drug in milk and the amount of milk consumed, which is usually 500–700 ml daily. The concentration of drug in milk depends on its transfer from plasma, which is the result of the influence of molecular weight, of fat and water solubility, of pKa, of protein binding, and of concentration gradient of the drug at the alveolar interface between plasma and milk.

The pH of milk is acidic (pH 6.6–7.3) with respect to plasma (pH 7.4). Drugs that are fat-soluble and are not bound to plasma proteins diffuse passively into milk with the concentration gradient. Basic drugs such as the antihistamines, theophylline, meperidine and opium alkaloids, imipramine, amitriptyline, isoniazid, erythromycin, and lincomycin tend to achieve concentrations in milk equal to or greater than unbound concentrations in plasma. Acidic drugs are more ionized in plasma and tend to pass less readily into milk than basic drugs.

Basic drugs often have very large volumes of distribution and therefore the amount in plasma represents only a small part of the total drug in the body. Some basic drugs are also highly protein bound. Therefore, although bases may cross more readily into milk than acidic drugs, the absolute amounts of both acids and bases that are transferred are usually very small.

For these reasons the total amount of drug in milk rarely represents a major threat to the baby, even when the drug is consumed in therapeutic amounts for long periods of time. Some drugs, nevertheless, have been reported to cause problems. Iodides and radioactive iodine are secreted by breast tissue and may cause goiter and thyroid dysfunction in the child. They are incompatible with breast-feeding. Propylthiouracil and other antithyroid drugs also may cause goiter and hypothyroidism in the baby. Mothers with migraine may take ergot preparations; in the baby ergot produces vomiting, diarrhea, cardiovascular instability, and convulsions, all of which are nonspecific and demand a high degree of suspicion of maternal ergot ingestion to determine the correct diagnosis.

The laxative dihydroxyanthraquinoline is often present in milk in sufficient concentration to produce loose bowel movements in suckling babies. Diazepam and its active metabolite, desmethyl-diazepam, both pass into breast milk, and although concentrations are relatively low, they are thought to produce drowsiness in babies. Reports of individual cases incriminate large doses of alcohol and the anticoagulant phenindione as potential risks to the baby if ingested in breast milk. The contraceptive pill has also been the subject of much discussion. Evidence that the pill in usual doses produces problems in the suckling infant is extremely limited, but there are some reports of vaginal hyperplasia and gynecomastia.

Excessive sensitivity of the baby to low concentrations of drugs remains an important theoretical risk. Deficiency of the enzyme glucose-6-phosphate dehydrogenase (G-6-PD) is manifested as hemolysis if the baby is exposed to certain chemicals such as sulfonamides, vitamin K analogues, nitrofurantoin, and nalidixic acid. Small doses of ingested sulfonamides seem to be capable of producing kernicterus in infants at risk by displacement of bilirubin from plasma proteins. Transmission of tetracyclines would be potentially hazardous to the development of teeth and bone, but there are no reports that these antimicrobials are transferred in milk to an extent adequate to produce these difficulties. Chloramphenicol similarly has never been reported to cause the gray syndrome in the newborn by its transmission in milk.

The evidence attributing discomfort or disease in the baby to the consumption of drugs in maternal milk is clearly rather slight. Indeed, in historical terms, the greatest catastrophe the world has known in this respect was related not to a medicine but to an agricultural chemical.

In 1956 an epidemic of papular skin rash, gastroenteritis, and death in young children occurred in a region of Turkey. The cause was thought initially to be an undetermined infectious agent but was later found to be hexachlorobenzene, a wheat fungicide, which had been transmitted in breast milk. The mothers, many of whom had tender, firm hepatomegaly, had eaten bread made from the flour of contaminated wheat grain. In the same decade Japanese children who were breast-fed by mothers exposed to organic mercurials suffered brain damage. However, it is probable that intrauterine exposure to mercury, the result of environmental pollution on a grand scale in Minamata Bay, played a more important role in their poisoning.

The clinician, nevertheless, must advise his patient or answer her questions about drug consumption during lactation. It must be emphasized that propylthiouracil, iodides, radioactive iodine, or other radioactive isotopes and ergot derivatives should not be given during lactation or that lactation be discontinued if their use for therapeutic or diagnostic purposes is imperative. In families with a history of G-6-PD deficiency, precipitating causes should be avoided. In general, short or intermittent use of most commonly used drugs including caffeine, nicotine, and alcohol appears to produce little risk to the newborn. The mother may be reassured that most commonly prescribed medications have not been incriminated as a cause of ill-health in babies because of breast-feeding. Much of the advice about not using drugs during lactation is based on legal precautions by pharmaceutical companies, and the subject of drug transfer in breast milk suffers generally from a lack of information.

The clinician should, nevertheless, advise the mother to take only essential medications, to note any possible untoward effects in her baby, and to report them for the clinician's consideration. The clinician should remember to tell the mother that toxic effects in the infant may not exactly resemble those in the adult. When there is uncertainty as to whether or not a significant change in the baby's health is related to a drug in breast milk, the mother should be advised to at least temporarily discontinue breast-feeding. In itself this maneuver may help clarify the problem. Measurement of drugs in milk or in plasma from the mother and baby is increasingly possible. Measurement of the prothrombin time in babies whose mothers receive oral anticoagulants is certainly indicated before any surgical procedure is undertaken. Since there is evidence that drugs diffuse back into plasma when the plasma concentration declines, a rational yet simple piece of advice to the mother is to feed the baby just before her medications are due or at least as long as possible after the previous dose.

Reviews

Catz, C. S., and Giacoia, G. P.   Drugs and breast milk. *Pediatr. Clin. North Am.* 19:151–166, 1972.

Knowles, J. A.   Breast milk: A source of more than nutrition for the neonate. *Clin. Toxicol.* 7:69–82, 1974.

Vorherr, H.   Drug excretion in breast milk. *Postgrad. Med.* 56:97–104, 1974.

Medication in
Children

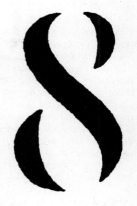

The use of drugs in children is difficult because of the continuous changes in body weight and composition during childhood growth. These changes significantly influence both the action and the kinetics of drugs. Most pediatric drug regimens have been obtained merely by fractionating the adult dose according to the weight, age, or body surface of the child. This approach has in many instances been very unsatisfactory, indicating that the child is not just a small adult. Many drugs have been approved for marketing without the necessary studies in children, making it difficult to administer many potentially valuable drugs in a rational manner. At present there is an enormous need for systematic clinical pharmacological studies in children to take them out of the shadows of the "therapeutic orphanage." Special problems exist in the neonate. In this period of human development the pharmacokinetic parameters change maximally and individual variability is very wide.

As in adults, rational pharmacotherapy in children should be based on controlled clinical trials; however, such trials are infrequent. Often the clinician and society decline to use children as experimental objects, presuming to protect the child but in fact depriving him of benefit derived from treatment based on thorough pharmacokinetic and pharmacodynamic information.

When available, exact dosage recommendations for each drug are given in Chapter 11. In this chapter a few general principles will be outlined.

Absorption

No differences seem to exist between the adult and the older child with regard to the efficiency of oral or parenteral absorption. In neonates, a decreased oral bioavailability has been shown for phenobarbital, nalidixic acid, rifampin, phenytoin, and acetaminophen, whereas the oral absorption of digoxin, phenylbutazone, diazepam, and several sulfonamides is comparable to that of adults, although clearly some of these drugs are rarely used in neonates. The bioavailability of antibiotics administered intramuscularly is the same in neonates and adults. As in adults, the intramuscular absorption of digoxin in neonates is slow and erratic. Vomiting, which is common in the neonate, may inadvertently prevent the oral absorption of any drug.

A very significant difference exists, however, in the percutaneous absorption of lipid-soluble drugs. The percutaneous absorption is much enhanced in the newborn, especially if an agent is applied to excoriated skin. Boric acid, although it has been shown to be therapeutically useless, has resulted in severe diarrhea and death when used for diaper rash, and aniline dyes from marking ink have caused methemoglobinemia. Babies with G-6-PD insufficiency do not tolerate clothes stored with mothballs composed of naphthalene.

Distribution

The body composition of the newborn and child is very different from that of the adult. Total body water in a premature infant is about 85% of the total body weight compared to about 70% in a full-term infant and 55% in an adult. This increase is mostly due to a large extracellular fluid volume that constitutes about 50% of the total body weight in a premature infant compared to about 40% in a full-term infant and only 20% in older children and adults.

This alteration primarily affects water-soluble drugs confined to the extracellular space such as the sulfonamides, penicillins, cephalosporins, and aminoglycosides. To achieve the same serum concentration as that of the adult a relatively larger loading dose is required. However, the dosage requirements may be modified during maintenance therapy by a concomitant decrease in the rate of elimination.

Protein binding is usually decreased in the newborn compared to the adult. This is partly due to a lower concentration of serum albumin but is also caused by a lower drug-binding capacity of fetal albumin. The protein binding seems to reach adult values after 1 year of age. Less protein binding in neonates compared to adults and older children has been shown for salicylates, ampicillin, phenytoin, several sulfonamides, phenylbutazone, phenobarbital, imipramine, and diazoxide.

In children, several of these drugs have a volume of distribution per kilogram of body weight far greater than that of adults. The volume of distribution for phenytoin in neonates is about 1.3 L/kg compared to about 0.6 L/kg in adults, and for salicylates the figures are 0.3 and 0.15 L/kg, respectively.

Interactions by displacement are important in neonates. Acidic drugs like the salicylates and sulfonamides, which are slowly eliminated in the newborn, have the ability to displace bilirubin from the serum albumin. The increased amount of free bilirubin may cross the blood-brain barrier, leading to brain damage (kernicterus) as the hepatic elimination of bilirubin is decreased in the newborn. Excessive doses of synthetic (not natural) vitamin K have the same capacity to compete for protein-binding sites with bilirubin. The integrity of the blood-brain barrier matures during the first month of life, but before that time the fetus is highly sensitive to many drugs acting on the central nervous system, e.g., several sedatives.

Metabolism

The rate of some oxidative processes and glucuronidation is often reduced in the newborn, whereas demethylation and sulfate conjugation seem to proceed at the adult level of activity. A decreased rate of oxidation in neonates has been demonstrated for acetaminophen, tolbutamide, nortriptyline, phenylbutazone, lidocaine, phenobarbital, phenytoin, and diazepam, and a decreased rate of glucuronidation has been demonstrated for chloramphenicol (gray syndrome), salicylate, and nalidixic acid. In the first month of life some drug metabolism processes increase dramatically in efficiency. Thereafter they increase more slowly, approaching the adult level during the first year.

Some drug metabolism processes in childhood may also be greater than in adults. Diazoxide, phenobarbital, theophylline, carbamazepine, ethosuximide, and several sulfonamides have a shorter half-life (termed the half-life dip) in 1- to 8-year-old children than in neonates or adults. This phenomenon is possibly due to a relatively larger liver volume in this age group. Children from 1 to 10 years of age often require higher doses of these drugs than adults on a milligram-per-kilogram basis to achieve the same steady-state serum concentration.

Induction of the drug-metabolizing enzyme system can take place in the fetal liver even before birth. The extent to which this occurs seems comparable to that of adults. Examples are the acceleration of bilirubin conjugation by phenobarbital treatment of neonatal hyperbilirubinemia and an increased rate of elimination of diazepam after administering phenobarbital to the mother.

Renal Excretion

The renal excretory capacity (per unit of body surface) is greatly diminished in newborns compared to adults. The glomerular filtration rate in newborns is about 10 ml/min/sq m reaching adult values after 2–4 months of age. Clearance of PAH is about 25 ml/min/sq m at birth and reaches adult values after about 6 months of age. These values seem independent of the gestational age, depending only on the length of extrauterine life.

Reduced renal function in the newborn will affect all drugs that are substantially eliminated by renal excretion of the unchanged drug or of active metabolites. Specifically, this applies to the sulfonamides, penicillins, cephalosporins, aminoglycosides, and digoxin, all of which have a much prolonged half-life in the first week of life; for example, the half-life of ampicillin is 6 hours, of carbenicillin 5–6 hours, and of gentamicin about 5 hours in the first week, and 1.5, 2–3, and about 3 hours, respectively, in the second to third week, rapidly becoming similar to those of adults. These values are averages. A large variation is always observed, especially during the first 8 days of life.

A "half-life dip" can also be observed for other drugs. The half-lives of several drugs are longer in neonates than in adults but are shorter in children than in adults. The same tendency is seen with digoxin, of which the weight-related dose is much higher in infants between 1 month and 2 years of age than in neonates and adults. A possible explanation may be that the volume of distribution is relatively larger in this age group than in adults (10–15 L/kg versus about 5 L/kg in adults); at the same time the half-life is decreased (18–20 hours at 1 year of age as opposed to 36 hours in young adults and about 70 hours in newborns).

Another special feature is the urinary pH, which is usually

more acidic in newborns than in older children. This will enhance the excretion of weak bases and delay the excretion of weak acids.

Pharmacodynamics

Clinically significant pharmacodynamic differences, i.e., differences between drug effects in children and adults with the same serum concentration, have been the subject of very few studies. Newborn babies appear to have increased sensitivity to non-depolarizing neuromuscular blocking agents like curare, while sensitivity to atropine, suxamethonium, and norepinephrine appears less in neonates and children than in adults. The therapeutic range of drugs with established concentration-effect relationships seems to be the same in children as in adults, although only a few studies have been performed.

Practical Considerations

The same basic principles of drug prescribing that apply to adults also apply to children (see Chapters 1 and 2). The simplest possible regimen should always be utilized, preferably avoiding the necessity of taking a dose at school. Dosage according to age, weight, or body surface by scaling down the adult dosage is recommended only as a preliminary approach when specific information is unavailable. Monitoring of plasma levels of drugs can be very helpful but is often not feasible. Compliance is also a problem in treating children. Careful instruction and adequate explanation about the illness to the parent and the child will help to ensure the patient's adherence to the regimen and may be just as important as the drug treatment itself, especially in many chronic diseases such as diabetes and epilepsy.

Reviews

Dancis, J., and Hwang, J. C. (Eds.). *Basic and Therapeutic Aspects of Perinatal Pharmacology.* New York: Raven Press, 1975.

Morselli, P. L.   Clinical pharmacokinetics in neonates. *Clin. Pharmocokin.* 1:81–98, 1976.

Pediatric pharmacology. *Practitioner* 204:1–176, 1970.

Rane, A., and Wilson, J. T.   Clinical pharmacokinetics in infants and children. *Clin. Pharmacokin.* 1:2–24, 1976.

Shirkey, H. C.   Clinical pharmacology in pediatrics. *Clin. Pharmacol. Ther.* 13:827–830, 1972.

Shirkey, H. C.   *Pediatric Therapy* (5th ed.). St. Louis: Mosby, 1975.

Yaffe, S. J. (Ed.).   Pediatric pharmocology. *Pediatr. Clin. North Am.* 19:1–259, 1972.

Yaffe, S. J., and Juchau, M. R.   Perinatal pharmacology. *Annu. Rev. Pharmacol.* 14:219–238, 1974.

Medication in the Elderly

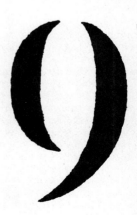

The proportion of the population above the age of 65 years is increasing in all countries. In the United States this proportion is now about 10%. However, this 10% of the population uses more than 25% of all medication prescribed.

Several problems are related to administration of drugs to elderly patients. A reduced rate of elimination, in particular a decreased rate of renal excretion, often makes a reduction in drug dosage necessary. Adverse reactions are more frequent in the elderly, and the signs are easily confused with aging processes. Multiple disorders occur frequently, thereby inviting polypharmacy and increasing the risk of adverse effects and drug interactions. Compliance is often a serious problem. Economic considerations in drug prescribing are especially important in this age group because the elderly are least able to spend large sums of money on expensive medication.

Although prescribing drugs for the elderly can be difficult, it is important to remember that old age per se is not a contraindication to drug therapy, provided that the therapy is well planned. Unfortunately, information is scanty; most drugs are tested primarily in younger persons. When information is available, specific dosage recommendations have been included in the text under individual drugs. The following review outlines some general principles about pharmacokinetics and pharmacodynamics in old age.

Absorption

Although age-dependent changes in several physiological parameters suggest that a reduced drug bioavailability should occur, none has ever been demonstrated. Gastric emptying rate, the secretion of hydrochloric acid, and gastrointestinal motility decrease with advancing age. Intestinal blood flow and many active transport systems are less effective in the elderly than in younger subjects. However, these factors appear to be of little significance since there are, by direct measurements, no age-dependent changes in the rate or extent of absorption of drugs given orally. The following drugs have been studied: acetaminophen, indomethacin, phenylbutazone, propylthiouracil, sulfamethizole, and propicillin. Higher plasma drug levels in elderly than in younger subjects have been reported, but they seem to be the result of a decreased rate of elimination or altered volume of distribution.

No systematic studies of the efficiency of parenteral absorption in different age groups have been done; the sparse information available does not suggest any age-dependent differences.

Volume of Distribution

No consistent relationship has been demonstrated between the volume of distribution and age. The most important factor to remember is that older people are, on the average, smaller than younger ones. Total body weight declines steadily after the age of 50–60 years, primarily because of a loss of intracellular water and lean body mass. The volume of distribution of diazepam (L/kg) is twice as large in the elderly as in younger subjects, a remarkable difference. The reason is not yet clarified; the plasma protein binding is unchanged.

Alteration in regional blood flow may affect the distribution of drugs, but no systematic studies have been performed. No data are available about the integrity of the blood-brain barrier in old age.

Protein Binding

The concentration of serum albumin decreases with advancing age. The concentration in subjects above the age of 70 years is about 3.5 g/dl opposed to a range of 4.0–4.5 g/dl in younger people. An increased unbound fraction of several drugs has been found in the elderly. Specifically, drugs such as warfarin, meperidine, phenylbutazone, and phenytoin have a free fraction in serum that is 1.2–3 times higher in elderly people than that in younger subjects. This increase seems to be explained by decreased concentration of serum albumin in older people, since the binding affinity between drug and serum albumin is independent of age after the first year.

The clinical significance of an increased free fraction depends on the therapeutic index of the drug and whether or not compensatory mechanisms decrease the steady-state concentration. Older people appear to be more sensitive to warfarin and meperidine, a fact that may be partly explained by a higher concentration of the unbound active drug.

A few studies have investigated age-related alterations in drug binding to erythrocytes. Although the binding of diazepam and pentazocine to erythrocytes is independent of age, the binding of meperidine to erythrocytes is much lower in elderly subjects than in younger people. This may imply that the binding of meperidine in other tissues is also decreased.

Metabolism

The common hepatic function tests, including the elimination of Bromsulphalein (BSP) and Rose-Bengal, are not age-dependent. However, as the hepatic blood flow decreases with age, a reduction of the rate of drug metabolism by the liver may be expected for drugs such as propranolol and lidocaine, since their elimination is highly flow-dependent. An age-dependent decrease in the activity of the hepatic microsomal drug-metabolizing enzyme system, with a decreased content of enzymes in biopsy tissue, has been demonstrated in rats. Data in humans are not available, but it is known that an age-related reduction in liver weight occurs and thus a loss of total enzyme activity is likely.

By measuring elimination half-lives, it has been demonstrated that the oxidative metabolism of antipyrine, aminopyrine, acetaminophen, and propranolol decreases with increasing age, while the metabolism of phenylbutazone, indomethacin, propylthiouracil, and warfarin is unrelated to age. In one study the body clearance of phenytoin in elderly subjects was higher than that in younger subjects. This could be due to reduced protein binding. The clinical significance of this observation is uncertain. The half-life of diazepam increases with age, but because of the concomitant increase in volume of distribution, clearance is unchanged. Consequently, dosage modifications based on pharmacokinetic considerations are not necessary.

Only a few metabolic processes other than oxidation have been investigated. In single studies the glucuronidation of indomethacin and the acetylation of sulfamethoxazole were shown to be age-independent.

It should be remembered that measurements of half-lives alone can be misleading. The total body clearance (volume of distribution × elimination rate constant) is the most important factor.

Renal Excretion

The renal function, which is evaluated by inulin clearance or endogenous creatinine clearance, decreases with age. Serum creatinine is age-independent, which means that the production and excretion of creatinine are reduced in elderly patients as compared with younger individuals. While the creatinine clearance in younger subjects with normal renal function varies between 80 and 120 ml/min, depending on body weight, many healthy octogenarians have a clearance of only 20–40 ml/min. The excretion of creatinine is 20–22 mg/kg/24 hr and about 10 mg/kg/24 hr, in young and old respectively.

A rapid estimation of the endogenous creatinine clearance, with an accuracy of about 80%, can be obtained from Figure 2 on page 29. The nomogram presumes only a knowledge of the weight, age, sex, and serum creatinine of the patient.

Dosage modifications are often necessary for the elderly because of the age-dependent decrease in renal function. (The decrease may be concealed by the absence of any increase in serum creatinine.) These modifications apply primarily to drugs for which the renal excretion of parent compound or active metabolites is a major part of elimination and is of special importance with drugs that have a small therapeutic index. An age-dependent reduction in the renal excretion rate has been demonstrated for digoxin, streptomycin, kanamycin, gentamicin, cephalothin, tetracycline, sulfamethizole, lithium, and phenobarbital and is to be expected for all drugs eliminated mainly unchanged by the kidneys.

The reduced renal excretion rate of pharmacologically active compounds seems to be by far the most important kinetic change in old age. The necessary dosage modifications may be calculated by using Table 1, page 30.

Pharmacodynamics

Very few investigations have demonstrated any pharmacodynamic differences between younger and older subjects. It seems, however, that there may be a reduced hepatic synthesis of blood-clotting factors, with a resulting greater sensitivity to the action of oral anticoagulants. Treatment with anticoagulants may be discouraging, since the risk of hemorrhagic episodes is considerable. Barbiturates and other psychotropic drugs often cause confusion in elderly patients and should be used sparingly. Treatment of hypertension should be carefully considered; many agents produce a large reduction in standing blood pressure, which may have disastrous effects on the cerebral blood supply in the presence of cerebrovascular insufficiency.

The use of oral hypoglycemic agents in the elderly is a particularly dubious practice. They may easily overdose accidentally or omit a meal, with resulting serious hypoglycemia from the sulfonylureas. Their reduced renal function creates a high risk of lactic acidosis from the biguanides, which should be avoided.

Conclusion

Proper drug treatment of the elderly can be extremely rewarding and may considerably improve the quality of life for them. However, it is important to remember that many disorders cannot be cured at the present time and can only be treated symptomatically. Therapeutic meddling may create more problems than relief at all ages, but the problem seems especially important in older patients. It is important to review all prescriptions carefully and frequently. Often, discontinuation of one or more drugs does not harm the patient but may actually improve well-being.

Practical considerations are extremely important in administration of drugs to the elderly. The simplest dosage schedule is preferable; daily changes in doses should be avoided. If possible, use tablets of different size or color. It must be remembered that the elderly often suffer from poor eyesight and lack of recent memory. Muscular weakness and arthritis make the opening of screwcap bottles difficult. Many patients of all ages find it a useful practice to make a daily ritual of having all their medications for that day placed in a convenient receptacle (away from children!). At mealtime and bedtime a simple check by the patient, a relative, or a friend helps ensure that the necessary medicines are taken.

Reviews

Crooks, J., O'Malley, K., et al.   Pharmacokinetics in the elderly. *Clin. Pharmacokin.* 1:280–296, 1976.

Davies, D. F., Shock, N. W., et al.   Age changes in glomerular filtration rate, effective plasma flow, and tubular excretory capacity in adult males. *J. Clin. Invest.* 29:496–507, 1950.

Ewy, G. A., Kapadia, G. G., et al.   Digoxin metabolism in the elderly. *Circulation* 39:449–453, 1969.

Hall, M. R. P.   Drug therapy in the elderly. *Br. Med. J.* 6:582–586, 1973.

O'Malley, K., Judge, T. G., et al.   Geriatric clinical pharmacology and therapeutics. In G. S. Avery (Ed.), *Drug Treatment.* Acton, Mass.: Adis Press, Sydney and Publishing Sciences Group, 1975.

Triggs, E. J., and Nation, R. L.   Pharmacokinetics in the ages: A review. *J. Pharmacokin. Biopharm.* 3:387–418, 1975.

Definition of Terms

10

Absorption

Absorption is the process by which a drug enters the body. The rate of absorption of a drug depends on the route of administration and a number of other factors, including the disintegration and dissolution rate if it is in a solid dosage form, the concentration of the drug and blood circulation at the site of absorption, and the location and the area of the absorbing surface. Absorption of drugs usually follows first-order kinetics. Absorption is usually passive, but absorption of some drugs, such as methyldopa and L-dopa, appears to be an active process.

Accumulation

When a drug is administered by continuous infusion or on a repetitive basis at regular intervals that are less than 4 or 5 half-lives (so that some drug remains from the previous dosage), there is exponential accumulation to a plateau. Drug accumulation will continue until the amount of drug eliminated per dosage interval equals the amount administered during that period. The time to maximum accumulation (steady state) depends on the half-life of the drug, irrespective of dosage interval and dosage. The time to 95% of maximum accumulation is between 4 and 5 half-lives. The extent of accumulation is a function of the ratio of the dosage interval (τ) and the half-life ($t_\frac{1}{2}$). When the drug is given intravenously or oral absorption is rapid, assuming a one-compartment model, the following formula describes the amount of accumulation (see also C_{max}):

$$\frac{\text{Concentration at steady state}}{\text{Concentration after first dose}} = \frac{1}{1 - e^{\frac{-0.693\tau}{t_\frac{1}{2}}}}$$

Adverse Reaction

An adverse reaction is any undesired effect of a drug or its metabolites. Most adverse reactions are extensions of a drug's major pharmacological effect or are secondary undesired pharmacological effects. These side-effects are predictable from a knowledge of the drug's action. Less common adverse reactions, which are more difficult to predict, occur when a patient is allergic to a drug or one of its constituents or when an idiosyncratic reaction occurs. The latter is defined as a genetically determined abnormal reactivity to a drug.

Agonist

An agonist is a drug or endogenous substance that produces some clearly defined biological response. It is assumed that the magnitude of the response is directly proportional to the occupancy of receptors by molecules of the particular agonist. The observed response is a sigmoid relationship to the plasma concentration. For practical purposes the logarithm of the plasma concentration of the agonist is directly proportional to effect between 20% and 80% of the maximum response.

Antagonist

When a drug inactivates the receptor, thus preventing an effective complex with and response to the agonist, this drug is known as an antagonist. Competitive or surmountable antagonism occurs when the antagonist combines reversibly with the same receptor site(s) as the agonist and may be overcome by increasing the dose of the agonist. Noncompetitive antagonism occurs when the agonist, irrespective of concentration, has no influence on the degree of antagonism or its reversibility. Noncompetitive antagonism may occur if the antagonist binds irreversibly to the same receptor as the agonist or causes a change in the receptor that prevents access of the agonist.

Pharmacological antagonism implies that the drugs act on the same receptor. Physiological antagonism involves antagonism of the activity of one effector system through an action at another receptor site. The decrease in heart rate produced by propranolol (beta-adrenoceptor antagonist) may be overcome by isoproterenol (beta-adrenoceptor agonist), which is pharmacological antagonism, or by atropine (muscarinic cholinergic antagonist), which is physiological antagonism.

Area Under the Curve (AUC)

If frequent plasma concentrations are measured after a drug is administered, a profile of plasma concentration versus time is obtained. When the two variables (time and plasma level) are plotted on rectilinear graph paper, the area under the curve may be obtained. AUC is expressed in units of concentration $\times$ time (e.g., $\mu g \cdot ml^{-1} \cdot min$, $mg \cdot l^{-1} \cdot hr$) and can be determined by several methods: by use of a planimeter; by the "cut and weigh" method, in which the entire area is cut out on rectilinear graph paper and weighed; by the trapezoidal rule; and by integration. The interval over which the AUC is measured must be defined, e.g., $AUC_{0 \to 6}$ hours, $AUC_{0 \to \infty}$. The AUC may be used to compare the bioavailability of two or more dosage forms of a drug. $AUC_{0 \to \infty}$ may be used to determine the volume of distribution of a drug after intravenous administration or by other routes when the bioavailability is known precisely.

$$\text{Clearance} = \frac{\text{fraction of dose absorbed (F)} \times \text{dose (D)}}{AUC_{0 \to \infty}}$$

$$\text{Volume of distribution} = \frac{\text{fraction of dose absorbed (F)} \times \text{dose (D)}}{k_{el} \times AUC_{0 \to \infty}}$$

Binding to Plasma Proteins

Most drugs are bound to plasma proteins, mainly to albumin. The binding is usually reversible and the extent of binding varies from drug to drug. Only the unbound drug is active and is available for glomerular filtration. The influence of protein binding on tubular secretion and biotransformation depends on the binding characteristics of individual drugs. Displacement of drug from albumin-binding sites by other drugs or endogenous substances may occur, resulting in a greater fraction of unbound drug. The clinical importance of this phenomenon will depend on the magnitude of redistribution of the unbound drug and its subsequent elimination.

Binding to Tissues

Many drugs achieve levels in cells that are higher than in the extracellular fluids. If the binding is readily reversible and the intracellular level is high, these tissues may act as an important reservoir. The presence of drug in cells is most commonly due to reversible tissue binding with proteins, phospholipids, or nucleoproteins. Many lipid-soluble drugs are stored in neutral fat by physical solution rather than by tissue binding.

Bioavailability

Bioavailability indicates the rate and relative amount of administered drug that is absorbed from a particular dosage form. Systemic bioavailability (θ) is best described by the measurement of the relative amount of an administered dose that reaches the general circulation ($AUC_{0 \to \infty}$ or drug excreted in urine), the maximum concentration achieved (C_{max}), and the time (t_{max}) at which this occurs. In general, with drugs given chronically the total amount of drug absorbed is usually more important than its rate of absorption. On the other hand, the t_{max} and C_{max} may be critical for drugs given infrequently or for drugs that depend on rapid achievement of high plasma and tissue concentrations for their effects.

Whereas availability depends on physical properties of a drug preparation, e.g., solubility, particle size, and excipient, systemic availability also depends on metabolism within the gut wall or liver, or both, before the drug gets into the systemic circulation.

It is important to note that bioavailability may vary substantially for different preparations of some drugs.

Biopharmaceutics

The study of the physical and chemical properties of a pharmaceutical preparation as these properties influence the manner in which the compound affects the body and is handled by the body is known as biopharmaceutics.

Such studies should include observations on the active drug itself and on the other compounds involved in its formulation. It should be recognized that few pharmaceutical preparations contain only the so-called active ingredient but have additional substances such as waxes, gelatin, syrups, ethanol, and various fillers or excipients of a supposedly inert nature. Parenteral solutions may contain solvents and stabilizers.

Biopharmaceutical observations therefore include information on these and other factors such as the acidic or basic nature of the drug and its solubility in water and lipids; the particle size, disintegration rate, and dissolution rate; the influence of gastric acid and gastrointestinal enzymes; and the sensitivity of the drug to heat, cold, light, and moisture.

C_{max}

C_{max} is the maximum plasma concentration of drug achieved after dosage. The term generally requires qualification with the dose, the dosage route (e.g., oral, rectal, inhalation, subcutaneous, or intramuscular), the number of doses given previously, and the time after dosage at which the concentration is achieved (t_{max}).

$(C_1)_{max}$ is the maximum concentration after the first dose. $(C_\infty)_{max}$ is the maximum concentration at steady state.

The relationship between $(C_1)_{max}$ and $(C_\infty)_{max}$ is an important fundamental consideration that depends on the ratio of the dosage interval to the half-life. When dosage occurs each half-life, the ratio of $(C_\infty)_{max}$ to $(C_1)_{max}$ is 2; that is, a twofold accumulation occurs with chronic administration. When dosage occurs only every 4 half-lives, the ratio of $(C_\infty)_{max}$ to $(C_1)_{max}$ is only 1.1, and accumulation is trivial (see the formula under Accumulation).

Clearance

Clearance is a concept used to describe the removal of a drug or endogenous substance from a biological system. Qualifications may include the plasma, blood, compartment, tissue, or whole body from which the drug is being cleared, the mechanism of clearance, and the tissue(s) or organ(s) responsible for clearance.

Clearance is measured as the apparent volume from which the drug or endogenous substance is cleared or removed in a given period of time. Conventional units are milliliters per minute (ml/min).

Total body clearance (Q_B) is a measure of the rate of removal of a drug from the body. Since clearance refers only to the specified drug, its calculation is not influenced by the presence of metabolites in the body. In kinetic terms, body clearance is the product of the volume of distribution (V_d) and the elimination rate constant (k_{el}). Elimination rate constant is the slope of the natural logarithm of the plasma concentration versus time curve and is equal to $0.693/t_\frac{1}{2}$.

$$Q_B = V_d \cdot k_{el}$$

$$Q_{B'} = V_d \cdot \frac{0.693}{t_\frac{1}{2}}$$

Compartment

Compartment, a mathematical rather than a physiological concept, is used to describe the distribution characteristics of a drug in the body.

The simplest kinetic model has one compartment, indicating that drug in plasma reaches instantaneous equilibrium with those tissues it enters. A simple monophasic decline in plasma concentration is observed. It should be appreciated that although there is equilibrium between plasma and one or more tissues, the concentration in each need not be, and rarely is, the same. In theory few drugs fit the one-compartment model concept, but in practice it is often a useful and simple clinical approximation.

The two-compartment model is convenient for describing the kinetic behavior of many drugs. A biphasic decline in plasma concentration is seen after IV dosage. In simple terms the *central compartment* may be assumed to represent the plasma and some tissues that the drug enters rapidly, while the *peripheral compartment* may represent other tissues that the particular drug enters more slowly.

It is occasionally necessary to use more complicated multicompartmental models to describe the elimination characteristics of some drugs. The term *deep compartment* indicates a tissue or tissues into which drug perfuses slowly in a multicompartmental model and from which it is also slow to leave during the elimination phase. The slow elimination of guanethidine from neuronal tissue is an example. Conversely, a *shallow compartment* describes a transient compartment at an early phase of a drug's distribution. This may represent temporary drug binding to intravascular components before distribution to the central compartment occurs.

Compliance

The ability of a patient to take medications as prescribed is called compliance. Problems of compliance include failure to take the correct medicine in the correct dose at the correct times.

Inadequate compliance should always be considered when the response to a drug appears inappropriate. It is a major difficulty of therapeutics, demanding the attention of all physicians and health care personnel, since even the best medicines are useless or potentially hazardous if used improperly.

Age, personality, socioeconomic factors such as poverty and isolation, and inadequate explanation of the purpose and possible effects of drugs to patients and those responsible for their care may lead to poor compliance. Large numbers of drugs, complexities of formulation and dosage times, a high incidence of side-effects, or a lack of apparent benefit combined with simple forgetfulness are other possible reasons for poor compliance. All patients are potential defaulters.

Disintegration

Disintegration is the process of physical reduction of a pharmaceutical preparation to particulate material prior to dissolution. Disintegration time, once thought to be the most important influence on the oral availability of a drug, is the time taken for the pill, tablet, or capsule to become particulate under certain defined in vitro conditions. It is now appreciated that disintegration, especially of water-insoluble preparations, may give little indication of the ultimate absorption in vivo.

Dissolution

In the process of solution in gastrointestinal juices, which is essential for absorption to occur, dissolution is the breaking down of fine particles to molecules or ions homogeneously dispersed in solution. Dissolution time is an expression of the rate at which the drug is dissolved under defined in vitro conditions, most of which aim to simulate in vivo activity.

Because dissolution appears to be a better measure of the oral availability of drugs than disintegration, it is increasingly used in industry to standardize preparation of those drugs that have known bioavailability problems, such as digoxin.

Distribution

Distribution is the dispersion of drug into body tissues. The extent and pattern of distribution depend on the molecular weight, pKa and lipid solubility of the drug, the binding to serum and tissue proteins, and on active transport processes, if these exist. Many acidic drugs are confined to the extracellular space, while most basic drugs are distributed throughout the body. Many very lipid-soluble drugs (thiopental and other inhalation anesthetics) accumulate to a large extent in body fat, including the brain. The passage of drugs to the central nervous system, to breast milk, and across the placenta is an important aspect of drug distribution. In general, biological membranes are much more permeable to unionized lipid-soluble molecules than to ionized hydrophilic molecules. Some drugs attain a very high level in specific tissues, e.g., digoxin in heart muscle, some antimalarials in the liver, and antithyroid compounds in the thyroid gland. A high level in a specific tissue does not necessarily imply that the drug is active in that tissue. *Disposition* is a term that denotes the sum of distribution and elimination, i.e., the postabsorptive fate of a drug (see also Compartment; Volume of Distribution [Apparent]: V_d).

Dose-Response Curve

More correctly termed the log dose-response curve, this is a graphic representation of the relationship between the dose administered (expressed in a logarithmic manner, x axis) and the biological effect observed (expressed in a linear manner, y axis). In general, if equilibrium is established between the amount of drug in plasma and receptor site and if the receptor response is a reversible one, a straight line relationship is obtained between 20% and 80% of the maximum response attainable. This maximum response is an expression of the *efficacy* of the drug and may be used to compare different drugs that produce the same response. Curves to the left on the graph indicate greater *potency* than curves to the right.

A "flat" dose-response curve denotes that large dosage increments produce little increase in effect, whereas a "steep" dose-response curve denotes that small increases in dosage substantially increase the response.

"Shifting" of the dose-response curve to the right is a reflection of the antagonism of the action of specific doses of the drug. For example, if a dose-response curve represented the increase in heart rate produced by doses of isoproterenol (agonist), pre-treatment with propranolol (antagonist) would necessitate giving larger doses of isoproterenol to produce the same tachycardia as before. The new dose-response curve would, therefore, be to the right of the old one,

Efficacy

The ability of a drug to carry out a given therapeutic action is called its efficacy. It is measured as the maximum response obtainable. This may be due either to flattening of the dose-response curve or to the development of intolerable side-effects. The comparative efficacy of drugs may be estimated by measuring their maximum tolerated clinical responses. Efficacy is dependent not only on absorption and rate of elimination but also on the affinity of a drug for its receptor site and its ability to produce a pharmacological response at the site.

Elimination

Elimination is the sum of all the processes that terminate the presence of a drug in the body. Drugs are eliminated from the body either unchanged (excretion) or as metabolites (biotransformation), or both. In general, more polar or highly ionized compounds, which are water-soluble but not lipid-soluble, are excreted relatively unchanged. Less polar, lipid-soluble drugs are not readily excreted because of back-diffusion through the renal tubular epithelium.

Elimination is usually characterized by the elimination rate constant (K or k_{el}), which is the sum of the rate constants of all the individual metabolic and excretory processes in the body. The elimination half-life ($t_\frac{1}{2}$) is related to the elimination rate constant by the following equation:

$$k_{el} = \frac{\ln 2}{t_\frac{1}{2}} = \frac{0.693}{t_\frac{1}{2}}$$

$$\text{or} \quad t_\frac{1}{2} = \frac{0.693}{k_{el}}$$

The terminal half-life and elimination rate constant are usually measured from a semilogarithmic plot of serum concentration versus time, preferably after intravenous administration so that the influence of absorption is avoided (see also Half-life).

Excretion

Excretion is removal of unchanged drug from the body, e.g., in urine, bile, saliva, and sweat. The fraction of drug that is excreted may vary from below 0.1 (lipid-soluble drugs) to above 0.9 (polar, water-soluble drugs).

Enterohepatic Recirculation (Biliary Recycling)

Drugs or metabolites excreted in bile into the intestine may be reabsorbed from the intestinal lumen into the portal circulation. Enterohepatic recirculation has clinical importance only if active drug or metabolite is reabsorbed or if an inactive metabolite is transformed to active drug during its passage along the intestine.

Drugs that undergo clinically important enterohepatic recirculation include digitoxin, sulfasalazine, indomethacin, morphine, and stilbestrol.

The rationale for the treatment of digitoxin toxicity with cholestyramine is thought to be the interruption of the enterohepatic recirculation of glycoside by binding to resin.

First-Order Kinetics

The transfer of a constant fraction, or percentage, of a drug or substrate per unit time is known as a first-order process. Examples are absorption and glomerular filtration, which are passive processes. The rate of transfer is directly proportional to the amount of drug remaining to be processed. The absolute rate of the process diminishes steadily.

Metabolism, renal tubular secretion, and biliary secretion are active processes, which are classically described by Michaelis-Menten kinetics. For practical purposes, however, these processes follow first-order kinetics within the therapeutic concentration range of most drugs. Exceptions are described under Zero-Order Kinetics.

Mathematically a first-order process is defined by the rate equation:

$$\frac{dA}{dt} = - kA$$

where

A = amount of drug
k = rate constant of the process

Integration and transformation of this expression produce the following equation, which is of more practical value, relating the amount of drug at time t (A_t) to the initial amount (A_o).

$$A_t = A_o \, e^{-kt}$$

In a one-compartment model it is possible to relate concentration at time t (C_t) to the initial concentration (C_o) by dividing both sides of the equation by the volume of distribution.

$$C_t = C_o \, e^{-kt}$$

This equation may be useful in predicting concentration changes in relation to time. When a first-order process is depicted graphically there is a straight line relationship with slope k between time and the logarithm of concentration or amount.

A simple example of a first-order process is seen in the observed decline of a drug with a 6-hour half-life. The initial concentration of 20 μg/ml falls to 10 μg/ml at 6 hours, 5 μg/ml at 12 hours, and 2.5 μg/ml at 18 hours. It is clear that the reduction in level is numerically less during successive intervals although the fractional reduction remains constant.

First Pass

All drugs taken orally must first pass through the gastrointestinal wall and then the portal system after their absorption. Most drugs undergo little metabolism at this stage. When extensive metabolism eliminates a large fraction of the drug during its first circulation through the gut wall or the liver, a first-pass effect is said to occur. The increased metabolism is due to a very high initial clearance fraction of drug by the gut or liver. The net result is a decreased systemic availability of drug with diminished therapeutic response. The first-pass effect may be bypassed by administration of the drug parenterally or sublingually. Larger oral doses may have the ability to saturate the metabolic capacity of the liver and the gut. A first-pass effect is suspected when there is a large difference between the oral and parenteral doses of the drug necessary to achieve similar effects or plasma levels, provided absorption is complete. In addition, the early urine after intravenous dosage may show a greater ratio of parent drug to metabolite compared with an equal oral dose. A reduction of the first-pass effect leading to greater drug availability may occur in patients with cirrhosis or portacaval anastomosis. Drugs with first pass include isoproterenol, terbutaline, alprenolol, propranolol, dopamine, methyldopa, levodopa, imipramine. desipramine, nortriptyline, morphine, meperidine, pentazocine, propoxyphene, naloxone, acetylsalicylic acid, phenacetin, atropine, lidocaine, nitroglycerin, and the natural estrogens.

If the metabolites are active the significance of the first-pass effect is diminished (propranolol, alprenolol, and acetylsalicylic acid).

Half-life: Alpha and Beta Phases

When a drug that fits a two-compartment open model is given intravenously and when the logarithm of the concentration is plotted against time, the resulting curve (Figure 3) has two clearly defined components.

After distribution the curve enters a slower, beta (β), or elimination, phase and represents predominantly irreversible elimination of drug from the central compartment. The beta half-life is defined as:

$$t_{\frac{1}{2}}\beta = \frac{\ln 2}{\beta} = \frac{0.693}{\beta}$$

where

β = the slope of the curve

B (in Figure 3) = the intercept

The units of β are the reciprocal of time, e.g., hour^{-1}.

The line described by the terminal or beta-elimination phase may be extrapolated to zero time. It clearly differs from the observed concentrations during the period of distribution. Subtracting the points on the extrapolated line from those on the observed line is a means of evaluating this distribution phase. The new line thus constructed by "feathering" or "peeling off" defines the alpha (α) phase. The initial fall in concentration is the alpha (α) or distribution phase and represents the rapid distribution of

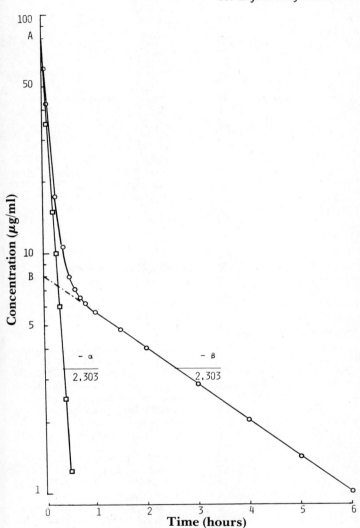

Figure 3   *Schematic two-compartment model.* $C = Ae^{-\alpha t} + Be^{-\beta t}$. *When concentration is plotted against time on the usual log scale (logarithm base 10) rather than the ln scale (natural logarithm), α and β must be determined by multiplying the slopes by 2.303.* $\bigcirc$ *= plasma concentration;* $\square$ *= residual concentration;* $A = 80$ $\mu g/ml$; $\alpha = 8.313\ hr^{-1}$; $t_{\frac{1}{2}}\alpha = 5\ minutes$; $B = 8\ \mu g/ml$; $\beta = 0.347\ hr^{-1}$; $t_{\frac{1}{2}}\beta = 2$ hours.

drug from the central to the peripheral compartments. The alpha half-life is defined as

$$t_{\frac{1}{2}}\alpha = \frac{\ln 2}{\alpha} = \frac{0.693}{\alpha}$$

where

α = the slope

A (in Figure 3) = the intercept of the line created by subtraction of extrapolated beta phase from observed plasma concentration data

The units of α are also the reciprocal of time.

$t_{\frac{1}{2}}\beta$ is the more important pharmacokinetic parameter of the two and is usually referred to as the half-life or elimination half-life. Each time an interval equal to $t_{\frac{1}{2}}\beta$ elapses, 50% of the drug present in the body at the beginning of that interval is eliminated. The area under the curve is described by the equation

$$AUC_{0\to\infty} = \frac{A}{\alpha} + \frac{B}{\beta}$$

The concentration (C) at any time (t) can be determined by the equation

$$C = Ae^{-\alpha t} + Be^{-\beta t}$$

Hypersensitivity (Allergy)

An allergic reaction is an adverse reaction not explained by the pharmacological properties of the drug and is assumed to be due to altered immunological sensitivity of the patient. It is usually associated with symptoms commonly ascribed to hypersensitivity (e.g., rash, fever, arthritis, eosinophilia, and asthma). It recurs on readministration of the drug and usually bears little relationship to dosage or drug accumulation. The reaction may be due to the drug or its metabolite(s), or both, forming an antigen complex in the body.

The type of hypersensitivity reaction may generally be classified according to the four classic types of Gell and Coombs, i.e., type 1, acute, anaphylactic type reactions in which the IgE antibody is fixed to cells and provocation promotes the release of histamine and histamine-like substances (urticaria, asthma, anaphylaxis); type 2, circulating antibodies attack cells (hemolytic anemia, aplastic anemia); type 3, circulating antigen-antibody complexes produce Arthus-type reactions (polyarthritis, nephritis); type 4, cell-mediated delayed hypersensitivity, tuberculin-like reaction. Sensitized lymphocytes react to antigen in fixed drug eruptions.

Many clinical syndromes, such as skin rashes and jaundice, are not easily categorized into any single type of reaction.

Induction and Inhibition of Enzyme Activity

Induction of enzyme activity is the increase in the rate of clearance of a drug by enhancement of its metabolism. Inhibition of enzyme activity is the decrease in the rate of clearance of a drug by reduction of its metabolism.

Enzyme induction is associated with a growth of the smooth endoplasmic reticulum (microsomal system) in the liver cells, which enlarge as a result. The number of liver cells is unchanged. Enhanced enzymatic activity is due to increased synthesis or reduced breakdown of cytochrome P-450, NADPH-cytochrome c reductase, and other enzymes involved in drug metabolism. Measurable changes in the rate of drug metabolism usually begin after administration of or exposure to the inducing drug or chemical. Enhanced enzyme activity may continue for 2–3 weeks after the inducing agent is discontinued. Enzyme induction is often variable and unpredictable, but as a rule susceptibility to inducing agents is greatest for individuals with the slowest initial rates of metabolism. Drug metabolizing activity may increase as much as fourfold, although a twofold increase is more common.

Common inducing agents are phenobarbital (and to a lesser extent other barbiturates), phenytoin, spironolactone, chlorophenothane (DDT), chlordane, cigarette-smoking (benzpyrene), and chronic ingestion of ethanol.

Enzyme inhibition may occur when two drugs compete for a common metabolic pathway. Reduction of metabolism usually starts immediately after exposure to the inhibiting agent and persists as long as the inhibiting drug is present in sufficient amount.

Common enzyme inhibitors are dicumarol, phenylbutazone, chloramphenicol, sulfaphenazole, sulfamethizole, chlorpromazine, sulthiame, disulfiram, and recent ethanol ingestion.

Induction and inhibition of drug-metabolizing enzymes are the basis for several interactions. Besides the extent and frequency of these interactions, their clinical relevance depends on the plasma concentration-response relationship of the drugs involved.

Metabolism

Metabolism is the process of biological transformation of a drug or endogenous substance. Metabolic pathways are usually in the liver but may be in plasma or other tissues. Metabolites may be active or inactive, toxic or nontoxic.

Four major types of metabolic reaction are described: oxidation, reduction, hydrolysis, and conjugation. The first three processes are sometimes known as phase 1 metabolism; conjugation may be described as phase 2 metabolism.

Oxidation is often mediated by a "mixed-function" enzyme system found in the smooth endoplasmic reticulum of liver cells, the cytochromes P-450, which depend on NADPH, magnesium ions, and oxygen. This system is capable of producing a wide variety of oxidative reactions, including aliphatic oxidation (to alcohols); aromatic hydroxylation; N-, O-, and S-dealkylation (the alkyl groups that are removed are oxidized to aldehydes); deamination (to ketones with release of ammonia); and sulfoxide formation and desulfuration. These processes should not be confused with the activities of xanthinoxidase, monoamine oxidase (MAO), and alcohol dehydrogenase, which exert specific oxidative functions.

Reduction, the addition of hydrogen across existing bonds, does not appear to be a major activity of mammalian tissue enzymes but is clinically relevant because it occurs in intestinal bacteria. The metabolism of sulfasalazine to 5-aminosalicylate and sulfapyridine by reduction of the azo bond is an important example. Chloral hydrate is reduced to trichloroethanol, the active chemical.

Hydrolysis is the splitting of molecules by the addition of water. Esters are hydrolyzed to acids and alcohols by esterases. Amides are hydrolyzed to acids and amines by amidases. Acetylcholinesterase and plasma cholinesterase are important specific esterases.

Conjugation or synthesis is the result of the addition of another molecule such as sulfuric or glucuronic acid to a drug or its metabolites. Enzymes called transferases are responsible for mediating the formation of sulfates and glucuronides, respectively. Conjugation succeeds oxidation in the metabolic process of many drugs.

In general, metabolic processes are slower at the extremes of life. Inadequate glucuronyl transferase activity in the newborn was responsible for deaths from inadvertent overdoses of chloramphenicol. The babies experienced concentration-related cardiorespiratory collapse (the gray syndrome).

Genetic and environmental factors both influence metabolic pathways. The genetic variation in plasma cholinesterase is an important clinical aspect of hydrolysis. People with abnormal variants of the enzyme suffer prolonged, potentially fatal apnea following exposure to the noncompetitive depolarizing muscle relaxant succinylcholine (suxamethonium). There is marked genetic variation with acetylation, a conjugation process. Individuals who have slow acetylation are homozygous autosomal recessive for the gene controlling acetylation, display diminished acetylation of drugs such as sulfonamides, procainamide, hydralazine, and isoniazid. Environmental factors are discussed under Induction and Inhibition of Enzyme Activity.

Michaelis-Menten Kinetics

Active transport and metabolic processes requiring enzyme activity display a limited capacity for the amount of substrate that they can handle. The maximum velocity (V_m) is a function of the particular enzyme or transport system.

The rate of decline of concentration of drug (dC/dt) is related to the concentration (C) and the maximum velocity (V_m) by the Michaelis-Menten equation:

$$- \frac{dC}{dt} = \frac{V_m \, C}{K_m + C}$$

K_m is the Michaelis constant. It is clear from the equation that when the rate of decline is $V_m/2$ that $C = K_m$. In other words, K_m is the concentration at which the rate is half maximal.

Two special situations should be considered.

(a) If the concentration C is very much less than K_m, the equation becomes

$$- \frac{dC}{dt} = \frac{V_m}{K_m} \cdot C$$

and the rate of decline is proportional to the concentration of drug, i.e., it is a first-order process. This is the situation with most drugs, since their therapeutic concentrations are usually well below K_m and the rate of enzyme or secretory activity is usually well below the maximum possible.

(b) When the concentration C is greatly in excess of the K_m, the equation resolves to

$$- \frac{dC}{dt} = V_m$$

and the rate of decline of concentration is steady at the maximum possible, irrespective of concentration (provided, of course, that concentration remains well above K_m). This is the description of a zero-order process.

The extreme examples of the Michaelis-Menten equation are described under First-Order Kinetics and Zero-Order Kinetics.

Pharmacodynamics

The measurement of the pharmacological, therapeutic, and toxic effects of drugs in the body, i.e., what the drug does to the body, is known as pharmacodynamics. This includes a description of the mechanism of drug action, the structure-activity relationship (SAR), and the relationship between response and dose or plasma concentration.

Pharmacokinetics

The time-dependent changes in the amount or serum concentrations of drugs and metabolites in the body, i.e., what the body does to the drug, are known as pharmacokinetics. These changes are usually divided into processes of liberation of active drug at the site of absorption, absorption, distribution, and elimination. Elimination is the sum of metabolism and excretion.

The study of pharmacokinetics is the basis for (1) the development of optimal dosage forms, (2) the establishment of dosage regimens, and (3) the understanding of many interactions.

pKa

The pH at which an acidic or basic group is 50% ionized is known as the pKa. For each unit change in pH away from the pKa, there will be a tenfold change in ionization according to the Henderson-Hasselbalch equation:

$$pH = pK' + \log \frac{[\text{proton acceptor}]}{[\text{proton donor}]}$$

pK' is the dissociation constant and is termed pKa when discussing the dissociation of a weak acid HA.

$$pH = pKa + \log \frac{[A^-]}{[HA]}$$

Note that a drug may have more than one acidic or basic substituent each with a different pKa. The degree of ionization at a given pH influences the drug's ability to interact with receptors and to cross biological membranes. In general, unionized molecules cross membranes easily, while ionized molecules do not. Renal elimination for many drugs depends on the fact that in urine they will be ionized and therefore unable to return to the bloodstream once they have been filtered.

The excretion of weak acids of pKa 3.5–7.5 will be increased in alkaline urine, since they will be increasingly ionized at higher pH. Weak bases of pKa 7.5–10.5 will be better excreted in acid urine. Practical examples include the forced alkaline diuresis of phenobarbital, a weak acid with a pKa of 7.2, and of salicylate, a weak acid with a pKa of 3.0.

Potency

Potency is the ratio of the dose of a drug that produces pharmacological effects equal to that of a reference compound. *Equal responses must be compared.* The dose of the drug under test may then be related to the dose of the standard that produces the same response. This dose may be derived empirically or by performing dose-response curves and estimating comparable doses from the curves.

Solubility

Solubility is the degree to which a compound will dissolve in a given volume of fluid under specified conditions of temperature and pH. Drugs cannot be absorbed from the gastrointestinal tract unless they are in solution. In general, the more soluble the dosage form of a drug, the greater the rate and extent to which it will be absorbed.

Summation (Addition)

Summation is the additive effect of two or more drugs on the same target organ or cell. The total effect equals the sum of the effects of the same doses of the individual drugs given separately. Pharmacological summation implies that the drugs involved act via the same mechanism or receptor sites, whereas physiological summation involves the activity of two or more effector systems that produce the same physiological response.

Synergism (Superaddition, Potentiation)

When two or more synergistic drugs are given together, the effect on the target organ or cell is greater than the sum of their separate effects. This result generally implies that the drugs achieve the same end point by different mechanisms, and it is the basis of many regimens of multiple chemotherapy as applied to cancer and to infections. In addition to the enhanced pharmacological effect, it is often also possible to use drugs in these regimens at a lower dosage and thus avoid the toxicity associated with higher doses of the individual drugs.

t_{max}

t_{max}

The time after administration of a drug when maximum plasma levels of the drug (C_{max}) are seen is known as t_{max}; t_{max} gives an estimate of how rapidly the drug is absorbed from a given site. It depends both on rate of absorption and on rate of elimination. In general the rate of absorption, being more rapid than the rate of elimination, is more important in determining the time when t_{max} occurs.

Therapeutic Index

In animal pharmacology, the therapeutic index implies the ratio between the lethal dose in 50% of a given species (LD_{50}) and the effective dose in 50% (ED_{50}). However, in clinical pharmacology, the therapeutic index has come to mean the ratio between the minimum toxic and maximum therapeutic plasma concentrations of a drug. Frequently, as in the case of digoxin and theophylline, these levels overlap to some extent and the drug is said to have a low therapeutic index. For other drugs, such as penicillin and propranolol, the therapeutic index is high because blood levels producing toxic and therapeutic effects are widely separated.

Therapeutic Range

The range of concentrations of drug in plasma required to achieve a satisfactory pharmacological response without significant toxicity is known as the therapeutic range. The upper limit of the therapeutic range is often defined by the onset of side-effects. The therapeutic range may be very wide, as in the case of penicillin, or very narrow, as in the case of digoxin, and may vary for a given drug according to which pharmacological effect is required, e.g., the use of aspirin as an analgesic requires lower plasma concentrations than when it is used as an anti-inflammatory agent.

Unbound ("Free") Drug

The unbound drug is that fraction of drug in plasma or tissues that is not bound to plasma or tissue proteins. A reversible equilibrium normally exists between the unbound drug and the protein-bound drug. Only the unbound drug is considered to be pharmacologically active and in equilibrium with the receptor site. This fraction appears to be responsible for the dose-related therapeutic effects and adverse reactions. The unbound fraction is also available for excretion and elimination.

Certain drugs (e.g., propranolol) have a marked hepatic uptake that is capable of rapidly shifting the equilibrium from bound to unbound drug. This creates the effect of so-called protein stripping by the liver. For these drugs increased protein binding results in enhanced hepatic clearance. Changes in their rate of metabolism depend mainly on hepatic blood flow. For other drugs an increase in unbound drug generally leads to increased hepatic metabolism. The rate of metabolism of such drugs is normally independent of liver blood flow. Protein binding limits glomerular filtration but generally does not influence renal tubular secretion, which also appears to "strip" bound drug.

The unbound fraction of some drugs, e.g., phenytoin, is dependent on the concentration of plasma proteins and may be altered in disease states that produce hypoalbuminemia. Throughout the therapeutic plasma concentration range, unbound drug is usually a constant fraction of total drug in plasma.

Interaction by displacement may temporarily increase the concentration of unbound drug. Redistribution and enhanced metabolism often modify this increase, but it may remain clinically relevant if the drug has a small volume of distribution. The interaction may be of little importance if the volume of distribution is very large.

Volume of Distribution (Apparent): V_d

$$V_d = \frac{\text{amount of drug in body}}{\text{concentration of drug in plasma}} = \frac{F \cdot D}{k_{el} \cdot AUC_{0 \to \infty}}$$

where

F = the fraction of the dose absorbed

D = the dose

k_{el} = the elimination rate constant

$AUC_{0 \to \infty}$ = the area under the plasma concentration–time curve between zero time and infinity

Volume of distribution (V_d) is that volume of fluid into which the drug appears to distribute with a concentration equal to that in plasma. It is a purely theoretical entity that gives an expression of the extent to which the drug passes from the plasma to peripheral tissues. In a one-compartment model this assumes that the body acts as a single homogeneous container with respect to the drug. Note that estimations of V_d can be made only if the drug is given intravenously or if its systemic bioavailability is known, since only under these circumstances can the amount in the body be known accurately. V_d may be used in the calculation of the drug dose (D) required to produce a given average plasma concentration ($\bar{C}$) if F is known. The average concentration is the AUC during a dosage interval, divided by that dosage interval (τ):

$$\bar{C} = \frac{AUC}{\tau}$$

since $\quad AUC = \frac{F \cdot D}{k_{el} \cdot V_d}, \quad \bar{C} = \frac{F \cdot D}{\tau \cdot k_{el} \cdot V_d}$

then $\quad D = \frac{C \cdot \tau \cdot k_{el} \cdot V_d}{F}$

or $\quad D = \frac{\bar{C} \cdot \tau \cdot V_d}{1.44 \cdot F \cdot t_{\frac{1}{2}}} \quad \left(\text{since } t_{\frac{1}{2}} = \frac{0.693}{k_{el}} \right)$

Zero-Order (Dose-Dependent or Capacity-Limited) Kinetics

Many of the body's enzyme systems, such as metabolic processes, renal and biliary excretion, and active and facilitated gastrointestinal absorption, are saturable processes. Although the plasma concentration of a drug in the clinical context generally falls within the capacity of the given system, this does not always occur. Then, instead of the reaction proceeding at a rate proportional to the concentration of substrate present, i.e., in a first-order fashion, the reaction proceeds at a fixed rate regardless of substrate concentration. Both of these processes occur together during the transition from first-order to zero-order kinetics. This phenomenon may be seen most clearly in the metabolism of phenytoin, acetylsalicylic acid, dicumarol, ethanol, and probenecid. Under these circumstances, the constant relationship between drug dosage and plasma concentration is lost and the plasma level rises disproportionately with increasing dosage. This is due to a progressively smaller increase in elimination rate relative to the increase in substrate concentration as enzyme systems become saturated (see Michaelis-Menten Kinetics).

An example of a zero-order process is a drug that has a plasma concentration of 24 μg/ml and then 20 μg/ml, 16 μg/ml, and 12 μg/ml at successive intervals of 6 hours.

Drug Profiles

II

ACETAMINOPHEN
(Paracetamol)

A metabolite of phenacetin and a relative of other aniline derivatives, most of which have been discontinued because of toxicity. Analgesic and antipyretic effects comparable to aspirin but devoid of anti-inflammatory action.

Absorption
Oral bioavailability: 100%. t_{max}: ½–1 hour, depending on preparation (see Interactions).

Distribution
V_d: 0.8–1.0 L/kg [7]. Protein binding: 25%, highest concentration in liver.

Elimination
$t_{\frac{1}{2}}$: 2–4 hours [2, 7]. Major metabolites (80%) are glucuronide and sulfate (both inactive). Minor deacetylation product (p-aminophenol) and intermediate N-hydroxyl derivative are relevant to toxicity. Drug (3–4%) and metabolites (probably active tubular secretion) are excreted in urine [1]. There is slight diurnal variation in metabolism [7]. Although $t_{\frac{1}{2}}$ is similar throughout life, the infant and young child produce relatively more sulfate than glucuronide [2].

Dosage Schedule
Oral use only. 300–600 mg every 4–6 hours as required. More than 3–4 g in 24 hours is considered unsafe.

Special Dosage Situations
If possible, prolonged administration of the drug should be avoided in patients with anemia or with cardiac, pulmonary, renal, or hepatic disease, since the effects from overdosage are potentially more serious in these individuals (see Adverse Reactions). Children: 10 mg/kg every 6–8 hours as required. No adjustment necessary in pregnancy or lactation.

Therapeutic Concentrations
Measurement of plasma levels appears to be relevant only in toxicity.

Adverse Reactions

Occasionally, rash and neutropenia. No clear association with analgesic nephropathy.

Hepatotoxicity, renal damage, respiratory depression, cardiovascular collapse, coma, and death in serious overdosage (e.g., single dose of 6 g or more). No absolute relationship between total dose and severity of poisoning. Plasma concentration greater than 250 μg/ml at 4 hours after ingestion is usually associated with hepatotoxicity. Liver damage generally is directly related to levels of transaminases, lactic dehydrogenase, and bilirubin and to the prothrombin time [6].

A useful index of liver injury is $t_{\frac{1}{2}}$ measured 4–12 hours after administration; $t_{\frac{1}{2}}$ greater than 4 hours suggests hepatocellular necrosis. The ratio of parent drug in plasma to its conjugated metabolites increases as the liver fails and urinary excretion of unchanged drug is increased.

An N-hydroxylated intermediate metabolite, which is normally inactivated by combining with glutathione, damages liver cells by covalent linkage [3]. Enzyme induction (e.g., prior alcohol or barbiturate use) and preexisting liver disease potentiate toxicity [3, 9]. Cysteamine (possibly by metabolite inactivation or inhibition of formation) may counteract toxicity in serious cases of acetaminophen overdosage if used early [4]; an IV dose of 3.2 g over 20 hours within 10 hours of acetaminophen overdose has been used successfully. Methionine and N-acetylcysteine (source of sulfhydryl group) may also play a part in therapy. Aminophenol may cause methemoglobinemia and, rarely, acute hemolysis.

Interactions

Propantheline delays and metoclopramide enhances the rate of absorption of acetaminophen. Acetaminophen may interfere with uric acid determination [8].

Review

Koch-Weser, J. Drug therapy. Acetaminophen. *N. Engl. J. Med.* 295:1297–1300, 1976.

References

1. Cummings, A. J., King, M. L., et al. A kinetic study of drug elimination: The excretion of paracetamol and its metabolites in man. *Br. J. Pharmacol.* 29:150–157, 1967.
2. Miller, R. P., Roberts, R. J., et al. Acetaminophen elimination kinetics in neonates, children, and adults. *Clin. Pharmacol. Ther.* 19:284–294, 1976.
3. Mitchell, J. R., Jollow, D. J., et al. Acetaminophen-induced hepatic necrosis. l. Role of drug metabolism. *J. Pharmacol. Exp. Ther.* 187:185–194, 1973.
4. Prescott, L. F., Swainson, C. P., et al. Successful treatment of severe paracetamol poisoning with cysteamine. *Lancet* 1:588–592, 1974.
5. Prescott, L. F., and Wright, N. The effects of hepatic and renal damage on paracetamol metabolism and excretion fol-

lowing overdosage. A pharmacokinetic study. *Br. J. Pharmacol.* 49:602–613, 1973.
6. Prescott, L. F., Wright, N., et al. Plasma-paracetamol half-life and hepatic necrosis in patients with paracetamol overdosage. *Lancet* 1:519–522, 1971.
7. Shively, C. A., and Vessell, E. S. Temporal variations in acetaminophen and phenacetin half-life in man. *Clin. Pharmacol. Ther.* 18:413–424, 1975.
8. Wilding, P., and Heath, D. A. Effect of paracetamol on uric acid determination. *Ann. Clin. Biochem.* 12:142–144, 1975.
9. Wright, N., and Prescott, L. F. Potentiation by previous drug therapy of hepatotoxicity following paracetamol overdosage. *Scot. Med. J.* 18:56–59, 1973.

ACETYLSALICYLIC ACID
(Aspirin)

A salicylate, possessing analgesic, antipyretic, and anti-inflammatory properties. Site of action for alleviation of fever and pain most probably located in the hypothalamic nuclei. Anti-inflammatory mechanism remains unresolved, but stabilization of lysosomes, inhibition of prostaglandins, and nonspecific reduction of capillary permeability are the most likely possibilities. Inhibits platelet aggregation, possibly by acetylation of the platelet cell membrane [10].

Major indication for use is for the symptomatic relief of fever and mild to moderate pain, such as headache or the pain accompanying arthritis, myalgia, or dysmenorrhea. Used as anti-inflammatory agent in rheumatic fever, rheumatoid arthritis, and radiation colitis.

The regular intake of aspirin has been associated with a decreased incidence of myocardial infarction [1].

Absorption

Oral bioavailability: 80–100%. t_{max}: 1–2 hours [8]. C_{max} and t_{max} vary with the preparation [3, 7], with buffered aspirin performing better than the unbuffered preparation or enteric-coated tablets [7]. The pH of stomach contents is also important [2]. Absorbed from the stomach and the small intestine and to some extent from the rectum.

Distribution

V_d for acetylsalicylic acid (ASA): 0.15–0.2 L/kg. V_d for salicylic acid (SA): 0.13 L/kg. Protein binding for ASA: 50–80%. Decreases with falls in serum albumin levels [10]. Fetal levels exceed maternal plasma concentrations [4]. Detected in breast milk, saliva, and spinal fluid at levels approximately 1.5 times those of blood. t_{max} in joints parallels that of blood [12].

Elimination

$t_{\frac{1}{2}}$ for ASA: 15–20 minutes [11]. Converted in liver and plasma to SA, which is pharmacologically active and exhibits dose-dependent kinetics in doses exceeding 300 mg of ASA, e.g., "$t_{\frac{1}{2}}$"

(apparent half-life) for 300 mg is 3 hours, for 1000 mg 5–6 hours, and for 10 g 20 hours [6]. SA is metabolized in the liver, the major metabolite being salicyluric acid, which is a glycine conjugate (70%). Other metabolites are salicyl phenolic glucuronide, salicyl acyl glucuronide, and gentisic acid [5]. Excretion of SA and metabolites in the urine is pH-dependent, with increased excretion in alkaline urine [9]. At pH 8, 80% of unchanged drug appears in urine, but at pH 4, only 10% is present [7]. Renal clearance involves glomerular filtration, tubular secretion, and tubular reabsorption. SA may compete with other drugs, e.g., probenecid, para-aminohippuric acid (PAH), and methotrexate, which are also eliminated by these mechanisms.

Dosage Schedule

Antipyretic and analgesic dose: usually given, as required, up to 10–15 mg/kg every 4–6 hours. Anti-inflammatory dose, e.g., rheumatic fever and rheumatoid arthritis in adults: 3–6 g/day in 4–6 divided doses. Children: 25 mg/kg/day for 1–2 days, 18 mg/kg/day for 7–10 days, and then 14 mg/kg/day for as long as necessary. Should be administered at 4- to 6-hour intervals.

Special Dosage Situations

Use cautiously in asthma, hepatic insufficiency, and bleeding diatheses. In hypoproteinemia, protein binding is decreased, with an increase in V_d and a decrease in plasma levels of drug. No adjustment required in renal disease if serum albumin normal. Although salicylates have uricosuric properties in large doses (more than 5 g/day), they decrease uric acid secretion in small doses (less than 2 g/day) and are therefore contraindicated in patients with gout. Children with fever and dehydration are especially prone to salicylate intoxication. No contraindication to use in pregnancy.

Therapeutic Concentrations

Antipyretic and analgesic: 20–100 μg/ml. Anti-inflammatory: 100–250 μg/ml.

Adverse Reactions

Toxicity is manifested by tinnitus and vertigo (plasma level above 200 μg/ml); reversible hepatotoxicity (200–400 μg/ml); and hyperventilation, respiratory alkalosis, metabolic acidosis, anemia, hypoprothrombinemia, fever, coma, cardiovascular collapse, and renal failure (400–900 μg/ml). Gastrointestinal bleeding occurs frequently, even with very small doses.

In minor poisoning, alkalinize the urine to hasten excretion. In more severe poisoning, the goals of treatment are to correct acidosis, hyperthermia, hypoglycemia, hypokalemia, and dehydration and to clear the plasma of salicylate. These effects may be achieved by gastric lavage, alkalinization of the urine, forced diuresis, and dialysis in comatose patients.

Aspirin intolerance is characterized by rhinitis, sinusitis, nasal polyposis, and asthma after exposure to aspirin, indomethacin, morphine, and codeine.

Interactions

Enhances anticoagulant effect of oral anticoagulants. Increases hypoglycemic effect of insulin and oral hypoglycemic agents. Interferes with uricosuric action of sulfinpyrazone and probenecid. Because renal clearance of PAH is decreased, avoid use of the drug in patients who have renal blood flow estimations. Concomitant administration of antacids decreases the drug's apparent systemic bioavailability because of enhanced excretion in alkaline urine. Severe bone marrow depression occurs when salicylates are administered with methotrexate.

Review

Levy, G., and Leonards, J. R. Absorption, Metabolism, and Excretion of Salicylates. In M. J. H. Smith and P. K. Smith (Eds.), *The Salicylates: A Critical Bibliographic Review*. New York: Interscience, 1966. Pp. 5–48.

References

1. Boston Collaborative Drug Surveillance Group. Regular aspirin intake and acute myocardial infarction. *Br. Med. J.* 1:440–443, 1974.
2. Hogben, C. A. M., Schanker, L. S., et al. Absorption of drugs from stomach. II. Human. *J. Pharmacol. Exp. Ther.* 120:540–545, 1957.
3. Hollister, L. E., and Kanter, S. L. Studies of delayed action medication. IV. Salicylates. *Clin. Pharmacol. Ther.* 6:5–11, 1965.
4. Levy, G., Procknal, J., et al. Distribution of salicylate between neonatal and maternal serum at diffusion equilibrium. *Clin. Pharmacol. Ther.* 18:210–214, 1975.
5. Levy, G., Tsuchiya, T., et al. Limited capacity for salicyl phenolic glucuronide formation and its effect on the kinetics of salicylate elimination in man. *Clin. Pharmacol. Ther.* 13:258–268, 1972.
6. Levy, G. Pharmacokinetics of salicylate elimination in man. *J. Pharm. Sci.* 54:959–967, 1965.
7. Levy, G., and Hayes, B. A. Physiochemical bases of the buffered acetylsalicylic acid controversy. *N. Engl. J. Med.* 262:1053–1058, 1960.
8. Levy, G., and Hollister, L. E. Inter- and intrasubject variations in drug absorption kinetics. *J. Pharm. Sci.* 53:1446–1452, 1964.
9. MacPherson, C. R., Milne, M. D., et al. Excretion of salicylate. *Br. J. Pharmacol.* 10:484–489, 1955.
10. Roth, G. J., and Majerus, P. W. The mechanism of the effect of aspirin on human platelets. I. Acetylation of a particulate fraction protein. *J. Clin. Invest.* 56:624–632, 1975.
11. Rowland, M., and Riegelman, S. Pharmacokinetics of acetylsalicylic acid and salicylic acid after intravenous administration in man. *J. Pharm. Sci.* 57:1313–1319, 1968.
12. Soren, A. Kinetics of salicylates in blood and joint fluid. *J. Clin. Pharmacol.* 15:173–177, 1975.

ALBUTEROL
(Salbutamol)

Noncatechol, highly selective (beta-2) adrenergic stimulant [5]. Indicated in the treatment of reversible obstructive airway disease. Bronchodilation is associated with little or no increase in heart rate at usual therapeutic doses. May also be effective in suppressing premature labor [6], thus permitting glucocorticoid administration to the mother for 24 hours to reduce the incidence of respiratory distress syndrome in the immature neonate [7]. Tolerance to the drug has not been observed [9].

Absorption

65–84% of oral dose absorbed. t_{max}: 1–3 hours [10]. 78–97% of inhaled dose absorbed. t_{max}: 3–5 hours [10]. Much of the inhaled dose appears to be swallowed and then absorbed from the gastrointestinal tract. There appears to be extensive first-pass metabolism [10].

Distribution

V_d: unknown. Protein binding: unknown. Maximum effect after oral dose occurs at 1–3 hours [10]. After inhalation maximum effect is observed at 10–15 minutes, indicating a direct action on the bronchi [10].

Elimination

$t_{\frac{1}{2}}$ for oral dose: 2.7–5 hours [10]. Salbutamol is not a substrate for catechol-O-methyltransferase (COMT). Hepatic transformation produces an unidentified, apparently inactive, metabolite. Metabolite (34–47% of dose) and parent drug are excreted in the urine. $t_{\frac{1}{2}}$ for inhaled dose: 1.7–7.1 hours [10]. At peak concentrations, ratio of metabolite to salbutamol is 4 : 1. Metabolite $t_{\frac{1}{2}}$ approximately the same as that of salbutamol.

Dosage Schedule

Oral: 6–16 mg/day in 3 or 4 divided doses for prophylaxis or continuous bronchodilation. Not very useful for acute asthmatic attacks.

Inhaler: 100–200 µg (1 or 2 puffs) by metered aerosol 3–4 times daily. In emergency repeat this dose every 4 hours at most.

Parenteral use: several regimens have been proposed. Optimal doses are 500 µg subcutaneously [2] and 8 µg/kg IM [4]. Single doses of 100–300 µg IV [3] and doses up to 25.0 µg/min by IV infusion have been safely used for bronchodilation [8]. Indeed, doses up to 76 µg/min have been used in obstetrics, but side-effects were common [6].

Special Dosage Situations

Increase dosage cautiously in elderly and in patients with known ischemic heart disease. Reduce dose in patients with severe renal disease, since 40–50% of the drug is excreted unchanged in urine (see Table 1, p. 30). Start with 4 mg daily in 4 divided doses for children and increase the dosage slowly. No available specific information about use in patients with hepatic disease or bronchodilating doses in pregnant women. Patients with extremely low pretreatment forced expiratory volume in 1 second (FEV_1) may respond better to inhalational therapy by intermittent positive pressure ventilation (IPPV) [1].

Therapeutic Concentrations

Not known. It is usual to assess changes in respiratory function by objective tests.

Adverse Reactions

Mainly signs of excessive sympathetic activity. Tremulousness, apprehension, tachycardia, palpitations, nausea, and sweating. Arrhythmias and angina may occur in individuals predisposed to these conditions. IV use of a beta-adrenergic blocking drug such as propranolol may be necessary to treat cases of serious overdose, but caution is advised, since beta-blocking drugs may aggravate airway obstruction if used in excess.

Interactions

Additive effects with other directly and indirectly acting sympathomimetics and theophylline.

References

1. Choo-Kang, Y. F. J., and Grant, I. W. B.   Comparison of two methods of administering bronchodilator aerosol to asthmatic patients. Br. Med. J. 1:119–120, 1975.
2. Coady, T. J., Stewart, C. J., et al.   Determination of the optimum dose of subcutaneous salbutamol in asthmatic patients. Br. J. Clin. Pharmacol. 3:239–242, 1976.
3. Fitchett, D. H., McNicol, M. W., et al.   Intravenous salbutamol in management of status asthmaticus. Br. Med. J. 1:53–55, 1975.
4. Ingram, J., Gaddie, J., et al.   The effect of intramuscular salbutamol in asthmatics. Br. J. Clin. Pharmacol. 2:263–266, 1975.
5. Kennedy, M. C. S., and Simpson, W. T.   Human pharmacological and clinical studies on salbutamol: A specific β-adrenergic bronchodilator. Br. J. Dis. Chest 63:165–174, 1969.
6. Korda, A. R., Lyneham, R. C., et al.   The treatment of premature labor with intravenously administered salbutamol. Med. J. Aust. 1:744–746, 1974.
7. Liggins, C. G., and Howie, R. N.   A controlled trial of antepartum glucocorticoids for prevention of the respiratory distress syndrome in premature infants. Pediatrics 50:515–525, 1972.
8. May, C. S., Paterson, J. W., et al.   Intravenous infusion of salbutamol in the treatment of asthma. Br. J. Clin. Pharmacol. 2:503–508, 1975.
9. Sims, B. A.   Investigation of salbutamol tolerance. Br. J. Clin. Pharmacol. 1:291–294, 1974.

10. Walker, S. R., Evans, M. E., et al. The clinical pharmacology of oral and inhaled salbutamol. *Clin. Pharmacol. Ther.* 13:861–867, 1972.

ALLOPURINOL

An analog of the naturally occurring purine hypoxanthine, which is successively oxidized to xanthine and uric acid by the enzyme xanthinoxidase. Allopurinol is a competitive inhibitor of xanthinoxidase at low concentrations; at higher concentrations direct noncompetitive enzyme inhibition is produced by allopurinol and its hydroxyl derivative alloxanthine or oxypurinol. Alloxanthine is itself the result of xanthinoxidase activity on allopurinol. The drug is indicated in the treatment of spontaneous gout (especially with coexistent renal disease), in hyperuricemia produced by thiazide diuretics, and in the prophylaxis of gout from the cellular destruction produced by cytotoxic drugs (note Interactions).

Absorption

Oral bioavailability: about 80%. t_{max}: 2–6 hours [4].

Distribution

V_d: unknown. Protein binding: unknown.

Elimination

$t_{\frac{1}{2}}$ of allopurinol: 2–3 hours. $t_{\frac{1}{2}}$ of alloxanthine: 18–30 hours [1]. Since alloxanthine and allopurinol inhibit xanthinoxidase, the amount of allopurinol excreted unchanged in urine varies from 10% at low plasma concentrations to 30% at higher concentrations. Alloxanthine is excreted entirely in urine, probably after substantial tubular reabsorption [2].

Dosage Schedule

Gout: 200–400 mg daily is usually satisfactory. Prophylaxis of hyperuricemia: 200–800 mg daily for several days when antimitotic drug is administered (note Interactions). A dose once daily is adequate [3]. In all cases a fluid intake in excess of 2 L daily is advisable.

Special Dosage Situations

Reduce dose in relation to creatinine clearance in renal disease. Children may require 100–200 mg daily.

Therapeutic Concentrations

The goals of therapy are the reduction of serum uric acid level below 5–6 mg/dl and the prevention of sudden, severe increases in serum uric acid levels during treatment of neoplasia. Dosage is individually determined by the patient's response to the drug.

Adverse Reactions

Fever, skin rashes, aching muscles, headache, vertigo, gastrointestinal disturbances, bone marrow depression, liver enlargement, and hepatitis may occur, but these reactions usually subside after discontinuing or reducing the dose.

Interactions
Azathioprine and 6-mercaptopurine are metabolized by xanthin-oxidase, and therefore enhanced toxicity of these antimetabo-lites should be expected. Reduce cytotoxic dosage to one-third or one-fourth of the usual dose. Other cytotoxic drugs, especially cyclophosphamide, may demonstrate enhanced toxicity for un-known reasons.

Special Note

Gout may actually be exacerbated during the early stages of treatment with allopurinol, and thus combined treatment with colchicine is indicated for at least a few weeks.

References
1. Elion, G. B., Kovensky, A., et al.   Metabolic studies of al-lopurinol, an inhibitor of xanthine oxidase. *Biochem. Phar-macol.* 15:863–880, 1966.
2. Elion, G. B., Yu, T. F., et al.   Renal clearance of oxypurinol. *Am. J. Med.* 45:69–77, 1968.
3. Rodnan, G. P., Robin, J. A., et al.   Allopurinol and gouty hyperuricemia. Efficacy of a single daily dose. *J.A.M.A.* 231:1143–1147, 1975.
4. Rundles, R. W., Metz, E. N., et al.   Allopurinol in the treatment of gout. *Ann. Intern. Med.* 64:229–258, 1966.

AMANTADINE
An antiviral agent, fortuitously found to be effective in the treat-ment of Parkinson's disease. Less effective than L-dopa, with which it has an additive effect. The effect of amantadine seems to diminish with time in some patients [4]. Mechanism of action appears to be promotion of dopamine release from nerve endings and a direct stimulant effect on dopamine receptors [1]. Useful as a prophylactic agent against A_2 influenza [13] and may be useful in the treatment of Jakob-Creutzfeldt's disease [11]. Effect on drug-induced dyskinesia has not been adequately determined [8].

Absorption
Oral bioavailability: 90–100%. t_{max}: 1–4 hours [8].

Distribution
V_d: about 6 L/kg [10]. Protein binding: unknown. Distribution into breast milk and fetus not known.

Elimination
$t_{\frac{1}{2}}$: about 22 hours [10]. Has a long duration of action, with usual doses effective for about 24 hours [3]. 90% of the drug excreted unchanged in the urine [2].

Dosage Schedule

For the treatment of Parkinson's disease, 200 mg daily in 2 divided doses; increasing the dose above 300 mg rarely improves the patient's condition and increases the risk of adverse reactions. For prophylaxis during influenza epidemics, the dose is 200 mg daily, continued for at least 10 days after a single exposure or for 90 days during an ongoing epidemic [13]. Continue prophylaxis for 2–3 weeks after influenza vaccination to permit antibody development.

Special Dosage Situations

Pregnancy: no special dosage seems necessary, although one case of cardiac malformation in the newborn has been reported after the use of amantadine [7]. Children: for influenza prophylaxis, about 6 mg/kg but should not exceed 150 mg/day. Children over 10 years: adult doses [13]. Renal disease [6]: use cautiously; reduce dose according to Table 1, page 30. Liver disease: no available information. Elderly: reduce dose according to the decrease in renal function.

Therapeutic Concentrations

No available information.

Adverse Reactions

Confusion, depression, nervousness, insomnia, dizziness, light-headedness, dry mouth, and skin rash [12]. Livedo reticularis, possibly due to vasoconstriction [9]. Peripheral edema, which responds to diuretics. Convulsions may occur with very large doses. All adverse reactions are reversible with the cessation of amantadine.

Interactions

Appears to enhance some of the side-effects of the anticholinergic agents used in the treatments of Parkinson's disease [5].

References

1. Bailey, E. V., and Stone, T. W. The mechanism of action of amantadine in parkinsonism: A review. *Arch. Int. Pharmacodyn. Ther.* 216:246–262, 1975.
2. Bleidner, W. E., Harmon, J. B., et al. Absorption, distribution, and excretion of amantadine hydrochloride. *J. Pharmacol. Exp. Ther.* 150:484–490, 1965.
3. Fahn, S., and Isgreen, W. P. Long-term evaluation of amantadine and levodopa combination in parkinsonism by double-blind crossover analyses. *Neurology* 25:695–700, 1975.
4. Forssman, B., Kihlstrand, S., et al. Amantadine therapy in parkinsonism. *Acta Neurol. Scand.* 48:1–18, 1972.
5. Harper, R. W., and Knothe, B. U. C. Coloured lilliputian hallucinations with amantadine. *Med. J. Aust.* 1:444–445, 1973.
6. Ing, T. S., Rahn, A. C., et al. Accumulation of amantadine

hydrochloride in renal insufficiency. *N. Engl. J. Med.* 291:1257, 1974.

7. Nora, J. J., Nora, A. H., et al.   Cardiovascular maldevelopment associated with maternal exposure to amantadine. *Lancet* 2:607, 1975.
8. Parkes, D.   Amantadine. *Adv. Drug Res.* 8:11–81, 1974.
9. Pearce, L. A., Waterbury, L. D., et al.   Amantadine hydrochloride: Alteration in peripheral circulation. *Neurology* 24:46–48, 1974.
10. Rizzo, M., Biandrate, P., et al.   Amantadine in depression: Relationship between behavioural effects and plasma levels. *Eur. J. Clin. Pharmacol.* 5:226–228, 1973.
11. Sanders, W. L., and Dunn, T. L.   Creutzfeldt-Jakob disease treated with amantadine. *J. Neurol. Neurosurg. Psychiatry* 36:581–584, 1973.
12. Schwab, R. S., Poskanzer, D. C., et al.   Amantadine in Parkinson's disease. *J.A.M.A.* 222:792–795, 1972.
13. Weinstein, L., and Chang, T. W.   Drug therapy: The chemotherapy of viral infections. *N. Engl. J. Med.* 289:725–730, 1973.

AMINOGLYCOSIDES
(Streptomycin, Gentamicin, Kanamycin, Tobramycin, Amikacin, Neomycin)

Water-soluble, stable, basic antibiotics. Bactericidal action by inhibition of bacterial protein synthesis. Used almost exclusively in the treatment of severe gram-negative and penicillinase-producing staphylococcal infections. Inactive against anerobic infections. Antibacterial spectrum similar for each drug; there is often, but not always, cross-resistance. Specifically, streptomycin is active against *Mycobacterium tuberculosis,* and kanamycin is inactive against *Pseudomonas* species. Neomycin is useful in hepatic failure (4–8 g daily orally) but has no proven value in preoperative bowel preparation. In general, the newer aminoglycosides should be reserved for specific organisms resistant to older members of the group.

Absorption

None is significantly absorbed when given orally. When given IM, t_{max} is about 1 hour.

Distribution

V_d: 0.25 L/kg. In CSF 5% (normal) to 20% (inflammation), in bile 75%, and in breast milk 100% of the concentration in serum. The fetus' serum concentration is about 50% of the mother's [2, 6]. Protein binding: see Table 7.

Elimination

$t_{\frac{1}{2}}$: See Table 7. Glomerular filtration with some tubular back-diffusion (10–30%) accounts for 70–90% of the dose. The fate of the rest is unknown, and no metabolites are isolated [1, 2, 5, 6].

Table 7. *Pharmacological Properties and Dosages of Aminoglycosides*

Pharmacological Property and Dose	Streptomycin	Gentamicin, Tobramycin	Kanamycin, Amikacin
$t_{1/2}$	2–3 hr	2 hr	3 hr
Protein binding	30%	10%	0%
Therapeutic concentration (peak)	15–20 μg/ml	4–9 μg/ml	15–25 μg/ml
Toxic concentration	50 μg/ml	12 μg/ml[a]	40 μg/ml
Dosage interval	12 hr	8 hr	12 hr
Adult dose	7.5–15 mg/kg	1–2 mg/kg	10–15 mg/kg
Pediatric dose	10–15 mg/kg	1–3 mg/kg	10–20 mg/kg

[a]Predose level should be below 2 μg/ml.
In renal disease the dose is directly proportional to creatinine clearance (normal value 120 ml/min), e.g., at clearance of 60 ml/min give half of normal dose or double usual dosage interval. Remember age-dependent reduction in clearance. In anuria $t_{1/2}$: 2–4 days [3, 4]. See also Table 1, p. 30.
Doses can be given IM or IV. For IV route, dissolve in 50 ml saline and inject over 10–30 minutes to avoid potential ototoxicity from high peak levels.
Note: These doses apply only if renal clearance is 100–120 ml/min.

Dosage Schedule, Special Dosage Situations, and Therapeutic Concentrations
Table 7 summarizes this and other information.

Adverse Reaction
Allergic skin eruptions. Ototoxicity (both acoustic and vestibular) and renal damage are common, especially when used for more than 7–10 days. All aminoglycosides exert a curare-like effect, which is important clinically only for patients who have myasthenia gravis or have recently undergone surgery involving the use of muscle relaxants. Cholinesterase inhibitors (e.g., neostigmine) improve muscle weakness. All aminoglycosides are effectively removed by hemodialysis.

Interactions
Increased ototoxicity when aminoglycosides are used in combination with ethacrynic acid and furosemide. Aminoglycosides potentiate all neuromuscular blocking agents. In vitro incompatibility with carbenicillin, cephalosporins, amphotericin B, and heparin.

Reviews
Ball, A. P., Gray, J. A., et al. Antibacterial drugs today: II. The aminoglycosides. *Drugs* 10:92–111, 1975.
Bunn, P. A. Kanamycin. *Med. Clin. North Am.* 54:1245–1256, 1970.
Cox, C. E. Gentamicin. *Med. Clin. North Am.* 54:1305–1315.
Finland, M., and Hewitt, W. L. (Eds.). Symposia on gentami-

100   11: Drug Profiles   Amitriptyline and Nortriptyline

cin. *J. Infect. Dis.* 119:332–540, 1969 and 124 (Suppl.):S1–S300, 1971.
Martin, W. J.   The present status of streptomycin in antimicrobial therapy. *Med. Clin. North Am.* 54:1161–1172, 1970.

References

1. Gingell, J. C., Chisholm, G. D., et al.   The dose, distribution, and excretion of gentamicin with special reference to renal failure. *J. Infect. Dis.* 119:396–401, 1969.
2. Kunin, C. M.   Absorption, distribution, excretion, and fate of kanamycin. *Ann. N.Y. Acad. Sci.* 132:811–818, 1966.
3. Lumholtz, B., Kampmann, J., et al.   Dose regimen of kanamycin and gentamicin. *Acta Med. Scand.* 196:521–524, 1974.
4. Mawer, G. E., Ahmad, R., et al.   Prescribing aids for gentamicin. *Br. J. Clin. Pharmacol.* 1:45–50, 1974.
5. Orme, B. M., and Cutler, R. E.   The relationship between kanamycin pharmacokinetics: Distribution and renal function. *Clin. Pharmacol. Ther.* 10:543–550, 1969.
6. Siber, G. R., Echeverria, P., et al.   Pharmacokinetics of gentamicin in children and adults. *J. Infect. Dis.* 132:637–651, 1975.

AMITRIPTYLINE
(and Nortriptyline)

A tricyclic dibenzazepine related to imipramine. Used in the management of endogenous depression and childhood enuresis. Mode of action probably related to inhibition of synaptic uptake of norepinephrine and 5-hydroxytryptamine in the brain.

Absorption
Systemic bioavailability: unknown. t_{max}: unknown.

Distribution
V_d: unknown. Protein binding: 95–98% [3].

Elimination
$t_{\frac{1}{2}}$: unknown. Metabolism appears to be essentially the same as that of imipramine: N-demethylation produces an active metabolite, nortriptyline; N-oxidation and C-hydroxylation also occur, the latter followed to a variable extent by glucuronide conjugation. Demethylation of the secondary amine is more pronounced than in imipramine metabolism (nortriptyline to desmethylnortriptyline) [6].
    For nortriptyline, the following pharmacokinetic figures apply. Bioavailability: 60%. t_{max}: 4–9 hours. V_d: 20–40 L/kg. Protein binding: 92–96% [3]. $t_{\frac{1}{2}}$: 14–93 hours [6]. Nortriptyline is available as an antidepressant agent. There is marked genetic variation in its metabolism [1].

Dosage Schedule
A single oral 50-mg dose daily at bedtime for 2 weeks. Increase by

50 mg daily at weekly intervals to 150 mg unless side-effects intervene. Larger doses, up to 300 mg daily, are occasionally required. Tolerance to minor side-effects may develop if dosage is increased gradually. Improvement in the patient's condition may require 3–30 days of drug therapy. For a single episode of severe depression, therapy for 3–6 months is usual.

Special Dosage Situations

Patients should not receive any tricyclic antidepressant within 2 weeks of treatment with a monoamine oxidase inhibitor (MAOI). Children under age 6: 10 mg in a single daily dose at bedtime for treatment of enuresis. Children ages 6–10: 10–20 mg. Children ages 11–15: 20–50 mg. Use with caution in the elderly and patients with known cardiovascular disease. Prostatic obstruction may be aggravated, with resulting urinary retention. No available information about dosages for women during pregnancy or lactation or in patients with renal or hepatic disease.

Therapeutic Concentrations

This topic has been controversial [5]. A combined plasma concentration of amitriptyline and nortriptyline greater than 120 ng/ml has been associated with improvement in patients with depression [4]. Improvement continued with combined concentrations of up to 250 ng/ml and was related to the total tricyclic and amitriptyline concentrations but not to nortriptyline levels [9]. However, studies of the administration of nortriptyline alone to patients with depression showed that the amelioration of depression was most pronounced in the nortriptyline plasma ranges 50–140 ng/ml [2] and 50–150 ng/ml [7]. Higher levels of nortriptyline were associated with less chance of recovery. Deaths have been reported with plasma levels of amitriptyline greater than 2 μg/ml [8].

Adverse Reactions

Just as for other tricyclic antidepressants, the anticholinergic effects of amitriptyline include dry mouth, blurred vision, urinary retention, and constipation. Cardiovascular effects include hypotension, dizziness, tachycardia, and other arrhythmias. Extrapyramidal reactions, confusion states with delusions, and hallucinations may occur, and severe toxicity is marked by hypertension, fever, serious arrhythmias, convulsions, and coma. Management includes symptomatic measures (diazepam IV for seizures and lidocaine or propranolol for arrhythmias) and specific treatment in the form of the anticholinesterase physostigmine (1–3 mg IV, repeated hourly if necessary). Dialysis is of no value.

Interactions

MAOI and amitriptyline taken together may produce a crisis of fever, hypertension, and coma. The antihypertensive action of guanethidine and bethanidine is reduced by amitriptyline.

Additive effects may be seen when amitriptyline is taken with anticholinergic drugs, sympathomimetics, thyroid hormone, and

other centrally acting drugs. Delirium may be produced by concurrent administration of ethchlorvynol.

References

1. Alexanderson, B. Pharmacokinetics of desmethylimipramine and nortriptyline in man after single and multiple
   oral doses—a crossover study. *Eur. J. Clin. Pharmacol.* 5:1–10,
   1972.
2. Åsberg, M., Crönholm, B., et al. Relationship between
   plasma level and therapeutic effect of nortriptyline. *Br. Med.
   J.* 3:331–334, 1971.
3. Borgå, O., Azarnoff, D. L., et al. Plasma protein binding of
   tricyclic antidepressants in man. *Biochem. Pharmacol.*
   18:2135–2143, 1969.
4. Braithwaite, R. A., Goulding, R., et al. Plasma concentration
   of amitriptyline and clinical response. *Lancet* 1:1297–1300,
   1972.
5. Glassman, A. H., and Perel, J. M. Plasma levels and tricyclic
   antidepressants. *Clin. Pharmacol. Ther.* 16:198–200, 1974.
6. Gram, L. F. Metabolism of tricyclic antidepressants. A review. *Dan. Med. Bull.* 21:218–231, 1974.
7. Kragh-Sørensen, P., Hansen, C. E., et al. Self-inhibiting action of nortriptyline's antidepressive effect at high plasma
   levels. *Psychopharmacologia* 45:305–312, 1976.
8. Munksgaard, E. C. Concentrations of amitriptyline and its
   metabolites in urine, blood and tissue in fatal amitriptyline
   poisoning. *Acta Pharmacol. Toxicol.* 27:129–134, 1969.
9. Ziegler, V. E., Bun Tee Co, et al. Amitriptyline plasma
   levels and therapeutic responses. *Clin. Pharmacol. Ther.*
   19:795–801, 1976.

AMPHOTERICIN B

A broad-spectrum, water-insoluble, unstable, polyene, antifungal
antibiotic that is chemically related to nystatin. Active against most
fungi that cause systemic mycoses except *Candida tropicalis* and
some strains of *Aspergillus*. Ineffective in the treatment of nocardiosis and actinomycosis. Inactive against bacteria, *Rickettsiae*, and
viruses. Mechanism of action is probably the changing of cell
membrane permeability after binding to sterols. No development
of resistance to this antibiotic.

Indicated in all serious mycotic infections, often in combination
with 5-fluorocytosine. The minimum period of treatment is usually 6 weeks.

Absorption

Oral bioavailability: probably below 3% and too small for any
clinical effect [3]. Amphotericin B is only administered locally or
by intravenous infusion.

Distribution

V_d: 0.5–1 L/kg [1]. Protein binding: 10%. The concentration in
CSF is less than 5% of the serum concentration [1, 3]. No available

information concerning distribution to breast milk or across placenta.

Elimination

$t_{\frac{1}{2}}$: about 24 hours [1]. Only about 5% is excreted unchanged in the urine [1, 3], but metabolic pathways are unknown.

Dosage Schedule

Marketed as a powder containing amphotericin B and sodium desoxycholate. The content of the vial is dissolved in 10 ml of sterile water, which is then added to a 5% dextrose solution for infusion over 4–6 hours. Solutions of electrolytes or acid solution (pH 5 or less) should not be used. Fresh solutions must be prepared before each infusion. The addition of 25–50 mg of hydrocortisone reduces the incidence of chills and fever. Protection of solution from light does not seem to be critical [4]. Several regimens have been proposed, but the main principle is to start with a small dose and then increase the dose to a maximum of about 1.0 mg/kg/day, observing carefully for deterioration of renal function. A usual initial dose is 0.25 mg/kg/day, which is increased by 0.1–0.25 mg/kg/day. Administration of a double dose every other day is equally effective and may cause fewer side-effects [1].

In fungal meningitis, intrathecal injection of 0.5 mg in 5–10 ml spinal fluid is given 2–3 times a week to a maximum of 15 g. Intra-articular doses of 5–15 mg may be used in coccidioidal arthritis.

Special Dosage Situations

Children: same schedule as for adults. Renal failure: normal doses [1, 2]. No available data about dosages for the elderly, for patients in hepatic failure, or for female patients during lactation or pregnancy.

Therapeutic Concentrations

Minimum inhibitory concentration (MIC) for *Blastomyces, Histoplasma, Coccidioides,* and *Cryptococcus* is 0.2–0.5 µg/ml. MIC for *Candida albicans* is up to 2 µg/ml.

Adverse Reactions

Almost all patients who take amphotericin B develop impaired renal function, including mild tubular acidosis and hypokalemia. With doses totaling over 4–5 g, permanent kidney impairment is common. Alkalinization of the urine seems to be helpful in preventing renal damage.

Infusion of the drug is often associated with chills, fever, nausea, phlebitis, and headache. Other side-effects are hepatic failure, blood dyscrasias, and cardiac arrhythmias. Allergic reactions include anaphylaxis, flushing, generalized pain, and convulsions. Intrathecal injections may produce headache, paresthesias, radiating pain along the lumbar nerves, and palsies. Amphotericin B is not removed significantly by hemodialysis [2].

Interactions

Hypokalemia with risk of digitalis intoxication.

Reviews

Bennett, J. E.   Chemotherapy of systemic mycoses. *N. Engl. J. Med.* 290:30–32, 1974.
Furcolow, M. L.   The use of amphotericin B in blastomycosis, cryptococcosus, and histoplasmosis. *Med. Clin. North Am.* 47:1119–1130, 1963.
Hildick-Smith, G.   Antifungal Therapy. In B. M. Kagan (Ed.), *Antimicrobial Therapy.* Philadelphia: Saunders, 1970. Pp. 120–126.
Winn, W. A.   Coccidiodomycosis and amphotericin B. *Med. Clin. North Am.* 47:1131–1148, 1963.

References

1. Bindschadler, D. D., and Bennett, J. E.   A pharmacologic guide to the clinical use of amphotericin B. *J. Infect. Dis.* 120:427–436, 1969.
2. Feldman, H. A., Hamilton, J. D., et al.   Amphotericin B therapy in an anephric patient. *Antimicrob. Agents Chemother.* 4:302–305, 1973.
3. Louria, D. B.   Some aspects of the absorption, distribution, and excretion of amphotericin B in man. *Antibiot. Med. Clin. Ther.* 5:295–301, 1958.
4. Shadomy, S., Brummer, D. L., et al.   Light sensitivity of prepared solutions of amphotericin B. *Am. Rev. Resp. Dis.* 107:303–304, 1973.

ATROPINE
(Hyoscyamine)

A widely distributed natural alkaloid usually associated with belladonna (deadly nightshade); an ester of tropic acid and tropine. Highly selective antagonist of acetyl choline (ACh) at muscarinic (postganglionic) nerve endings and other sites where ACh has muscarinic activity. Parasympathetic blocking activity produces widespread effects: initial slowing of heart rate with atrioventricular (A-V) dissociation followed by tachycardia; reduction of secretions of salivary and sweat glands, bronchi, and gastrointestinal tract; reduced gastrointestinal motility and urinary bladder contractility; reduced airway resistance; and pupillary dilatation and ciliary paralysis. Used in preparation for general anesthesia, in the treatment of bradycardia that causes diminished cardiac output, in combination with opiates for the management of biliary and renal colic (not very effective), and topically as a mydriatic, although its analogue, homatropine, is usually preferable because of shorter action.

Absorption

t_{max}: 15–50 minutes after IM injection [5]; 1 hour after oral dose [1].

Atropine appears to be absorbed completely [1], but evidence of possible first-pass metabolism includes the clinical observations that the oral dose necessary to produce a certain tachycardia must be twice the IV dose [3, 6] and that the ratio of parent drug to metabolites in urine is much higher after IV dosage than after oral dosage [2].

Distribution
V_d: about 2–4 L/kg [1]. Protein binding: 50%.

Elimination
Distribution phase: about 6 hours. $t_{\frac{1}{2}}$: 13–38 hours [5]. Atropine is partly N-demethylated and glucuronidated [1]. Hydrolysis of the ester bond does not appear significant [4]. 33–50% appears in urine as parent drug, the rest as metabolite [4, 5].

Dosage Schedule
0.3–0.6 mg IV, IM, or subcutaneously for preoperative management and in the treatment of bradyarrhythmia due to excessive vagal activity. A dose of 0.04 mg/kg parenterally totally blocks vagal activity on the heart [2]. In organic phosphate poisoning, doses of 1 mg may be repeated at 15- to 30-minute intervals, according to the patient's response.

Special Dosage Situations
Used topically in ophthalmology when iridoplegia is indicated in treatment of iridocyclitis. Homatropine is preferable to atropine when short-term mydriasis is required.

Atropine is combined with the opiate diphenoxylate in a mixture (Lomotil) that is used to treat diarrhea. There are special problems with this preparation (see Adverse Reactions), especially in children.

In patients with glaucoma, especially those with narrow-angle glaucoma, anticholinergic drugs are relatively contraindicated, since a sustained rise in intraocular pressure may occur.

Therapeutic Concentrations
No available data because of inadequate assay techniques.

Adverse Reactions
Dry mouth and skin, thirst, flushing, blurring of vision, difficulty in micturition, tachycardia, marked pupillary dilatation, skin rash, restlessness, excitement, confusion, delirium, hallucinations, and convulsions may accompany overdose or ingestion of nightshade shrub berries containing belladonna alkaloids. Poisoning from the mixture Lomotil (atropine and diphenoxylate) also displays features of opiate poisoning. Severe atropine poisoning produces cardiovascular and respiratory collapse, coma, and death.

Physostigmine (a cholinesterase inhibitor) together with symptomatic management of fever, convulsions, and respiratory failure is the specific treatment. Physostigmine, 0.01–0.05 mg/kg, should be given slowly by intravenous route and should be repeated as necessary, since its effects are of much shorter duration than those of atropine.

Interactions

Absorption of drugs that require prolonged dissolution in the gastrointestinal tract, e.g., digoxin preparations, may be enhanced. Atropine possibly has additive effects when used with antihistamines, anti-parkinsonian drugs, tricyclic antidepressants, and other drugs with anticholinergic activity.

Review

Kalser, S. C.   The fate of atropine in man. *Ann. N.Y. Acad. Sci.* 179:667–683, 1971.

References

1. Beermann, B., Hellström, K., et al.   The gastrointestinal absorption of atropine in man. *Clin. Sci.* 40:95–106, 1971.
2. Chamberlain, D. A., Turner, P., et al.   Effects of atropine on heart rate in healthy man. *Lancet* 2:12–15, 1967.
3. Cullumbine, H., McKee, W. H. E., et al.   The effects of atropine sulfate upon healthy male subjects. *Q. J. Exp. Physiol.* 40:309–319, 1955.
4. Gossellin, R. E., Gabourel, J. D., et al.   The fate of atropine in man. *Clin. Pharmacol. Ther.* 1:597–603, 1960.
5. Kalser, S. C., and McLain, P. L.   Atropine metabolism in man. *Clin. Pharmacol. Ther.* 11:214–227, 1970.
6. Möller, J., and Rosen, A.   Comparative studies on intramuscular and oral effective doses of some anticholinergic drugs. *Acta Med. Scand.* 184:201–209, 1968.

AZATHIOPRINE

Methyl-nitro-imidazolyl derivative of 6-mercaptopurine, used as an immunosuppressive agent. Although developed as a slow releaser of 6-mercaptopurine, the intact compound also appears to have an effect of its own. The mechanism of action is unknown, but it has been suggested that it is the inhibition of the proliferation of immunocompetent cells by interference with DNA synthesis. The action is most pronounced in immunological disorders involving T cells. The main established indication is as an adjunct for the prevention of rejection in renal transplantation. Other indications are unsettled. The drug appears to be valuable in some cases of rheumatoid arthritis, pemphigus, systemic lupus erythematosus, and other collagen diseases. May be valuable in the treatment of Crohn's disease but seems ineffective in chronic active hepatitis and glomerulonephritis. In all cases, azathioprine is rarely the drug of first choice, and the treatment should be initiated only in centers in which immunology specialists are available. It is particularly difficult to evaluate the merits of azathioprine in comparison with other immunosuppressants such as cyclophosphamide, methotrexate, and corticosteroids.

Absorption

Oral bioavailability: 85–90% [5]. t_{max}: ½–1 hour [2].

Distribution

V_d: unknown. Protein binding: unknown. The concentration of azathioprine and 6-mercaptopurine in the fetal circulation is about 10% of the maternal serum concentration [9].

Elimination

$t_{\frac{1}{2}}$: unknown. Appears to be almost completely converted to 6-mercaptopurine ($t_{\frac{1}{2}}$ is about 1 hour) within a few hours after administration [5, 8]. About 1% of this compound is excreted unchanged in the urine [5]; the rest is metabolized by methylation, by desulfuration, and in particular, by oxidation to the inactive 6-thiouric acid, the latter process being catalyzed by xanthinoxidase [4]. Mercaptoimidazole is a minor metabolite [3]. Only a small percentage of unchanged azathioprine is excreted in the urine [2].

Dosage Schedule

Highly individual, adjusted in relation to development of side-effects, especially leucopenia. Most common initial dose is 1–3 mg/kg/day in 2 or 3 divided doses. A hydrocortisone-stimulating test to determine those patients likely to develop leucopenia may be helpful [6].

Special Dosage Situations

Children: initially 3–5 mg/kg/day, reduced to a maintenance dose of 1–2 mg/kg/day. Renal failure: no dosage adjustments seem necessary, since the rates of elimination of azathioprine and 6-mercaptopurine are unchanged [1]. Sulfur-containing inactive metabolites accumulate. Hepatic failure: no available information, but the conversion to 6-mercaptopurine has been decreased in some patients with severely reduced liver function [2]. Pregnancy: the frequency of abortions is increased, but there is no evidence of a higher rate of infants born with malformations [7].

Therapeutic Concentrations

Unknown, but probably irrelevant (has hit-and-run activity).

Adverse Reactions

Toxic anemia, leucopenia, and thrombocytopenia, all of which can be fatal, are the most important adverse reactions. Megaloblastic anemia is rare. Infections are common; *Pneumocystis carinii* pneumonia has often been described. The frequency of malignancies in patients who are receiving cytotoxic immunosuppressant therapy, especially intracranial lymphoma, may be higher than that in control groups. Ovarian function is decreased, although several successful pregnancies have been reported. Azoospermia is frequent. Chromosomal anomalies have been demonstrated, but long-term genetic effects are unknown.

Nausea, vomiting, diarrhea, and obstructive liver damage are common. Eliminated well by hemodialysis.

Interactions

Allopurinol inhibits the metabolism of 6-mercaptopurine and azathioprine by inhibition of xanthinoxidase. Patients treated simultaneously with both allopurinol and azathioprine should receive 25–33% of the usual dose of azathioprine.

Reviews

Avery, G. S. (Ed.).   Focus on immunosuppressive drugs. *Drugs* 11:1–35, 1976.
Bach, J. F., Dardenne, M., et al.   Dosage des métabolites actifs des immunosuppresseurs dans le sérum. *Nouv. Presse Med.* 35:2293–2298, 1972.
Rosman, M., and Bertino, J. R.   Azathioprine. *Ann. Intern. Med.* 79:694–700, 1973.

References

1. Bach, J. F., and Dardenne, M.   The metabolism of aziathio-prine in renal failure. *Transplantation* 12:253–259, 1971.
2. Bach, J. F., and Dardenne, M.   Serum immunosuppressive activity of azathioprine in normal subjects and patients with liver diseases. *Proc. R. Soc. Med.* 65:260–263, 1972.
3. Chalmers, A. H.   Studies on the mechanism of formation of 5-mercapto-1-methyl-4-nitroimidazole, a metabolite of the immunosuppressive drug azathioprine. *Biochem. Pharmacol.* 23:1891–1901, 1974.
4. Elion, G. B.   Biochemistry and pharmacology of purine analogues. *Fed. Proc.* 26:898–903, 1967.
5. Elion, G. B.   Significance of azathioprine metabolites. *Proc. R. Soc. Med.* 65:257–260, 1972.
6. Fisher, K. A., Mahajan, S. K., et al.   Prediction of azathio-prine intolerance in transplant patients. *Lancet* 1:828–830, 1976.
7. Goldby, M.   Fertility after renal transplantation. *Transplantation* 10:201–207, 1970.
8. Loo, T. L., Luce, J., et al.   Clinical pharmacologic observa-tion on 6-mercaptopurine and 6-methylthiopurine ribonu-cleoside. *Clin. Pharmacol. Ther.* 9:180–194, 1968.
9. Saarikoski, S., and Seppälä, M.   Immunosuppression during pregnancy: Transmission of azathioprine and its metabolites from the mother to the fetus. *Am. J. Obstet. Gynecol.* 115:1100–1106, 1973.

BECLOMETHASONE

A topical steroid, 5000 times as potent as hydrocortisone as a topical anti-inflammatory agent [1]. Usual therapeutic doses do not suppress adrenal cortical function. Given by metered aerosol in the management of chronic asthma as a prophylaxis against acute exacerbations. May be used in combination with bronchodilators or with systemic steroids in order to reduce the dose and side-effects of the latter. Also indicated in the treatment of allergic rhinitis and of nasal polyps. Most likely to be effective in patients with a history of atopy, elevated serum IgE levels, and positive skin tests and in those who would otherwise require 5–10 mg prednisone daily for control of their symptoms. Available as dipropionate. Betamethasone valerate has similar properties.

Absorption

When inhaled, 10–25% of the dose enters the respiratory tract, and the rest is swallowed. When very fine particles are used (diameter = 7 μm), 90% of the swallowed dose is absorbed from the gastrointestinal tract. Larger particles are absorbed less well, since they are only sparingly soluble in water. t_{max}: 3–5 hours [2, 3].

Distribution

V_d: unknown. Protein binding: 87% [4].

Elimination

$t_{\frac{1}{2}}$: unknown. Completely metabolized to inactive metabolites. Has possible large first-pass effect, which may limit its systemic bioavailability and therefore its toxicity. 65% of metabolites appear in bile and 10–15% in urine [4]. Beclomethasone dipropionate appears to be hydrolyzed in the gut to beclomethasone monopropionate and beclomethasone [4, 5].

Dosage Schedule

Generally 200–800 μg/day (1 puff = 50 or 100 μg). Doses greater than 1600 μg/day associated with adrenal cortical suppression [1]. May be introduced in patients who have not taken steroids previously, although it is generally better to optimize the patient's condition first with oral steroids, since the aerosol will not penetrate well to the lower lung if bronchospasm is present. May also be given to patients already taking systemic steroids, with the object of decreasing their dose. Reduction of systemic steroids should not take place until the patients have taken beclomethasone for 10–14 days. For patients who are taking 10 mg/day or less of prednisone, it is frequently possible to suspend systemic steroids altogether, and in other patients worthwhile reductions may be obtained. Reduction of steroid dose should be undertaken with caution. Nasal drops of beclomethasone in a dose of 200–800 μg/day relieve allergic rhinitis and reduce nasal polyps when used for several months. Will also prevent recurrence of polyps after surgery.

Special Dosage Situations

Should be used only as a prophylactic; *of no value in acute attack.* Patients taking beclomethasone should be transferred to systemic steroids during an acute attack. Children appear to obtain no increased benefit from doses greater than 400 μg/day [2]. Use cautiously in patients who have a past history of tuberculosis.

Therapeutic Concentrations
Not relevant.

Adverse Reactions
May provoke oral moniliasis, especially with large doses. If dose cannot be reduced, nystatin usually clears fungal infections rapidly.

Interactions
None known.

Review
Brogden, R. M., Pinder, R. M., et al.   Beclomethasone dipropionate inhaler. A review of its pharmacology, therapeutic value, and adverse effects. I. Asthma. II. Allergic rhinitis and other conditions. *Drugs* 10:166–210, 1975.

References
1. Gaddie, J., Petri, G. R., et al.   Aerosol beclomethasone dipropionate: A dose-response study in chronic bronchial asthma. *Lancet* 2:280–281, 1973.
2. Gwynn, C. M., and Smith, J. M.   A one year follow-up of children and adolescents receiving regular beclomethasone dipropionate. *Clin. Allergy* 4:325–330, 1974.
3. Harris, D. M.   Some properties of beclomethasone dipropionate and related steroids in man. *Postgrad. Med. J.* 51(Suppl. 4):21–25, 1975.
4. Martin, L. E., Harrison, C., et al.   Metabolism of beclomethasone dipropionate by animals and man. *Postgrad. Med. J.* 51(Suppl. 4):11–20, 1975.
5. Martin, L. E., Tanner, R. J. N., et al.   Absorption and metabolism of orally administered beclomethasone dipropionate. *Clin. Pharmacol. Ther.* 15:267–275, 1974.

BETA-ADRENERGIC BLOCKING AGENTS
Propranolol

Beta-adrenergic blocking agent, nonspecific, devoid of intrinsic sympathomimetic activity and possessing local anesthetic or quinidine-like activity, which is probably unimportant in usual pharmacological concentrations. In the heart, reduces automaticity of pacemaker cells, conduction velocity, and height and rate of rise of muscle action potential and prolongs effective refractory period. Hypotensive effect is multifactorial—involves diminution of cardiac output by production of bradycardia, central effect, and suppression of plasma renin and angiotensin II levels.

Indicated for therapy of angina pectoris, hypertension, cardiac arrhythmias (especially supraventricular and digitalis-induced), hypertrophic obstructive cardiomyopathy, tetralogy of Fallot, aortic dissection, hyperthyroidism, pheochromocytoma, and essential tremor.

Absorption

Oral bioavailability: 90%. t_{max}: 60–90 minutes [5]. With oral dose the first-pass effect in liver is very high initially, saturated with approximately 30 mg of propranolol. After this initial effect, drug begins to accumulate in the plasma.

Distribution

V_d: 3 L/kg. Protein binding: 90–95%.

Elimination

$t_{\frac{1}{2}}$: 3 hours. Numerous metabolites, which are not all well defined. Some are active, e.g., 4-OH propranolol [3]. Metabolites appear in urine, with only very small quantities of parent drug.

Dosage Schedule

For antihypertensive, antianginal, and antiarrhythmic effect, most common initial dose is 40–160 mg/day in 2–4 divided doses. This dose may be increased to 3000 mg/day if side-effects do not supervene. In thyrotoxicosis, higher initial dose may be needed. When used intravenously, give boluses of 1 mg, repeated as necessary, each bolus separated by a period of 10–20 minutes. Do *not* discontinue long-term beta-blockade abruptly, since severe rebound angina or myocardial infarction may develop.

Special Dosage Situations

Absolutely contraindicated in obstructive airway disease, congestive cardiac failure, and first- or second-degree heart block, since all are exacerbated by beta blockade. If cardiac failure is due to severe hypertension or arrhythmia, patient may benefit from treatment of these underlying conditions by beta blockade. No contraindications to use in elderly or in patients with liver disease; however, in patients with renal disease, higher plasma levels of the drug are obtained for a given dose, and the dose may need to be decreased [4]. Avoid use in pregnant women unless absolutely essential.

Therapeutic Concentrations

50–100 ng/ml [1]. Although good correlation exists between the plasma level of the drug and the degree of beta blockade as measured by the chronotropic response to isoproterenol [7], the plasma level does not correlate so well with the hypotensive effect. However, the plasma level does correlate well with the antianginal and antiarrhythmic effects.

Adverse Reactions

Bronchospasm, left ventricular failure, bradycardia, diarrhea, drowsiness, inversion of sleep pattern, hallucinations, and hypoglycemia. In overdose, use isoproterenol or atropine. Propranolol should not be discontinued suddenly, since serious worsening of angina or sudden death may occur.

Interactions

Enhanced hypoglycemia with oral hypoglycemic agents. The clinical signs of hypoglycemia may be suppressed by beta blockade. Cardiac asystole may occur in patients given propranolol and verapamil concurrently. Concurrent use of propranolol and clonidine should be avoided because hypertensive control may be lost and hypertensive overshoot due to clonidine may be aggravated.

Special Note

Note the following useful combinations.

Propranolol + hydralazine + diuretic in hypertension [6].
Propranolol + phenoxybenzamine in pheochromocytoma.
Propranolol + digoxin or nitroglycerin in angina [2].
Propranolol + reserpine in dissecting aneurysm.

Review

Nies, A. S., and Shand, D. G.   Clinical pharmacology of propranolol. *Circulation* 52:6–15, 1975.

References

1.   Coltart, D. J., and Shand, D. G.   Plasma propranolol levels in the quantitative assessment of β-adrenergic blockade in man. *Br. Med. J.* 3:731–734, 1970.
2.   Crawford, M. H., LeWinter, M. M., et al.   Combined propranolol and digoxin therapy in angina pectoris. *Ann. Int. Med.* 83:449–455, 1975.
3.   Fitzgerald, J. D., and O'Donnell, S. R.   Pharmacology of 4-hydroxypropranolol, a metabolite of propranolol. *Br. J. Pharmacol.* 43:222–235, 1971.
4.   Lowenthal, D. T., Briggs, W. A., et al.   Pharmacokinetics of oral propranolol in chronic renal disease. *Clin. Pharmacol. Ther.* 16:761–769, 1974.
5.   Paterson, J. W., Connolly, M. E., et al.   The pharmacodynamics and metabolism of propranolol in man. *Eur. J. Clin. Pharmacol.* 2:127–133, 1970.
6.   Zacest, R., Gilmore, E., et al.   Treatment of essential hypertension with combined vasodilation and beta-adrenergic blockade. *N. Engl. J. Med.* 286:617–622, 1972.
7.   Zacest, R., and Kock-Weser, J.   Relation of propranolol plasma level to β-blockade during oral therapy. *Pharmacology* 7:178–184, 1972.

Oxprenolol, Sotalol, Pindolol, Alprenolol, Atenolol, Metoprolol, Timolol

Competitive antagonists at beta-adrenergic receptors. The primary member of this family of drugs, dichloroisoproterenol (DCI), is an analogue of the beta-adrenergic agonist isoproterenol. DCI was succeeded by pronethalol and then by propranolol, which is currently the only beta blocker available in the United States. Propranolol is described separately on p. 110.

Table 8. *Some Properties of Beta-Adrenergic Blocking Drugs*

Drug	Cardio-selectivity (Relative)	Partial Agonist Activity	V_d (L/kg)[a]	$t_{\frac{1}{2}}$ (hr)[a]	Oral Dose (mg/day)[a]
Propranolol	−	−	3.0	3	60–480
Oxprenolol	−	+	1.5	2	120–480
Sotalol	−	−	0.7	13	120–600
Pindolol	−	+	2.0	4	7.5–45
Alprenolol	−	+	3.3	3	100–600
Atenolol	+	−	0.7	7	200–800
Metoprolol	+	−	5.6	3	50–300
Timolol	−	−	8.0	5	20–60

[a]These are average values. Substantial variation has been noted.
Key: −, absent; +, present.

The other drugs listed in Table 8 have not been evaluated as extensively as propranolol. There are differences among them in lipid/water partition, potency, protein binding, and ancillary pharmacological effects such as cardioselectivity, partial agonist activity, and local anesthetic activity, but it appears that indications and effects are similar for all of them. However, it should be noted that pronethalol has produced thymic tumors in mice and that practolol, another early beta blocker, has produced a serious oculocutaneous syndrome in a small number of patients; thus, structural differences may have an important influence on toxicity.

Absorption

With the exception of atenolol (50%), all other drugs listed are completely absorbed. Propranolol and alprenolol undergo extensive dose-dependent first-pass metabolism. The systemic availability of atenolol (about 50%) does not appear to be dose-dependent. t_{max}: 1–3 hours.

Distribution

V_d: see Table 8. Protein binding: propranolol 95%, alprenolol 85%, and metoprolol 11%. No available information about the other beta blockers.

Elimination

Propranolol, alprenolol, and metoprolol undergo extensive hepatic metabolism, followed by renal elimination of metabolites. 4-Hydroxy propranolol and 4-hydroxy alprenolol are active beta blockers, as potent as their parent drugs.

Oxprenolol, sotalol, pindolol, and atenolol are eliminated in urine, mainly as unchanged drug.

Dosage Schedule

Usual daily doses are indicated in Table 8. Doses twice daily are often adequate. It is best to start with a low dose and adjust according to the drug's effect. Occasionally patients may need much larger doses than the doses indicated in Table 8.

Special Dosage Situations

Cardioselective beta-adrenergic blocking drugs may be used cautiously in patients with obstructive airway disease. Contraindicated in patients with congestive heart failure and first- or second-degree heart block, since all are exacerbated by beta blockade. If cardiac failure is due to severe hypertension or arrhythmia, patient may benefit from beta blockade. Little information about use in patients with renal or hepatic disease, in pregnant women, or in the elderly.

Therapeutic Concentrations

Little available information relating plasma concentrations of these drugs to their therapeutic effects.

Adverse Reactions

Bronchospasm, left ventricular failure, and bradycardia are potential side-effects of all beta-adrenergic blocking agents. In overdose, use isoproterenol or atropine. If cutaneous or ocular disturbances occur, the drug should be discontinued immediately.

Interactions

The signs of hypoglycemia may be masked by beta blockade. The other interactions reported with propranolol may also occur.

Reviews

Johnsson, G., and Regårdh, C.-G.   Clinical pharmacokinetics of β-adrenoceptor blocking drugs. *Clin. Pharmacokin.* 1:233–263, 1976.

Oxprenolol

Brunner, L., Imhof, P., et al.   Relation between plasma concentrations and cardiovascular effects of oral oxprenolol in man. *Eur. J. Clin. Pharmacol.* 8:3–9, 1975.

Mason, W. D., and Winer, N.   Pharmacokinetics of oxprenolol in normal subjects. *Clin. Pharmacol. Ther.* 20:401–412, 1976.

Motolese, M., Muiesan, G., et al.   Hypotensive effect of oxprenolol in mild to moderate hypertension: A multicentre controlled study. *Eur. J. Clin. Pharmacol.* 8:21–31, 1975.

Sotalol

Brown, H. C., Carruthers, S. G., et al.   Observations on the efficacy and pharmacokinetics of sotalol after oral administration. *Eur. J. Clin. Pharmacol.* 9:367–372, 1976.

Sundqvist, H., Anttila, M., et al.   Antihypertensive effects of practolol and sotalol. *Clin. Pharmacol. Ther.* 16:465–472, 1974.

Pindolol

Aellig, W. H.   β-Adrenoceptor blocking activity and duration of action of pindolol and propranolol in healthy volunteers. *Br. J. Clin. Pharmacol.* 3:251, 257, 1976.

Gugler, R., Herold, W., et al. Pharmacokinetics of pindolol in man. *Eur. J. Clin. Pharmacol.* 7:17–24, 1974.

Alprenolol

Regårdh, C.-G. Pharmacokinetics and biopharmaceutics of some adrenergic beta-receptor antagonists with special emphasis on alprenolol and metoprolol. *Acta Pharmacol. Toxicol.* 37 (Suppl. 1): 3–39, 1975.

Atenolol

Brown, H. C., Carruthers, S. G., et al. Clinical pharmacologic observations on atenolol, a beta-adrenoceptor blocker. *Clin. Pharmacol. Ther.* 20:524–534, 1976.

Metoprolol

Johnsson, G., Regårdh, C.-G., et al. Combined pharmacokinetic and pharmacodynamic studies in man of the adrenergic β_1-receptor antagonist metoprolol. *Acta Pharmacol. Toxicol.* 36(Suppl. 5): 7–23, 1975.

Timolol

Brogden, R. N., Pheight, T. M., et al. Timolol: A preliminary report on its pharmacological properties and therapeutic efficacy in angina and hypertension. *Drugs* 9:164–177, 1975.

BETHANIDINE

An antihypertensive, postganglionic adrenergic blocking agent from the same family as guanethidine and debrisoquine. Transported into peripheral nerve endings, where it is bound to norepinephrine storage sites and may act either as a "false" neurotransmitter or by persistent nerve depolarization. Indicated in all forms of hypertension *except* pheochromocytoma.

Absorption

Oral absorption: 50–100%, apparently greater with lower doses. t_{max}: 1–5 hours, parallels rate of onset of antihypertensive effect [3].

Distribution

V_d: about 6 L/kg. Protein binding: about 8% [3].

Elimination

$t_{\frac{1}{2}}$: 7–11 hours. Not metabolized, appears unchanged in urine. Clearance approximates renal blood flow; it therefore involves both glomerular filtration and tubular secretion. Elimination curve is triexponential, suggesting, as for guanethidine, a "deep" tissue store [3].

Dosage Schedule

No fixed dose; adjust dose against blood pressure level. Usual starting dose is 20 mg twice daily but may be increased to 700 mg twice daily. Approximately equivalent to guanethidine as antihypertensive agent. However, because of shorter $t_{\frac{1}{2}}$, maximum action occurs within 2 days, and it is possible to minimize postural hypotension by giving smaller doses more frequently.

The following b.i.d. regimen has been recommended for loading in emergencies [2]:

Day 1	50 mg	0 mg
Day 2	50 mg	20 mg
Day 3	50 mg	50 mg
Day 4	50 mg	100 mg

This regimen may be suspended when blood pressure reaches the required level, and the maintenance dosage is continued.

Special Dosage Situations

Avoid use in patients with cardiac or cerebrovascular disease because of postural hypotensive effect (see Adverse Reactions). Dose may need to be decreased in renal failure because of lengthened $t_{\frac{1}{2}}$. Avoid use in males because of poor compliance due to high incidence of failure of ejaculation.

Therapeutic Concentrations

Adjust dose according to patient's response.

Adverse Reactions

Same as those for guanethidine (failure of ejaculation, postural hypotension, dry mouth, and diarrhea), with the exception that diarrhea is much less common [1].

Interactions

Uptake into nerve endings is blocked by tricyclic antidepressants, cocaine, and amphetamine.

References

1. Gifford, R. Q.   Bethanidine sulfate—a new antihypertensive agent. *J.A.M.A.* 193:901–905, 1965.
2. Gupta, N., and McNay, J. L.   Rapid control of hypertension with oral bethanidine. *Eur. J. Clin. Pharmacol.* 4:417–421, 1972.
3. Shen, D., Gibaldi, M., et al.   Pharmacokinetics of bethanidine in hypertensive patients. *Clin. Pharmacol. Ther.* 17:363–373, 1975.

CARBAMAZEPINE

A dibenzazepine derivative, structurally related to tricyclic antidepressants. Used in the treatment of tonic-clonic seizures, partial epilepsy, and trigeminal neuralgia and potentially useful in the treatment of diabetes insipidus [8].

Absorption

Bioavailability: unknown. t_{max}: after 400 mg approximately 8 hours [4].

Distribution

V_d: 0.8–1.4 L/kg [9]. Protein binding: 65–83% [3]. CSF concentration 15% of plasma concentration [5]. Fetal plasma level of the drug is 50% and breast milk level is 60% of maternal plasma level [7].

Elimination

$t_{\frac{1}{2}}$: 24–48 hours. At least seven metabolites formed, probably in the liver; the epoxide metabolite is probably active. Extent of formation of this metabolite is not known.

Dosage Schedule

10–20 mg/kg, once daily if tolerated.

Special Dosage Situations

Children: 10–20 mg/kg. Pregnancy: drug to be avoided (because of fetal abnormalities in mice). Elderly: no available information. Renal and liver disease: no precautions required.

Therapeutic Concentrations

6–10 μg/ml [2].

Adverse Reactions

Nystagmus, diplopia, slurred speech, and drowsiness in 50% of patients with plasma levels in excess of 8.5 μg/ml [5]. Bone marrow depression and systemic lupus erythematosus are rare. Water retention may occur, presumably because of antidiuretic activity.

Interactions

Plasma levels of phenytoin are lowered with concomitant carbamazepine administration, and vice versa [1, 6].

References

1. Christiansen, J., and Dam, M.   Influence of phenobarbital and diphenylhydantoin on plasma carbamazepine levels in patients with epilepsy. *Acta Neurol. Scand.* 49:543–546, 1973.
2. Eadie, M. J., and Tyrer, J. H.   *Anticonvulsant Therapy.* Edinburgh and London: Churchill/Livingstone, 1974. Pp. 101–107.
3. Hooper, W. D., Dubetz, D. K., et al.   Plasma protein binding of carbamazepine. *Clin. Pharmacol. Ther.* 17:433–440, 1975.
4. Levy, R. H., Pitlick, W. H., et al.   Pharmacokinetics of carbamazepine in normal man. *Clin. Pharmacol. Ther.* 17:657–668, 1975.
5. Meinardi, H.   Carbamazepine. In D. M. Woodbury, J. K. Penry, and R. P. Schmidt (Eds.), *Antiepileptic Drugs.* New York: Raven Press, 1972. Pp. 487–496.
6. Mølholm Hansen, J., Siersbaek-Nielsen, K., et al. Carbamazepine-induced acceleration of diphenylhydantoin and warfarin metabolism in man. *Clin. Pharmacol. Ther.* 12:539–543, 1971.

7. Pynnönen, S., and Sillanpää, M. Carbamazepine and mother's milk. Lancet 2:563, 1974.
8. Radó, J. P. Clinical use of additive antidiuretic action of carbamazepine and chlorpropamide. Horm. Metab. Res. 5:309, 1973.
9. Rawlins, M. D., Collste, P., et al. Distribution and elimination kinetics of carbamazepine in man. Eur. J. Clin. Pharmacol. 8:91-96, 1975.

CARBENOXOLONE

A triterpine, the disodium salt of the succinic acid ester of enoxolone (18 beta-glycerrhetic acid), a derivative of licorice root, and long used as a folk remedy in the treatment of dyspepsia. Possible mechanisms of action are enhanced gastric mucus secretion, prolonged survival of the gastric epithelium, reduced back-diffusion of hydrogen ions, and diminished peptic activity. Increased rate of healing and relief of symptoms in ambulatory patients with benign gastric ulcers are comparable to that achieved by bed rest and hospitalization.

Absorption

Rapid, complete, mainly in the stomach. t_{max}: 1-2 hours when fasting, but incomplete. t_{max}: 6-10 hours when even a light meal is taken first [2]. Absorption does not occur when gastric pH is greater than 2 [1].

Distribution

After absorption, about 60% is within the intravascular space [1]. V_d: therefore about 0.1 L/kg. Protein binding: 99-100%.

Elimination

$t_{\frac{1}{2}}$: 13-16 hours. Hydrolysis of ester bond, possibly in the intestine, with subsequent metabolism of succinate to carbon dioxide, accounts for 10-20% of a single oral dose [2]. Following biliary excretion, 70-80% eliminated unchanged in the feces. Less than 1% excreted in urine. An enterohepatic circulation is proposed because of a secondary peak of radioactivity at 3-6 hours [1]. Carbenoxolone glucuronide is detected in bile [1]. Metabolites are inactive.

Dosage Schedule

200-300 mg daily in 3 divided doses at least 1 hour before meals for 4-6 weeks.

Special Dosage Situations

There appears to be no advantage in using the drug in gastric ulcer patients who are treated with bed rest, since the effects of both treatments are comparable and are not additive. Chinese and possibly other Orientals show no response, for unknown reasons [3]. The treatment of acute duodenal ulcer with special intraduodenal release preparations has shown no clear success to date. Weekly examination of weight, blood pressure, and electrolytes is desirable in all patients. Use cautiously in patients with hypertension and congestive heart failure.

Therapeutic Concentrations

Apparently not relevant, because carbenoxolone is thought to act during passage through the gastric mucosa.

Adverse Reactions

Hypertension, salt and water retention, and hypokalemia and its associated effects are common major side-effects related to the aldosterone-like activity of the drug. Mild dyspepsia, diarrhea, flushing, headache, and abdominal discomfort have been occasionally reported.

Interactions

Spironolactone, an aldosterone antagonist, prevents major side-effects but also prevents the therapeutic effect. Thiazides prevent hypertension and fluid retention without inhibiting the therapeutic action of carbenoxolone, but patients may require additional potassium supplements.

Reviews

Baron, J. H., and Sullivan, F. M. *Carbenoxolone Sodium.* London: Butterworth, 1970.

Lewis, J. R. Carbenoxolone sodium in the treatment of peptic ulcer. A review. *J.A.M.A.* 229:460–462, 1974.

Robson, J. M., and Sullivan, F. M. *A Symposium on Carbenoxolone Sodium.* London: Butterworth, 1967.

References

1. Downer, H. D., Galloway, R. W., et al. The absorption and excretion of carbenoxolone in man. *J. Pharm. Pharmacol.* 22:479–487, 1970.
2. Parke, D. V., Hunt, T. C., et al. The fate of ^{14}C-carbenoxolone in patients with gastric ulcer. *Clin. Sci.* 43:393–400, 1972.
3. Wye-Poh, F., Kho, K. M., et al. Carbenoxolone sodium in the treatment of gastric ulceration in Chinese. *Med. J. Aust.* 2:919–922, 1974.

CARBIMAZOLE

A mercaptoimidazole used in the treatment of hyperthyroidism. Inhibits the synthesis of thyroid hormones but does not interfere with the iodine uptake or release of hormones.

Absorption

Oral bioavailability: unknown. t_{max} (methimazole): about 1 hour [3].

Distribution

V_d: unknown. Protein binding: unknown. Accumulates in the thyroid gland as methimazole [1], usually producing a response in 5–10 days. Passes easily to breast milk and fetal circulation (potentially goitrogenic).

Elimination

$t_{\frac{1}{2}}$: unknown. Transformed rapidly and completely to the active compound methimazole. Half-life of methimazole is about 7 hours. Metabolism unknown; about 10% excreted unchanged in the urine [2, 4].

Dosage Schedule

Only used orally. Initially, 20–60 mg in 3 daily doses; reduce dosage after 3–6 weeks to 5–20 mg daily, according to laboratory and clinical response of the patient. Thyroxine is often added in doses of 0.1–0.3 mg to prevent thyroid enlargement. Maintain treatment for 18–24 months. Relapse to hyperthyroidism is frequent, usually 20–50%. Patients with large and nodular goiters and those who have had previous iodine treatment show a diminished response to carbimazole and methimazole.

Special Dosage Situations

Children: 0.3–0.5 mg/kg/day in 3 divided doses. Pregnancy: reduce dose, keeping serum thyroxine at the physiologically slightly elevated level to avoid fetal goiter. Contraindicated during lactation. Probably no dose adjustment required in patients with renal disease or in the elderly. No available information about dose adjustment in patients with liver disease. A large intrathoracic goiter is a contraindication to use of this drug, especially without concurrent thyroxine treatment.

Therapeutic Concentrations

Not known. Probably not relevant.

Adverse Reactions

Nausea, epigastric discomfort, arthralgia, skin rashes, and occasional alopecia. Bone marrow suppression is rare and unpredictable. Goiter may develop with large doses.

Interactions

None demonstrated.

Review

Mills, L. C.   Drug treatment in thyroid disease. *Semin. Drug Treat.* 3:377–402, 1974.

References

1. Marchant, B., Alexander, W. D., et al.   The accumulation of ^{35}S-antithyroid drugs by the thyroid gland. *J. Clin. Endocrinol. Metab.* 34:847–851, 1972.
2. Pitman, J. A., Beschi, R. J., et al.   Methimazole: Its absorp-

tion and excretion in man and tissue distribution in rats. *J. Clin. Endocrinol. Metab.* 33:182–185, 1971.

3. Skellern, G. G., Stenlake, J. B., et al. Plasma concentrations of methimazole, a metabolite of carbimazole, in hyperthyroid patients. *Br. J. Clin. Pharmacol.* 1:256–269, 1974.

4. Vesell, E. S., Shapiro, J. R., et al. Altered plasma half-life of antipyrine, propylthiouracil, and methimazole in thyroid dysfunction. *Clin. Pharmacol. Ther.* 17:48–56, 1975.

CEPHALOSPORINS

Water-soluble, broad-spectrum, semisynthetic bactericidal antibiotics derived from 7-aminocephalosporanic acid. Active against *Staphylococci,* including penicillin-resistant strains, and the majority of cultures of *Salmonella, Shigella, Escherichia coli, Proteus mirabilis, Klebsiella,* and *Hemophilus influenzae.* Inactive against *Pseudomonas, Enterococci,* and *Enterobacter.* Only minor differences exist between different cephalosporins in antibacterial activity. Mechanism of action is inhibition of bacterial wall synthesis. Cephalosporins do not cross blood-brain barrier; therefore they are not useful in the treatment of meningitis except when given intrathecally [2].

Absorption

Oral bioavailability: 90–95%. t_{max} for oral preparations: about 1 hour. t_{max} for intramuscular preparations: 0.5–1 hour.

Distribution, Elimination, and Dosage Schedule

See Table 9.

Concentrations in bile and fetal circulation are about the same as in serum [4, 9]. Cephalosporins are excreted 90–100% unchanged in the urine except for cephalothin and cephapirin, which are partly metabolized (30%) by desacetylation to compounds with less antimicrobial activity. The metabolites are also excreted in the urine. Cephaloridine and cefazolin are excreted mainly by glomerular filtration; the other cephalosporins are secreted by the renal tubule.

Hemodialysis decreases the half-life of all cephalosporins. $t_{\frac{1}{2}}$ in anuria is about 24 hours; during hemodialysis it is 2–4 hours.

Special Dosage Situations

Children: see Table 9. Renal failure: cephaloridine contraindicated. For other cephalosporins, increase dosage intervals according to Table 1 on page 30, e.g., if clearance is below 50 ml/min, dose should be given every 6–12 hours; if clearance is below 10 ml/min, dose should be given every 12–24 hours. No dosage adjustments necessary in the elderly, in patients with hepatic disease, or in women during pregnancy or lactation.

Therapeutic Concentrations

Gram-positive organisms: 0.5–3 μg/ml. Gram-negative organisms: 1.0–12 μg/ml.

Table 9. *Some Properties of the Cephalosporins*

Cephalosporin	Route	$t_{\frac{1}{2}}$ (min)	Protein Binding (%)	V_d (L/kg)	Daily Dose (mg) Adults	Daily Dose (mg) Children
Cephaloridine [5, 10]	IM IV	60–90	10–30	0.25	250–500 q6h	. . .
Cephalothin [5, 10, 12]	IM IV	20–40	65–80	0.25	500–1000 q3–6h	10–20/kg q6h
Cephalexin [5, 7, 11]	PO	20–60	10–15	0.25	250–1000 q6h	6–12/kg q6h
Cefazolin [10]	IM IV	90–120	75–85	0.15	500–1000 q8h	6–12/kg q8h
Cephradine [3]	IM PO	40–50	5–20	0.25	250–1000 q6h	6–12/kg q6h
Cephapirin [1]	IM IV	40–50	40–50	0.15	500–2000 q4–6h	10–20/kg q6–8h

Adverse Reactions

Drug fever, eosinophilia, positive Coombs' reaction, serum sickness, urticaria, rashes, and anaphylactic shock are side-effects common to all cephalosporins. Penicillin allergy is not a contraindication to the use of cephalosporins, although patients who are sensitive to penicillin are more frequently allergic to cephalosporins than patients who are not sensitive to penicillin. Overall allergy incidence is 2–3% in those patients not sensitive to penicillin and about 8% in those patients allergic to penicillin [8]. Intramuscular injection of cephalothin, cephaloridine, and cephapirin is painful. Nephrotoxicity is frequent with cephaloridine (almost inevitable with daily dose above 6 g) but infrequent with other cephalosporins [6].

Interactions

Increased risk of nephrotoxicity when a cephalosporin is used in combination with gentamicin. Probenecid inhibits the tubular secretion of cephalothin, cephalexin, cephradine, and cephapirin.

Reviews

Benner, E. J., Lewis, A. A. G., et al. (Eds.). Symposium on cephalosporin antibiotics. *Postgrad. Med. J.* 47(Feb. suppl.):1–142, 1971.

Moellering, R. C., and Swartz, M. N.   The newer cephalosporins. *N. Engl. J. Med.* 254:24–28, 1976.

Weinstein, L., and Kaplan, K.   The cephalosporins. *Ann. Intern. Med.* 72:729–739, 1970.

References

1. Axelrod, J., Meyers, B. R., et al. Cephapirin: Pharmacology in normal human volunteers. *J. Clin. Pharmacol.* 12:84–88, 1972.
2. Fisher, L. S., Chow, A. W., et al. Cephalothin and cephaloridine therapy for bacterial meningitis. *Ann. Intern. Med.* 82:689–693, 1975.
3. Harvengt, C., DeSnepper, P., et al. Cephradine absorption and excretion in fasting and nonfasting volunteers. *J. Clin. Pharmacol.* 13:36–40, 1973.
4. Hirsch, H. A. The use of cephalosporin antibiotics in pregnant women. *Postgrad. Med. J.* 47(Feb. suppl.):90–93, 1971.
5. Kirby, W. M. M., DeMaine, J. B., et al. Pharmacokinetics of the cephalosporins in healthy volunteers and uremic patients. *Postgrad. Med. J.* 47(Feb. suppl.):41–46, 1971.
6. Mandell, G. L. Cephaloridine. *Ann. Intern. Med.* 79:561–565, 1973.
7. Meyers, B. R., Kaplan, K., et al. Cephalexin: Microbiological effect and pharmacologic parameters in man. *Clin. Pharmacol. Ther.* 10:810–816, 1969.
8. Petz, L. D. Immunologic reactions of humans to cephalosporins. *Postgrad. Med. J.* 47 (Feb. suppl.): 64–69, 1971.
9. Ratzan, K. R., Ruiz, C., et al. Biliary tract excretion of cefazolin, cephalothin, and cephaloridine in the presence of biliary tract disease. *Antimicrob. Agents Chemother.* 6:426–431, 1974.
10. Regamey, C., Gordon, R. C., et al. Cefazolin vs. cephalothin and cephaloridine. *Arch. Intern. Med.* 133:407–410, 1974.
11. Thornhill, T. S., Levison, M. E., et al. *In vitro* antimicrobial activity and human pharmacology of cephalixin, a new orally absorbed cephalosporin C antibiotic. *Appl. Microbiol.* 17:457–461, 1969.
12. Wick, W. E. *In vitro* and *in vivo* laboratory comparison of cephalothin and desacetylcephalothin. *Antimicrob. Agents Chemother.* 870–875, 1965.

CHLORAL HYDRATE

A condensation of chloral and water: $CCl_3CH(OH)_2$. A rapidly acting hypnotic that has little analgesic activity but is effective against both experimental seizures and grand mal epilepsy. However, the ratio of anticonvulsant to sedative effect is much smaller than for barbiturates, diazepam, and phenytoin. The hypnotic mechanism is unknown. Depresses rapid eye movement (REM) sleep only slightly.

Absorption

Systemic bioavailability: 0, due to a large first-pass effect that transforms chloral hydrate to trichlorethanol. t_{max} for trichlorethanol: about 30 minutes.

Distribution

V_d for trichlorethanol: about 0.6 L/kg. Protein binding: about 40% [5]. The concentration of trichlorethanol in CSF is from 5–50% of the concentration in serum [3]. In maternal and fetal blood, the concentrations of trichlorethanol are equal [1]. After rectal administration, the concentration of trichlorethanol in breast milk is 50–75% of the maternal serum concentration [2].

Elimination

$t_{\frac{1}{2}}$ of trichlorethanol: 4–8 hours. Most of the trichlorethanol is inactivated by glucuronidation to urochloralic acid. 20–40% of trichlorethanol is oxidized to inactive trichloracetic acid [5].

Dosage Schedule

Only used orally and as an enema. 500–1500 mg orally before sleep. If taken in solution, the drug should be well diluted with water or milk. Rectal suppositories: 600–1800 mg.

Special Dosage Situations

Children: 50 mg/kg with a maximum of 1 g in a single dose. No information about regimens in patients with hepatic or renal failure. Seems to be safe for use in the elderly. No adverse effects in nursing infants when given to mothers [2].

Therapeutic Concentrations

Not established. After about 1000 mg orally, a maximum concentration of 10–20 μg/ml is obtained.

Adverse Reactions

Metallic taste, epigastric pain, nausea, vomiting, and flatulence; and light-headedness, ataxia, nightmares, and hangover. Allergic reactions are seen (urticaria and exanthemata). Leucopenia is rare.

An average toxic dose is about 10 g. Poisoning resembles acute barbiturate intoxication, with the addition of severe gastric irritation. Pinpoint pupils are often seen. Hepatic and renal damage may be seen later. Treat symptomatically; hemodialysis may be used in severe poisoning.

Chronic intake can result in tolerance and physical dependence. Sudden withdrawal results in symptoms of abstinence.

Interactions

Decreases the effects of dicumarol and warfarin by hepatic enzyme induction. During the first few days of concurrent administration, an increased anticoagulant effect, caused by displacement of the coumarin anticoagulants by trichloracetic acid, may be evident [4].

Ethanol increases the serum concentration of trichlorethanol by stimulation of NADH (reduced nicotinamide adenine dinucleotide) production [6].

References

1. Bernstine, J. B., Meyer, A. E., et al. Maternal and fetal blood estimation following the administration of chloral hydrate during labor. *J. Obstet. Gynaecol. Br. Empire* 61:683–685, 1954.
2. Bernstine, J. B., Meyer, A. E., et al. Maternal blood and breast milk estimation following the administration of chloral hydrate during the puerperium. *J. Obstet. Gynaecol. Br. Empire* 63:228–231, 1956.
3. Bernstine, J. B., Meyer, A. E., et al. Maternal blood and cerebrospinal fluid estimation following the administration of chloral hydrate during the puerperium. *J. Obstet. Gynaecol. Br. Empire* 64:801–804, 1957.
4. Koch-Weser, J., and Sellers, E. M. Drug interactions with coumarin anticoagulants. *N. Engl. J. Med.* 285:547–558, 1971.
5. Marshall, E. K., Jr., and Owens, A. H., Jr. Absorption, excretion, and metabolic fate of chloral hydrate and trichloroethanol. *Bull. Johns Hopkins Hosp.* 95:1–18, 1954.
6. Sellers, E. M., Lang, M., et al. Interaction of chloral hydrate and ethanol in man. I. Metabolism. *Clin. Pharmacol. Ther.* 13:37–49, 1972.

CHLORAMPHENICOL

An almost water-insoluble, stable, bacteriostatic antibiotic. Active against most gram-negative and gram-positive bacteria and several species of *Rickettsia, Chlamydia,* and *Mycoplasma.* Inactive against *Pseudomonas aeruginosa.* Mechanism of action is inhibition of microsomal protein synthesis (50 S subunit of RNA). The development of resistance is rare. Because of severe side-effects the drug should be used only in serious infections caused by susceptible organisms that cannot be treated more safely and effectively with other agents. In practice the indications are (1) acute typhoid fever and other systemic *Salmonella* infections (inactive against carriers, in whom ampicillin is the drug of choice); (2) *Hemophilus influenzae* meningitis; and (3) rickettsial diseases when tetracyclines are contraindicated. Recent investigations suggest, however, that the better-absorbed ampicillin derivatives, e.g., amoxycillin and pivampicillin, are valuable alternatives to chloramphenicol in typhoid fever [5].

Absorption

Oral bioavailability: 75–90%. t_{max}: about 2 hours [3].

Distribution

V_d: about 0.6 L/kg [3]. Protein binding: 60–80%. The concentration in CSF is 25–50% of the blood concentration and is probably more in inflammation [9]. The placental transfer is 50–75% [7].

Elimination

$t_{\frac{1}{2}}$: 2–3 hours [3]. 90% is inactivated in the liver by glucuronidation and hydrolysis. The glucuronidated compound is excreted by tubular secretion. Unchanged drug is excreted by glomerular filtration.

Dosage Schedule

Typhoid fever: 2 g initially, followed by 1 g every 6 hours for 4 weeks. Rickettsial diseases: 0.5–1 g every 4–6 hours. IM administration should be avoided, since absorption is erratic.

Special Dosage Situations

Infants below 1 month of age: 25 mg/kg/day in 2–3 divided doses. Children above 1 month of age: 50 mg/kg/day in 2–3 divided doses. Older children: up to 100 mg/kg/day. Hepatic diseases: dosage reduction seems appropriate, but no information is available. No special dosage adjustments in patients with renal disease, for women during pregnancy or lactation, or in the elderly.

Therapeutic Concentrations

Serum concentrations above 10 μg/ml are associated with a higher risk of toxicity. Most strains of *Salmonella* are susceptible to concentrations of 2–10 μg/ml.

Adverse Reactions

Dose-related side-effects: gastrointestinal disturbances such as nausea, vomiting, diarrhea, and pruritus ani. Neuritis is rare, usually affecting the optic nerve. Reversible anemia, with high serum iron and reticulocytopenia, occurs frequently if the serum concentration exceeds 25 μg/ml. When neonates are given daily doses larger than 100–200 mg/kg, the gray syndrome may occur. Main symptoms are vomiting, diarrhea, cyanosis, hypotonia, irregular respiration, and an ashen-gray color. Mortality is about 40%, but no sequelae are seen in infants who recover. The gray syndrome results from inadequate elimination of chloramphenicol during the first months of life [1].

Allergic reaction: bone marrow depression, progressing to aplastic anemia, leucopenia, and thrombocytopenia [6, 8]. Frequency of allergic reaction is about 1 : 40,000. The interval between exposure and symptoms may exceed 6 months. The mortality appears to be greater with longer intervals between exposure and symptoms. No adequately documented cases have been described after parenteral administration, perhaps because there are fewer cases and also because bacterial metabolism of the drug in the intestine may cause the formation of haptens [4]. However, no studies are available to ascertain this point. Other allergic reactions include skin rashes, atrophic glossitis, and Herxheimer's reaction.

Superinfection with *Candida* and *Staphylococci* may occur after oral administration.

Chloramphenicol is not eliminated by dialysis.

Interactions

Inhibits the metabolism of phenytoin, tolbutamide, chlorpropamide, and dicumarol [2].

Reviews

Brock, T. D. Chloramphenicol. *Bacteriol. Rev.* 25:32–48, 1961.
Snyder, M. J., and Woodward, T. E. The clinical use of chloramphenicol. *Med. Clin. North Am.* 54:1187–1197, 1970.

References

1. Burns, L. E., Hodgman, J. E., et al. Fetal circulatory collapse in premature infants receiving chloramphenicol. *N. Engl. J. Med.* 261:1318–1321, 1959.
2. Christensen, L. K., and Skovsted, L. Inhibition of drug metabolism by chloramphenicol. *Lancet* 2:1397–1399, 1969.
3. Glazko, A. J., Wolf, L. M., et al. Biochemical studies on chloramphenicol (Chloromycetin). *J. Pharmacol. Exp. Ther.* 96:445–459, 1949.
4. Holt, R. The bacterial degradation of chloramphenicol. *Lancet* 1:1259–1260, 1967.
5. Pillay, N., Adams, E. B., et al. Comparative trial of amoxycillin and chloramphenicol in treatment of typhoid fever in adults. *Lancet* 2:333–334, 1975.
6. Polak, B. C. P., Wesseling, H., et al. Blood dyscrasias attributed to chloramphenicol. *Acta Med. Scand.* 192:409–414, 1972.
7. Scott, W. C., and Warner, R. F. Placental transfer of chloramphenicol (Chloromycetin). *J.A.M.A.* 142:1331–1332, 1950.
8. Wallerstein, R. O., Condit, P. K., et al. Statewide study of chloramphenicol therapy and aplastic anemia. *J.A.M.A.* 208:2045–2050, 1969.
9. Williams, B., Jr., and Dart, R. M. Chloramphenicol (Chloromycetin) concentration in cerebrospinal, ascitic, and pleural fluid. *Boston Med. Quar.* 1:7–10, 1950.

CHLOROQUINE

A 4-aminoquinoline derivative that has been developed as an antimalarial agent. Apart from its usefulness in the treatment and prophylaxis of malaria when the plasmodium is sensitive, it may also be recommended for the management of rheumatoid arthritis, systemic lupus erythematosis (SLE), discoid lupus, erythematosis (DLE), and other forms of disseminated collagen disorders; polymorphic light eruptions; solar urticaria; porphyria cutanea tarda; and amebic liver abscess.

Multiple pharmacological actions include enzyme inhibition, melanin binding, porphyrin binding, nucleic acid binding, antihistamine effects, and lysosomal stabilization, including ultraviolet-induced release of enzymes from lysosomes. The DNA binding probably explains its antibacterial and antimalarial properties and may be part of its activity in SLE. The antihistaminic effect may underlie its usefulness in solar urticaria and as an anti-inflammatory agent, and the porphyrin binding probably explains its value in porphyria cutanea tarda. It has been shown to increase fragmentation of phytohemagglutinin-treated chromosomes in lymphocytes in vitro.

Absorption
Oral bioavailability: 90% [1]. t_{max}: 6 hours [4].

Distribution
V_d: probably large but no available good data. Protein binding: 55% [1]. Concentrated twofold in red cells [5] and approximately tenfold in liver, lung, kidneys, and heart [4]. Crosses placenta. Penetrates blood-brain barrier poorly [4].

Elimination
$t_{\frac{1}{2}}$: 5 days [1]. Extensively metabolized by N-desethylation, 25% appearing unchanged in the urine. This percentage is increased as the urine becomes more acidic [2]. Patients with rheumatoid arthritis appear to develop higher plasma levels of the drug than normal subjects given the same dose, but the mechanism for this effect is not clear [5].

Dosage Schedule
Malaria prophylaxis: 5 mg/kg chloroquine phosphate once weekly; maximum dose should not exceed 500 mg/week. Regimen must be commenced at least 4 weeks before entering an area where malaria is endemic for the prophylaxis to be effective, and this dosage should be continued for 8 weeks after leaving the area.

Treatment of an acute attack of malaria: a dose of as little as 200 mg has been shown to be effective [1], although the usual schedule is 600 mg base immediately, followed by 300 mg 6 hours later. Thereafter, 300 mg daily for 2 days, assuming that there is no *Plasmodium falciparum* malaria resistant to chloroquine in the area. *Plasmodium malariae, vivax,* and *ovale* are all sensitive to chloroquine, but their treatment should always be followed by primaquine base, 15 mg daily for 10–14 days, to eliminate the extra-erythrocytic phase of the plasmodium cycle.

Collagen diseases: up to 250 mg daily long-term. Doses in excess of 100 g/year have a high incidence of retinopathy. Hepatic amebic abscess: 500 mg/day for 10 weeks.

Special Dosage Situations
Because of chromosome breakage and sporadic cases of ototoxicity in infants whose mothers took chloroquine in high doses in the first trimester of pregnancy, ensure that potential benefit outweighs risk in pregnant women. However, if acute treatment of malaria is necessary, chloroquine should be used, because it has been used frequently without side-effects in the fetus. Maximum dose in children is 4 mg/kg/day [3]. Contraindicated in patients with psoriasis.

Therapeutic Concentrations
10 ng/ml clears parasites from the blood at 14 days follow-up for *Ps. vivax* and 21 days for *Ps. falciparum.* Maximum safe level in collagen disorders is 250–280 ng/ml [3].

Adverse Reactions

Gastrointestinal disturbances and pigment changes, which may be expressed as generalized loss of hair pigment or as blue-black pigmentation of the skin and oral mucosa. Keratopathy and retinopathy, with peripheral constriction of the visual fields and impairment of central vision, occur in patients taking 250 mg/day for a prolonged period of time. Retinopathy is reversible in the early stages, but it may occur months after drug therapy has ceased. Therefore patients at risk should have regular ophthalmological examinations. Ototoxicity that causes sensorineural deafness occurs rarely in children whose mothers consume high doses during pregnancy. Myopathy, asymptomatic T-wave flattening on ECG, and a lichen planus type of skin eruption may occur. Overdose may cause fatal cardiorespiratory collapse, especially in children. Deaths have been recorded with blood levels of 1 μg/ml.

Interactions

Chlorpromazine interferes with the melanin binding of chloroquine. Although not proved, administration of this drug combination may be useful in the prevention of retinopathy. However, it is not recommended at present. Concurrent use of gold and phenylbutazone may increase the likelihood of exfoliative dermatitis.

Reviews

Sams, W. M. Chloroquine: Its therapeutic use in photosensitive eruptions. *Int. J. Dermatol.* 15:99–111, 1976.
Sams, W. M. Chloroquine: Mechanism of action. *Mayo Clin. Proc.* 42:300–309, 1967.

References

1. Berliner, R. W., Earle, D. P., Jr., et al. Studies on the chemotherapy of the human malarias. VI. The physiological disposition, antimalarial activity, and toxicity of several derivatives of 4-aminoquinoline. *J. Clin. Invest.* 27:98–107, 1948.
2. Jailer, J. W., Rosenfeld, M., et al. The influence of orally administered alkali and acid on the renal excretion of quinacrine, chloroquine and santoquine. *J. Clin. Invest.* 26:1168–1172, 1947.
3. Laaksonen, A. L. Dosage of antimalarial drugs for children with juvenile rheumatoid arthritis and systemic lupus erythematosus. *Scand. J. Rheumatol.* 3:103–108, 1974.
4. Maio, V. J., and Henry, L. D. Chloroquine poisoning. *South. Med. J.* 67(9):1031–1035, 1974.
5. Zvaifler, N. J., and Rubin, M. The metabolism of chloroquine (abstract). *Arthritis Rheum.* 5:330, 1962.

CHLORPROMAZINE

A phenothiazine, with antipsychotic, antiemetic, hypothermic, sedative, antidopaminergic, and anticholinergic actions and weak alpha-adrenergic blocking activity. Antipsychotic actions may be mediated by increasing turnover rate of dopamine in the basal ganglia. Inhibits the release of adrenocorticotropic hormone (ACTH) and of growth hormone. Increases the secretion of prolactin, presumably by the inhibition of the prolactin-inhibiting factor activity. Used in the treatment of psychotic disorders (especially schizophrenia), as an antiemetic, and in the suppression of hiccups. Reduces growth hormone levels in patients with acromegaly [8].

Absorption
Systemic bioavailability: about 25% [7]. Attributed to a high degree of first-pass metabolism, possibly in the gut wall [2]. t_{max}: 3–4 hours orally and 1–2 hours intramuscularly [1].

Distribution
V_d: 10–20 L/kg [9]. Protein binding: 95–98% [1]. No information on the distribution to the fetus. Sedation starts within 15 minutes after intramuscular injection and about 2 hours after oral administration of usual therapeutic doses [3]. Antipsychotic effect may take 1–3 weeks to appear [13, 14].

Elimination
$t_{\frac{1}{2}}$: 16–30 hours [9]. It is believed that there are more than 100 metabolites of chlorpromazine, and approximately 70% of the drug can be recovered from the urine as conjugated metabolites [6]. About 1% of a dose is recovered unchanged from the urine [1].

Dosage Schedule
Control of psychosis: 200–800 mg/day [12], taken as a single dose at bedtime; when the dose is divided, systemic bioavailability may be less than when the drug is taken as a single dose. Doses of 100–200 mg IV or IM may be necessary in acute psychotic states. Emesis: 25–50 mg intramuscularly. Acromegaly: 100 mg daily orally.

Special Dosage Situations
Pregnancy: no information. Old age: use cautiously and avoid parenteral use because of tendency to produce hypotension and hypothermia. Children: use carefully because of the higher incidence of acute dystonic reactions in children than in adult patients. Liver disease: in cirrhosis, $t_{\frac{1}{2}}$ is similar to that in normal subjects. However, patients with cirrhosis, especially those with a previous history of encephalopathy, appear more susceptible to the sedating effect of the drug than do other patients [9]. Renal disease: no available information.

Therapeutic Concentrations
Plasma levels of 50–300 ng/ml are associated with improvement of psychotic states, especially thought disorder and paranoid delusions, but the drug is not effective for depression or retarded

withdrawal states [12]. The correlation between dose and plasma level is quite weak [12].

Adverse Reactions

Parkinsonian syndrome characterized by rigidity and tremor; akathisia; acute dystonic reactions; tardive dyskinesia, especially in elderly patients; orthostatic hypotension common, being correlated to plasma level of the drug [13]; tachycardia and dry mouth; and hypothermia; urticaria, dermatitis, and abnormal skin pigmentation. Deposits of the drug in the lens and cornea in the majority of the patients who receive a mean dose of 325 mg daily for 3½ years appear to be irreversible, but these deposits do not interfere with vision [10]. Galactorrhea and gynecomastia occur rarely. Hypersensitivity reactions include jaundice, which is caused by intrahepatic cholestasis in approximately 2% of patients, and blood dyscrasias, which are rare. High serum levels are associated with convulsions [11]. Procyclidine, benztropine, diphenhydramine, or other antiparkinsonian agents given parenterally are useful in treating acute extrapyramidal disturbances.

Interactions

Trihexyphenidyl is associated with decreased plasma chlorpromazine levels of about 40% [12]. Lithium may also lower plasma chlorpromazine levels [12]. Alcohol potentiates chlorpromazine's sedative effects [15], as do other sedatives. Antacids may decrease the plasma level of chlorpromazine [4]. Chlorpromazine may potentiate the anticholinergic effects of tricyclic antidepressants; it may antagonize the hypotensive effect of guanethidine [5]; and it may potentiate the hypotensive effect of methyldopa, reserpine, and beta blockers.

References

1. Curry, S. H., Davis, J. M., et al. Factors affecting chlorpromazine plasma levels in psychiatric patients. *Arch. Gen. Psychiatry* 22:209–215, 1970.
2. Curry, S. H., D'Mello, A., et al. Destruction of chlorpromazine during absorption by rat intestine *in vitro. Br. J. Pharmacol.* 40:538P–539P, 1970.
3. Curry, S. H., Marshall, J. H. L., et al. Chlorpromazine plasma levels and effects. *Arch. Gen. Psychiatry* 22:289–296, 1970.
4. Fann, W. E., Davis, J. M., et al. The effect of antacids on the blood levels of chlorpromazine. *Clin. Pharmacol. Ther.* 14:135, 1973.
5. Fann, W. E., Janowski, D. S., et al. Chlorpromazine reversal of the antihypertensive action of guanethidine. *Lancet* 2:436–437, 1971.
6. Hollister, L. E., and Curry, S. H. Urinary excretion of chlorpromazine metabolites following single doses and in steady-state conditions. *Res. Commun. Chem. Pathol. Pharmacol.* 2:330–338, 1971.
7. Hollister, L. E., Curry, S. H., et al. Studies of delayed

action medication. V. Plasma levels and urinary excretion of four different dosage forms of chlorpromazine. *Clin. Pharmacol. Ther.* 11:49–59, 1970.

8.   Kolodny, H. D., Sherman, L., et al.   Acromegaly treated with chlorpromazine. *N. Engl. J. Med.* 284:819–822, 1971.

9.   Maxwell, J. D., Carrella, M., et al.   Plasma disappearance and cerebral effects of chlorpromazine in cirrhosis. *Clin. Sci.* 43:143–151, 1972.

10.   Rasmussen, K., Kirk, L., et al.   Deposits in the lens and cornea of the eye during long-term chlorpromazine medication. *Acta Psychiat. Scand.* 53:1–6, 1976.

11.   Rivera-Calimlim, L., Castañeda, L., et al.   Effects of mode of management on plasma chlorpromazine in psychiatric patients. *Clin. Pharmacol. Ther.* 14:978–986, 1973.

12.   Rivera-Calimlim, L., Nasrallah, H., et al.   Clinical response and plasma levels: Effects of dose, dosage schedules, and drug interactions on plasma chlorpromazine levels. *Am. J. Psychiatry* 133:646–652, 1976.

13.   Sakalis, G., Curry, S. H., et al.   Physiologic and clinical effects of chlorpromazine and their relationship to plasma level. *Clin. Pharmacol. Ther.* 13:931–946, 1972.

14.   Simpson, G. M., Varga, E., et al.   Bioequivalency of generic and brand-named chlorpromazine. *Clin. Pharmacol. Ther.* 15:631–641, 1974.

15.   Zirkle, G. A., King, P. D., et al.   Effects of chlorpromazine and alcohol on coordination and judgment. *J.A.M.A.* 171:1496–1499, 1959.

CHLORPROPAMIDE

A sulfonylurea that mediates hypoglycemic action, at least initially, through the stimulation of pancreatic insulin release. Used in adult onset of nonketotic diabetes, with functioning islet tissue, in patients for whom weight control and carbohydrate restriction alone have been unsuccessful in controlling hyperglycemia. Also used in steroid-induced hyperglycemia when steroids must be continued. Has antidiuretic activity in the management of partial pituitary diabetes insipidus.

Absorption

t_{max}: usually 1–2 hours for complete absorption but may be delayed to 5–7 hours in some patients.

Distribution

V_d: 0.1–0.2 L/kg [5]. Protein binding: 5–10% [2]. Maximum effect on fasting blood glucose is seen in responsive diabetics 4–6 hours after oral dosage. This response is much later than the response in normal individuals.

Elimination

$t_{\frac{1}{2}}$: 25–40 hours, unchanged by diabetes [5]. Approximately 80% of the drug is metabolized with 2-OH chlorpropamide, accounting for about 50% of the drug in urine. Metabolites have much shorter half-lives and represent only a small fraction of drug in plasma; their activities are unknown but are probably unimportant. Metabolites and parent drug are excreted entirely in urine [5].

Dosage Schedule

Usual starting dose is 125–250 mg orally daily as a single dose. The dose may be increased every 10–14 days, according to blood glucose response, up to 750 mg daily. A dose of 8 mg/kg is adequate for most patients.

Special Dosage Situations

Not indicated in juvenile diabetes mellitus, after pancreatectomy, or in patients with ketoacidosis. Care is required in patients with extensive liver disease because of reduced metabolism. The elderly appear to be particularly at risk of hypoglycemic coma [4]. During periods of stress such as accidents, operations, and infections, it may be necessary to use insulin instead of oral hypoglycemic agents.

Therapeutic Concentrations

Maximum therapeutic response occurs with plasma concentrations up to 150 μg/ml [1]. It is common to simply measure blood glucose levels of the drug, a procedure that should be performed frequently after treatment is started and during dosage adjustments.

Adverse Reactions

Skin rashes and hypersensitivity cholestasis occur infrequently. Hypoglycemia is potentially the most serious effect because of prolonged drug activity. Observation of the patient and blood glucose monitoring may therefore be necessary for 2–4 days after overdosage or inadvertent fasting. A reversible granulomatous reaction associated with anicteric hepatitis and exfoliative dermatitis may be related to chlorpropamide [3]. Cardiovascular mortality may be increased [6].

Interactions

The Antabuse (disulfiram) reaction is especially important: vomiting, flushing, hypotension, and palpitations may occur in patients who ingest alcohol. Dicumarol and chloramphenicol inhibit chlorpropamide metabolism and enhance its hypoglycemic action. Beta blockers and acetylsalicylic acid may enhance the drug's hypoglycemic action. Thiazides and corticosteroids may antagonize the hypoglycemic effect.

Review

Goldner, M. G. (Ed.). Chlorpropamide and diabetes mellitus. *Ann. N.Y. Acad. Sci.* 74:407–1028, 1959.

References

1. Gorman Hills, A., and Abelove, W. A. Clinical experience with chlorpropamide in the management of diabetes mellitus. *Ann. N.Y. Acad. Sci.* 74:845–857, 1959.

2. Johnson, P. C., Hennes, A. R., et al.   Metabolic fate of chlor-propamide in man. *Ann. N.Y. Acad. Sci.* 74:459–472, 1959.
3. Rigberg, L. A., Robinson, M. J., et al.   Chlorpropamide-induced granulomas. A probable hypersensitivity reaction in liver and bone marrow. *J.A.M.A.* 235:409–410, 1976.
4. Schen, R. J.   Chlorpropamide: Dangerous hypoglycemia in old age. *Lancet* 1:1121, 1973.
5. Taylor, J. A.   Pharmacokinetics and biotransformation of chlorpropamide in man. *Clin. Pharmacol. Ther.* 13:710–718, 1972.
6. University Group Diabetes Program.   A study of the effects of hypoglycemic agents on vascular complications in patients with adult-onset diabetes. *Diabetes* 19 (Suppl. 2):747–830, 1970.

CLINDAMYCIN

Clindamycin, 7-deoxy-7-chlorolincomycin, is an acid-stable antibiotic related to lincomycin. Bacteriostatic—in higher concentrations bacteriocidal—by inhibition of bacterial protein synthesis. Active against most gram-positive species, including penicillinase-producing staphylococci. Inactive against enterococci. Inactive against all gram-negative species except obligate anaerobes such as *Bacteroides*. Often cross-resistant with erythromycin.

Absorption

Oral bioavailability: 90–100%, unaffected by food. t_{max}: about 1 hour. Intramuscular t_{max}: about 3 hours (phosphate salt) [4], 1–2 hours in children [3].

Distribution

V_d: about 1.2 L/kg. Protein binding: 95% [2]. No passage to CNS, even in inflammation. Concentration in fetal circulation 100% of maternal serum concentration. No available data on distribution to breast milk. Concentration in bile equal to or slightly above serum concentration in normal gallbladders, often below serum concentration in gallbladder disease, but therapeutic concentrations are obtained most of the time [4]. Distribution to bone comparable to that of lincomycin.

Elimination

$t_{\frac{1}{2}}$: 2–3 hours. Mainly metabolized in the liver to N-demethyl-clindamycin and clindamycinsulfoxide. 10% excreted unchanged by the kidneys [1, 5]. Possibly dose-dependent metabolism [3].

Dosage Schedule

Oral: 150–300 mg 6 hourly. IM: 1–3 g daily in 2–4 divided doses. IV: same dose as IM but dissolved in 250 ml isotonic glucose or saline and infused over at least 1 hour because of risk of cardiopulmonary arrest.

Special Dosage Situations

Children's V_d is one-third of adults', and they have shorter $t_{\frac{1}{2}}$ than adults [3]. Oral: 8–16 mg/kg/day in 3–4 divided doses. Infants who weigh less than 10 kg should receive at least 37.5 mg every 8 hours. IM: 10–40 mg/kg/day in 3–4 divided doses. No dosage adjustment is necessary in patients with renal failure, in the elderly, or for women during pregnancy or lactation. No contraindications to use except for patients who are allergic to clindamycin and lincomycin.

Therapeutic Concentrations

2–10 μg/ml of clindamycin and active metabolite, depending on bacterial strain.

Adverse Reactions

Especially with oral dosage, diarrhea (20%), pseudomembranous colitis (10% of cases may be fatal), glossitis, and stomatitis; skin rashes, vaginitis, leucopenia, and thrombocytopenia. Cross-allergy with lincomycin. Drug not removed by dialysis.

Interactions

Clindamycin, chloramphenicol, and erythromycin mutually antagonize each other's antibiotic effect. Clindamycin potentiates neuromuscular blocking agents.

Review

DeHaan, R. M., Metzler, C. M., et al.   Pharmacokinetic studies of clindamycin hydrochloride in humans. *Int. J. Clin. Pharmacol.* 6:105–119, 1972.

References

1. DeHaan, R. M., Metzler, C. M., et al.   Pharmacokinetic studies of clindamycin phosphate. *J. Clin. Pharmacol.* 13:190–209, 1973.
2. Gordon, R. C., Regamey, C., et al.   Serum protein binding of erythromycin, lincomycin, and clindamycin. *J. Pharm. Sci.* 62:1074–1077, 1973.
3. Kauffman, R. E., Shoeman, D. W., et al.   Absorption and excretion of clindamycin-2-phosphate in children after intramuscular injection. *Clin. Pharmacol. Ther.* 13:704–709, 1972.
4. Sales, J. E. L., Sutcliffe, M., et al.   Excretion of clindamycin in the bile of patients with biliary tract disease. *Chemotherapy* 19:11–15, 1973.
5. Wagner, J. G., Novak, E., et al.   Absorption, excretion, and half-life of clindamycin in normal adult males. *Am. J. Med. Sci.* 256:25–37, 1968.

CLOFIBRATE

Ethyl ester of *p*-chlorophenoxyisobutyric acid. The acid CPIB is the active form of the drug. Enhances removal of very low-density lipoproteins (VLDL) from circulation; lowers plasma triglycerides predominantly. Also has cholesterol-lowering effect by inhibiting cholesterol synthesis and increasing excretion of neutral sterols. Used in the treatment of types IIb, III (particularly effective), IV, and V hyperlipoproteinemias; also useful in the treatment of pituitary diabetes insipidus [5]. Increases uric acid elimination.

Absorption
Oral bioavailability: 90–100%. If CPIB is given, bioavailability decreases to 60%, thus indicating that the ester is necessary for complete absorption to occur. The ester is subsequently split, leaving the active CPIB [4]. t_{max}: 2–8 hours [4].

Distribution
V_d: unknown. Protein binding: 96% [3]. No available information about distribution to fetus, breast milk, brain, or other regions.

Elimination
One study reports biphasic, 10½ hours distribution (alpha) phase, and 54 hours elimination (beta) phase (as CPIB) [4]. Other authors report an 18-hour half-life [3]. Excreted 40% as CPIB and 40% as CPIB glucuronide.

Dosage Schedule
1.0 g twice daily for maintenance therapy. Loading not necessary.

Special Dosage Situations
No available information about use in the elderly or in women during pregnancy, or lactation. Renal disease: when creatinine clearance is reduced below 20 ml/min, dose should not exceed 0.5 g/day (see Table 1 on p. 30). Toxicity may be related to increased amount of free drug; in patients with nephrosis, protein binding is decreased to 89%, but dosage need not be reduced unless creatinine clearance is below 50 ml/min [3]. Contraindicated in hepatic failure.

Therapeutic Concentrations
Not known, but response is associated with levels above 100 μg/ml. 1 g daily produces levels of 65–80 μg/ml [1].

Adverse Reactions
Nausea, diarrhea, myositis, impotence, and increased muscle enzymes (creatine phosphokinase), with or without clinical myositis [6]; and increased incidence of gallstones [2] and pulmonary emboli.

Interactions
Increases the action of coumarin anticoagulants.

References
1. Berlin, A.   Quantitative gas chromatographic determination of clofibrinic acid in plasma. *J. Pharm. Pharmacol.* 27:54–55, 1975.
2. Cooper, J., Geizerova, H., et al.   Clofibrate and gallstones. *Lancet* 1:1083, 1975.
3. Gugler, R., Shoeman, D. W., et al.   Pharmacokinetics of

drugs in patients with the nephrotic syndrome. *J. Clin. Invest.* 55:1182–1189, 1975.
4. Männistö, P. T., Tuomisto, J., et al. Pharmacokinetics of clofibrate and chlorophenoxy isobutyric acid. I. Cross-over studies on human volunteers. *Acta Pharmacol. Toxicol.* 36:353–365, 1975.
5. Moses, A. M., Howanitz, J., et al. Clofibrate-induced antidiuresis. *J. Clin. Invest.* 52:535–542, 1973.
6. Schneider, J., and Kaffarnik, H. Impotence in patients treated with clofibrate. *Atherosclerosis* 21:455–457, 1975.

CLONAZEPAM

A benzodiazepinone; a chlorinated derivative of nitrazepam. Has been shown to suppress artificially induced seizure activity in animals [7]. Used in the treatment of absence seizures, tonic-clonic seizures, status epilepticus, myoclonic-akinetic petit mal, myoclonic seizures, and akinetic seizures [4]. After several months of regular use, a reduction in efficacy has been noted [4].

Absorption

Oral bioavailability: 80–100% [1]. t_{max}: 1–2 hours [6]. No available data on intramuscular administration.

Distribution

V_d: 1.5–4.4 L/kg [1]. Protein binding: about 45% [8]. No available data on distribution to breast milk, CSF, or across placenta.

Elimination

$t_{\frac{1}{2}}$: 22–33 hours [2]. Metabolism involves reduction, acetylation, and hydroxylation, which result in metabolites that are probably inactive [3].

Dosage Schedule

Start with 0.02 mg/kg/day; increase dosage by 0.015 mg/kg/day every 3–4 days to a maximum of 0.3 mg/kg/day [8]. For status epilepticus, 1.0 mg may be given intravenously and repeated if necessary within 15 minutes.

Special Dosage Situations

Children: start with 0.01–0.03 mg/kg/day; increase every 3–4 days by 0.015 mg/kg/day to a maximum dose of 0.1–0.2 mg/kg/day. No available information at present on dosage for women during pregnancy, for the elderly, or for patients with liver or renal disease.

Therapeutic Concentrations

Not clearly established, but plasma drug levels of 13–72 ng/ml have been associated with a reduction in seizure frequency [2]. There is a linear relationship between dose and plasma concentration of the drug in children; 0.05 mg/kg/day yields a plasma level of 25 ng/ml, and a dose of 0.10 mg/kg/day results in a plasma level of 55 ng/ml [2].

Adverse Reactions

Ataxia, drowsiness, and dysarthria [5]; hyperactivity, personality change [2]; and weight gain [5]. Exacerbation of preexisting or appearance of new seizure types (e.g., tonic-clonic) have been reported in 2–10% of patients [5]. Sialorrhea, increased bronchial secretions, elevated liver enzymes, and blood dyscrasias occur rarely.

Interactions

None has been reported. Doses of other antiepileptic drugs may have to be adjusted.

Reviews

Browne, T. R.   Clonazepam: A review of a new anticonvulsant drug. *Arch. Neurol.* 33:326–332, 1976.

Pinder, R. M., Brogden, R. N., et al.   Clonazepam: A review of its pharmacological efficacy in epilepsy. *Drugs* 12:321–361, 1976.

References

1.   Berlin, A., and Dahlström, H.   Pharmacokinetics of the anticonvulsant drug clonazepam evaluated from single oral and intravenous doses and by repeated oral administration. *Eur. J. Clin. Pharmacol.* 9:155–159, 1975.
2.   Dreifuss, F. E., Penry, J. K., et al.   Serum clonazepam concentrations in children with absence seizures. *Neurology* 25:255–258, 1975.
3.   Eschenhof, E.   Untersuchungen über das Schicksal des Antikonvulsivums Clonazepam im Organismus der Ratte, des Hundes, und des Menschen. *Arzneim. Forsch.* 23:390–400, 1973.
4.   Fazio, C., Manfredi, M., et al.   Treatment of epileptic seizures with clonazepam. *Arch. Neurol.* 32:304–307, 1975.
5.   Hanson, R. A., and Menkes, J. H.   A new anticonvulsant in the management of minor motor seizures. *Dev. Med. Child Neurol.* 14:3–14, 1972.
6.   Kaplan, S. A., Alexander, K., et al.   Pharmacokinetic profiles of clonazepam in dogs and humans and of flunitrazepam in dogs. *J. Pharm. Sci.* 63:527–532, 1974.
7.   Lipp, J. A.   Effect of small doses of clonazepam upon soman-induced seizure activity and convulsions. *Arch. Int. Pharmacodyn. Ther.* 210:49–54, 1974.
8.   Müller, W., and Wollert, U.   Characterization of the binding of benzodiazepines to human serum albumin. *Naunyn-Schmiedeberg's Arch. Pharmacol.* 280:229–237, 1973.

CLONIDINE

An imidazoline derivative, which acts as an alpha-adrenoceptor agonist. Developed as a nasal decongestant, it was found to have a potent hypotensive action, with both peripheral [8] and CNS [1] effects. Generally produces no postural hypotension. Has the advantage of maintaining the glomerular filtration rate and renal blood flow while lowering the blood pressure. Suppresses renin release [5]. Indicated in the management of all forms of hypertension *except* pheochromocytoma, with the proviso that its toxicity (see Adverse Reactions) frequently makes it a second-line drug. Also indicated for the treatment of migraine [7].

Absorption
Oral bioavailability: 65–95% [6]. t_{max}: 2–4 hours [3].

Distribution
V_d: probably large, but no available data. Protein binding: unknown. In animal studies, highest tissue concentrations appear in kidneys, liver, and brain [2].

Elimination
$t_{\frac{1}{2}}$: 6–24 hours [3]. Metabolism unknown but may be metabolized to p-OH-clonidine. Plasma clearance: 200–500 ml/min, excreted in urine [3].

Dosage Schedule
Most common starting dose is 150–300 μg orally 3–4 times daily. Dose must be adjusted in relation to blood pressure response.

Special Dosage Situations
The drug should not be given to patients who are unreliable medicine takers (see Adverse Reactions). Effects in the elderly not known. No evidence of hepatotoxicity or nephrotoxicity [2].

Therapeutic Concentrations
Not known (assay difficult because of low plasma concentrations of the drug).

Adverse Reactions
Sedation and a dry mouth occur very frequently in the therapeutic dose range and limit the use of the drug [5]. After sudden discontinuation of the drug, an acute hypertensive overshoot may occur, which on occasion may be severe. The treatment for such an overshoot is the use of an alpha blocker such as phenoxybenzamine [4].

Interactions
Action blocked by alpha-adrenoceptor blocking drugs such as phentolamine and phenoxybenzamine and possibly by beta-adrenergic blocking agents. Desipramine abolishes hypotensive effect [1]. Other tricyclic antidepressants should be used with care, since they may also block hypotensive action of clonidine.

Review
Pettinger, W. A. Clonidine, a new antihypertensive drug. *N. Engl. J. Med.* 293:1179–1180, 1975.

References

1. Bousquet, P., and Guertzenstein, P. G.   Localization of the central cardiovascular action of clonidine. *Br. J. Pharmacol.* 49:573–579, 1973.
2. Conolly, M. E.   Clonidine in the Treatment of Hypertension. In D. S. Davies and J. L. Reid (Eds.), *Central Action of Drugs in Blood Pressure Regulation.* London: Pitman, 1975. Pp. 268–275.
3. Dollery, C. T., Davies, D. S., et al.   Clinical pharmacology and pharmacokinetics of clonidine. *Clin. Pharmacol. Ther.* 19:11–17, 1976.
4. Hunyor, S. N., Hansson, L., et al.   Effects of clonidine withdrawal: Possible mechanisms and suggestions for management. *Br. Med. J.* 2:209–211, 1973.
5. Onesti, G., Paz-Martinez, V., et al.   Effect of Clonidine on Renin Release. In G. Onesti, K. E. Kim, et al. (Eds.), *Hypertension.* New York: Grune & Stratton, 1973. Pp. 405–409.
6. Rehbinder, D., and Deckers, W.   Untersuchungen zur Pharmakokinetik und zum Metabolismus des 2-(2,6-dichlorphenylamino)-2-imidazoline hydrochloride (ST 155). *Arzneim. Forsch.* 19:169–176, 1969.
7. Shafer, J., and Tallett, E. R.   Evaluation of clonidine in prophylaxis of migraine. *Lancet* 1:403–406, 1972.
8. Zaimis, E.   On the Pharmacology of Catapres. In M. E. Conolly (Ed.), *Catapres in Hypertension.* London: Pitman, 1970. P. 155.

CODEINE

A narcotic alkaloid analgesic isolated from opium; 3-0-methyl morphine. Has the same pharmacological properties as morphine: analgesia, respiratory and circulatory depression, sedation, change in mood, mental clouding, nausea, vomiting, increase of biliary tract pressure, and atony of the bowel. Analgesic potency is about one-sixth to one-twelfth that of morphine. May be used to suppress cough and control diarrhea.

Absorption

Systemic bioavailability: not known absolutely but approximately two-thirds as effective orally as parenterally. t_{max}: 1–2 hours [2].

Distribution

V_d: unknown. Protein binding: unknown. No available data on distribution to breast milk and fetus.

Elimination

$t_{\frac{1}{2}}$: 3–4 hours [2]; 6 hours after overdosage [3], possibly indicating saturable metabolism [3, 4]. Metabolized by the liver and excreted chiefly in the urine, 37% as glucuronide and 10% unchanged drug [1]. Approximately 10% of codeine is demethylated to form morphine.

Dosage Schedule

For analgesia, 15–60 mg orally every 4–6 hours, depending on response. For cough suppression and control of diarrhea, 15–30 mg orally every 4–6 hours.

Special Dosage Situations

Children: 0.2–0.3 mg/kg every 6–8 hours for cough suppression. Should be avoided in patients with decreased respiratory reserve; $t_{\frac{1}{2}}$ may be prolonged in patients with acute liver disease [3].

Therapeutic Concentrations

Not known. Respiratory arrest was associated with a plasma concentration of 5 μg/ml [3].

Adverse Reactions

Nausea, vomiting, dizziness, mental clouding, dysphoria, constipation, epigastric distress, biliary colic, respiratory depression, and hypotension. Tolerance and drug dependence may develop. Naloxone, 0.4–0.8 mg IV or IM, may be repeated at 30- to 60-minute intervals while signs of serious overdosage persist.

Interactions

The depressant effects of codeine may be exaggerated and prolonged by phenothiazines, monoamine oxidase inhibitors (MAOI), and tricyclic antidepressants.

References

1. Adler, T. K., Fujimoto, J. M., et al. The metabolic fate of codeine in man. *J. Pharmacol. Exp. Ther.* 114:251–262, 1955.
2. Brunson, M. K., Nash, J. F. Gas-chromotographic measurement of codeine and norcodeine in human plasma. *Clin. Chem.* 21:1956–1960, 1975.
3. Huffman, D. H., and Ferguson, R. L. Acute codeine overdose: Correspondence between clinical course and codeine metabolism. *Johns Hopkins Med. J.* 136:183–186, 1975.
4. Nomof, N., Parker, K. D., et al. Metabolism of codeine administered by intravenous infusion. *Clin. Pharmacol. Ther.* 15:215–216, 1974.

COLCHICINE

An alkaloid isolated from autumn crocus. Provides relief from acute attacks of gout and is also effective as a prophylactic. No effect on pseudogout (articular chondrocalcinosis). May be used in sarcoid arthritis [2]. May prevent attacks of familial Mediterranean fever [7]. Mechanism of action is probably inhibition of migration and phagocytosis of urate by granulocytes. The antimitotic effect has no therapeutic significance but may be important in the development of adverse reactions. No influence on the serum level or excretion of uric acid.

Absorption

Systemic bioavailability: unknown, but probably small [5, 6]. Oral t_{max}: ½–2 hours.

Distribution

V_d: about 2 L/kg [5]. Protein binding: unknown.

Elimination

$t_{\frac{1}{2}}$: about 90 minutes [5]. Extensively metabolized by the liver, probably by deacetylation, to inactive metabolites, which are mainly eliminated by the feces. 5–20% excreted unchanged by the kidneys [3, 4].

Dosage Schedule

Acute gouty attacks: 1 mg orally as an initial dose followed by 0.5 mg every 2–3 hours until pain disappears or gastrointestinal symptoms develop. Total amount of drug taken should not exceed 10 mg.

Can be used for prophylaxis during initiation (first 1–2 months) of chronic medication with allopurinol or probenecid [1], in frequent attacks, before operations, and during prolonged bed rest in a dose of 0.5 mg 2–3 times daily.

IV administration in acute attacks: 2 mg as a single dose diluted in 20 ml of isotonic saline.

Special Dosage Situations

Renal failure: clearance below 20 ml/min; increase dose intervals by 50%. Hepatic failure: shortened half-life and decreased V_d [5]; dose should probably be decreased slightly. No available information concerning use of drug in children or in women during pregnancy or lactation.

Therapeutic Concentrations

After 1 mg is given orally, a maximum concentration of about 3 ng/ml is obtained [6]. Activity is probably not related to serum levels of the drug but to the higher concentrations of it in the leucocytes.

Adverse Reactions

Frequent dose-related gastrointestinal symptoms are nausea, vomiting, diarrhea, and abdominal pain. These effects are seen both after oral and IV administration. After higher doses, hemorrhagic diarrhea caused by severe gastroenteritis, kidney impairment with hematuria and oliguria, shock, neuromuscular depression, and burning of skin and throat may occur. During chronic administration of the drug, agranulocytosis, aplastic anemia, megaloblastic anemia, and alopecia are rare side-effects.

Interactions

Not known.

References

1. Goldfinger, S. E. Drug therapy: Treatment of gout. *N. Engl. J. Med.* 285:1303–1306, 1971.
2. Kaplan, H. Further experience with colchicine in the treatment of sarcoid arthritis. *N. Engl. J. Med.* 268:761–764, 1963.
3. Walaszek, E. J., Kocsis, J. J., et al. Studies on the excretion of radioactive colchicine. *Arch. Int. Pharmacodyn. Ther.* 125:371–382, 1960.
4. Walaszek, E. J., LeRoy, G. V., et al. Renal excretion of radioactive colchicine in patients with and without neoplastic disease. *Fed. Proc.* 13:413–414, 1965.
5. Wallace, S. L., Omokoku, B., et al. Colchicine plasma levels. *Am. J. Med.* 48:443–448, 1965.
6. Wallace, S. L., and Norman, H. E. Plasma levels of colchicine after oral administration of a single dose. *Metabolism* 22:749–753, 1973.
7. Zemer, D., Revach, M., et al. A controlled trial in preventing attacks of familial Mediterranean fever. *N. Engl. J. Med.* 291:932–937, 1974.

COLISTIN
(Polymyxin E)

A basic bactericidal polypeptide closely related to polymyxin B. Impairs the integrity of the bacterial membrane. Active against most gram-negative microorganisms except *Proteus* and gram-negative cocci. Indicated in severe gram-negative infections; especially valuable in *Pseudomonas* and *Klebsiella* infections. Development of bacterial resistance is infrequent. Complete bacterial cross-resistance occurs between polymyxin B and E.

Absorption

Neither colistin nor any of its salts is absorbed from the gastrointestinal tract. t_{max}: 1–2 hours after IM administration [2].

Distribution

V_d: about 0.5 L/kg [2]. Protein binding: unknown. No distribution to CNS, even in inflammation.

Elimination

$t_{\frac{1}{2}}$: 1.5–3 hours. About 80% excreted unchanged by glomerular filtration [2]. $t_{\frac{1}{2}}$ in anuria: 2–3 days.

Dosage Schedule

For parenteral administration the water-soluble colistin sodium methanesulfonate, colistimethate sodium, is used. Colistin sulfate only is used intrathecally.

IM or IV dose is 2.5–5 mg/kg daily in 2–3 divided doses.

In *Pseudomonas* meningitis additional colistin sulfate can be given intrathecally, with a dose of 2–10 mg daily for 3 days and then every other day for 1–2 weeks. Do not use colistimethate sodium intrathecally.

Special Dosage Situations

Children: parenterally, same as adults; orally (colistin sulfate), 3–5 mg/kg daily in 3 divided doses for bacterial enterocolitis [4]. Renal failure and elderly: adjust dose intervals or dose according to the decrease in renal function, e.g., if the clearance is below 50 ml/min, the dosage interval should be 1–1.5 days; if the clearance is below 20 ml/min, the dosage interval should be about 3 days [1, 3, 6]. Also see Table 1, page 30.

Therapeutic Concentrations

1–5 μg/ml, depending on species and strain. Toxic concentration: 8–10 μg/ml.

Adverse Reactions

Paresthesiae, pruritus, rashes, dizziness, flushing, gastrointestinal pain, and diarrhea. Leucopenia is rare. Kidney impairment and respiratory paralysis. Most symptoms are reversible [5]. Colistin is removed by hemodialysis [1].

Interactions

Potentiates all neuromuscular blocking agents.

Review

Goodwin, N. J.   Colistin and sodium colistimethate. *Med. Clin. North Am.* 54:1267–1276, 1970.

References

1. Curtis, J. R., and Eastwood, J. B.   Colistin sulphomethate sodium administration in the presence of severe renal failure and during hemodialysis and peritoneal dialysis. *Br. Med. J.* 1:484–485, 1968.
2. Froman, J., Gross, L., et al.   Serum and urine levels following parenteral administration of sodium colistimethate to normal individuals. *J. Urol.* 103:210–214, 1970.
3. Goodwin, N. J., and Friedman, E. A.   The effects of renal impairment, peritoneal dialysis, and hemodialysis on serum sodium colistimethate levels. *Ann. Intern. Med.* 68:984–994, 1968.
4. Greengard, J., and Alisdea, A. F.   Treatment of acute diarrhea of infancy with oral colistin sulfate. *Antibiotics Annu.* 101–106, 1959–1960.
5. Koch-Weser, J., Sidel, V. W., et al.   Adverse effects of sodium colistimethate. *Ann. Intern. Med.* 72:857–868, 1970.
6. MacKay, D. N., and Kaye, D.   Serum concentration of colistin in patients with normal and impaired renal function. *N. Engl. J. Med.* 270:394–397, 1964.

CONTRACEPTIVES, ORAL

Combination of synthetic estrogen and progestogen or progestogen alone. Estrogens inhibit follicle-stimulating hormone (FSH) and midcycle luteinizing hormone (LH) secretion with suppression of ovulation. Progestogens alter properties of cervical mucus, making it less permeable to penetration by spermatozoa. Estrogens used are ethinyl estradiol (EE_2) and mestranol, while the most common progestogens used are norgestrel, norethisterone, and norethindrone, which are 19-nortestosterone derivatives. Estrogens used alone are unsatisfactory as contraceptives, but very small doses combined with progestogens are effective if judged by suppression of ovulation and FSH and LH secretion. Failure rate is about 1–3 pregnancies per 100 woman years.

Indicated in the prevention of pregnancy, for the regulation of the menstrual cycle in dysmenorrhea and menorrhagia, and in the treatment of endometriosis.

Absorption

Bioavailability: unknown. t_{max}: no data. An enterohepatic recirculation exists. Progestogens probably completely absorbed [6]. Absorption is apparently decreased during gastroenteritis, since pregnancy has been reported to follow ingestion of the "pill" during this illness [13].

Distribution

V_d: unknown. Protein binding: unknown. EE_2 is bound to uterine muscle. Estrogens and progestogens cross the placenta.

Elimination

Estrogens $t_{\frac{1}{2}}$: EE_2, 6–10 hours. EE_2 is extensively metabolized, 10–20% appearing in urine as EE_2 glucuronide [1]. Metabolites have not been completely identified but include 2-methoxy-EE_2, 16β-hydroxy-EE_2, 2-hydroxy-EE_2, 6α-hydroxy-EE_2, D-homestradiol-17$\alpha\beta$, 2-hydroxy-mestranol, estrone, estradiol-17β, estriol, and 2-methoxyestradiol-17β [24]. 50% is excreted in the bile, and a large enterohepatic recirculation appears to exist [3].

Progestogens $t_{\frac{1}{2}}$: norethisterone, 19 hours; norgestrel, 24 hours [8]. Metabolized by reduction to tetrahydrosteroids and by hydroxylation, with subsequent hepatic conjugation. 25% of norgestrel [7] and 25–28% of norethisterone [9] appear in urine as the reduced metabolites. 30% of norgestrel appears in urine as 16β-hydroxy-norgestrel [18]. 20–30% of norgestrel and 35–43% of norethisterone appear in feces.

Dosage Schedule

Formulations of the oral contraceptives contain varying amounts of estrogen and progestogen. 50 μg of EE_2 or of mestranol is adequate to suppress ovulation and is associated with a lower incidence of adverse reactions. The optimal dose of progestogen has not yet been established, but it appears to be about 0.35–1 mg norethindrone or 0.3–0.5 mg of norgestrel, either in combination with estrogen or alone. The combined pill may be obtained in either a continuous formulation, in which both estrogen and progestogen are taken for 21 days, or in a sequential form, in which progestogen is added for only the last 7 days of the menstrual cycle.

In the treatment of endometriosis, dosage may need to be higher in order to suppress menstruation altogether.

Special Dosage Situations

Contraindicated in patients with a history of deep venous thrombosis, pulmonary embolism, myocardial infarction, stroke, retinal venous or arterial thrombosis, cholestasis of pregnancy, hypertension, severe liver disease, undiagnosed abnormal vaginal bleeding, and hormone-dependent tumors. Use cautiously in patients with migraine, hyperlipemia, depression, and recurrent urinary tract infection.

All women who take oral contraceptives long-term should have their blood pressure checked and a Papanicolaou smear done at least yearly.

Therapeutic Concentrations

No available data.

Adverse Reactions

Venous Thromboembolism

Oral contraceptives increase ninefold or tenfold the incidence of deep venous thrombosis and vascular pulmonary embolism, especially in older women [20]. These disorders are associated with the estrogen; the mechanism is believed to be due in part to the elevation of plasma fibrinogen and Factors VII, IX, and X and the depression of plasma antithrombin III. Susceptibility may be predicted by obtaining a measurement of high molecular weight complexes of fibrinogen in the patient's blood [2]. Estrogens also cause increased venous distensibility [10]. Venous thromboembolism appears to occur more frequently in women of blood group A and less frequently in women of blood group O [12].

Myocardial Infarction

Occurs 2½ times more frequently in premenopausal women taking oral contraceptives [14, 15], but contraceptives are not a factor in this disorder after menopause [4, 16]. The pill appears to act synergistically with other risk factors in predisposing women who take the pill regularly to myocardial infarction.

Cerebrovascular Accident

Incidence of both strokes and transient ischemic attacks is increased in women taking oral contraceptives [20], with a greater incidence of thrombotic rather than hemorrhagic stroke [4]. This increase is very small numerically (1/10,000), although population studies show a relative risk of 9.5 in women taking the pill. The risk of stroke is also increased synergistically by hypertension and possibly by migraine [5].

Hypertension

Blood pressure is increased in women taking the pill, although the increase may not be very great and the blood pressure may still be within the normal range [22]. The increase in blood pressure is greater in older patients than in younger women. About 5% of those whose blood pressure increases become clinically hypertensive [17], and occasionally malignant hypertension occurs but subsides after suspension of the pill [11]. The mechanism for the increase in blood pressure is not known precisely, but it may be related to changes in the renin-angiotensin-aldosterone system or to salt and water retention.

Neoplasm

In the United States, there has been a sharp increase in the incidence of endometrial cancer since 1969 [19]. This increase can be correlated in part to the use of estrogens in menopausal and postmenopausal women, but endometrial cancer has also occurred in patients who have never taken these medications. In these patients, it has been suggested that the oral contraceptive used by women during their reproductive years may be a causative agent.

Angiomatous liver tumors occasionally occur in association with the use of oral contraceptives. The importance of these tumors is that they may rupture and hemorrhage into the peritoneum and that some are malignant.

There is no evidence of an increase in the incidence of breast malignancy with the use of oral contraceptives [21].

Miscellaneous

There has been an increased incidence of limb reduction defects in male infants of mothers who had taken oral contraceptives.

Cholestatic jaundice, gallbladder disease, hyperlipemia, acute pancreatitis, facial chloasma, urinary tract infection, and spider nevi are other possible side-effects. Amenorrhea may follow discontinuation of the pill. No evidence of an increase in the incidence of depression.

Migraine has been found to be exacerbated by some authors [23]. Carpal tunnel syndrome, chorea, optic neuritis, ocular palsies, and retinal artery and vein thrombosis have been reported in association with use of the pill in a few cases.

Alterations in Laboratory Tests

Elevation of blood glucose, triglycerides, thyroid-binding globulin and thyroxine (T_4), cortisol, iron, iron-binding capacity, coagulation factors, and renin substrate. Decrease in albumin, triiodothyronine (T_3) resin, 17-OH corticosteroids, 17-ketogenic steroids, and bromosulfthalein excretion.

Interactions

Metabolism of oral contraceptives is induced by rifampin. Pregnancy may ensue.

Reviews

Fotherby, K.: Metabolism of synthetic steroids by animals and man. *Acta Endocrinol.* [Suppl.](Kbh)185:119–147, 1974.

Heyman, A., and Hurtig, H. I.   Clinical complications of oral contraceptives. *Disease-A-Month*, August 1975. Pp. 3–34.

References

1. Abdel-Aziz, M. T., and Williams, K. I. H.   Metabolism of radioactive 17 α-ethinylestradiol by women. *Steroids* 18:695–710, 1970.
2. Alkjaersig, N., Fletcher, A., et al.   Association between oral contraceptive use and thromboembolism: A new approach to its investigation based on plasma fibrinogen chromatography. *Am. J. Obstet. Gynecol.* 122:199–209, 1975.
3. Cargill, D. I., Steinetz, B. G., et al.   Fate of ingested radiolabeled ethynylestradiol and its 3-cyclopentyl ether in patients with bile fistulas. *J. Clin. Endocrinol. Metab.* 29:1051–1061, 1960.
4. Collaborative Group for the Study of Stroke in Young Women.   Oral contraceptives and stroke in young women. *J.A.M.A.* 231:718–722, 1975.
5. Collaborative Group for the Study of Stroke in Young Women.   Oral contraception and increased risk of cerebral ischemia or thrombosis. *N. Engl. J. Med.* 288:871–878, 1973.
6. Fotherby, K.   Contraceptiver Steroide. In H. Kewitz (Ed.), *Nebenwirken.* Berlin: Westkreuz Verlag, 1971. P. 18.
7. Fotherby, K., Kamyab, S., et al.   Metabolism of synthetic progestational compounds in humans. *J. Reprod. Fertil.* 17(Suppl. 5):51–61, 1968.
8. Fotherby, K., and Keenan, C. A.   Metabolism of D-, L- and DL-norgestrel in man. *Acta Endocrinol.* [Suppl.] (Kbh) 138:83, 1969.
9. Gerhards, E., Hecker, W., et al.   Zum Stoffwechsel von Norethisteron (17α-äthinyl-4-östren-17β-ol-3-on) und DL-sowie D-norgestrel (18-methyl-17α-äthinyl-4-östren-17β-ol-3-on) beim Menschen. *Acta Endocrinol.* (Kbh.) 68:219–248, 1971.
10. Goodrich, S. M., and Wood, J. E.   Peripheral venous distensibility and velocity of venous flow during pregnancy or during oral contraceptive therapy. *Am. J. Obstet. Gynecol.* 90:740–744, 1964.
11. Harris, R. W. R.   Malignant hypertension associated with oral contraceptives. *Lancet* 2:466–467, 1960.
12. Jick, H., Westerholm, B., et al.   Venous thromboembolic disease and ABO blood type. *Lancet* 1:539–542, 1969.
13. John, A. H., and Jones, A. J.   Gastroenteritis causing failure of oral contraception. *Br. Med. J.* 3:207–208, 1975.
14. Mann, J. I., and Inman, W. H. W.   Oral contraceptives and death from myocardial infarction. *Br. Med. J.* 2:245–248, 1975.
15. Mann, J. I., Vessey, M. P., et al.   Myocardial infarction in young women with special reference to oral contraceptive practice. *Br. Med. J.* 2:241–245, 1975.
16. Rosenberg, L., Armstrong, B., et al.   Myocardial infarction and estrogen therapy in post-menopausal women. *N. Engl. J. Med.* 294:1256–1259, 1976.
17. Royal College of General Practitioners.   Oral Contraceptives and Health (an interim report). London: Pitman, 1974.
18. Sisenwine, S. F., Kimmel, H. B., et al.   Urinary metabolites

of DL-norgestrel in women. *Acta Endocrinol.* (Kbh.) 73:91–104, 1973.

19. Smith, D. C., Prentice, R., et al. Association of exogenous estrogens and endometrial carcinoma. *N. Engl. J. Med.* 293:1164–1167, 1975.

20. Vessey, M. P., and Doll, R. Investigation of relation between use of oral contraceptives and thromboembolic disease. A further report. *Br. Med. J.* 2:651–657, 1969.

21. Vessey, M. P., Doll, R., et al. Oral contraceptives and breast cancer. *Lancet* 1:941–944, 1975.

22. Weir, R. J., Riggs, E., et al. Blood pressure in women taking oral contraceptives. *Br. Med. J.* 1:533–535, 1974.

23. Whitty, C. W. M., Hockaday, J. M., et al. The effect of oral contraceptives on migraine. *Lancet* 1:856–859, 1966.

24. Williams, M. C., Helton, E. D., et al. The urinary metabolites of 17 α-ethynylestradiol-9,11ϵ-^{3}H in women. Chromatographic profiling and identification of ethinyl and non-ethinyl compounds. *Steroids* 25:229–246, 1975.

CORTISOL
(Hydrocortisone)

A natural hormone of adrenal cortex. Essential to most, if not all, body systems, especially carbohydrate, protein, and fat metabolism, and to a lesser extent, water and electrolyte balance. Antagonism or enhancement of catecholamines and other hormone systems may be involved. Therapeutic indications include suppression of adrenocorticotropic hormone (ACTH) activity in certain congenital adrenogenital syndromes, replacement of glucocorticoid activity in adrenal destruction or absence due to disease or surgery, palliative suppression of harmful inflammatory or immunological activity, and depression of lymphocyte activity in transplant surgery and reticuloendothelial tumors.

Absorption
Complete absorption by oral route. Variable absorption from skin and mucous membranes, depending on concentration, formulation, area, occlusion, and duration of application. Parenteral forms, including salts, esters, and cortisol analogues, are well absorbed from the site of injection.

Distribution
V_d: about 0.3 L/kg [3]. Protein binding: 95%. Bound to protein of the alpha$_1$ globulin class (transcortin), which is saturated at cortisol levels of 20 μg/ml [4]. Albumin binding is only 70–80%, permitting more unbound cortisol at higher concentrations in plasma.

Elimination
$t_{\frac{1}{2}}$: about 1½–2 hours [2]. Extensively metabolized by reduction, followed by glucuronide or sulfate conjugation. Parent hormone (1%) and metabolites excreted in urine [2].

Dosage Schedule

Adrenogenital Syndrome

Children with the usual 21-hydroxylase form of deficiency require cortisol, 0.6 mg/kg daily in 4 equally divided, evenly spaced doses.

Replacement Therapy

Acute addisonian crisis requires immediate intravenous cortisol in doses of 100–200 mg repeated every 6–8 hours as required. Treatment of aggravating factors and regulation of glucose, fluids, and electrolytes are essential. Chronic deficiency generally requires 37.5 mg cortisol daily for life of the patient. Cortisol is often given in a dose of 20–25 mg on waking and 10–12.5 mg 8–12 hours later to simulate physiological diurnal variation. Additional cortisol is required during critical periods, e.g., operations, accidents, and infections. Mineralocorticoids, e.g., fludrocortisone, are added when required.

Other disorders that respond to steroids are generally treated with prednisone or prednisolone, which have 5 times more antiinflammatory activity than cortisol. In life-threatening exacerbations of such disorders (e.g., severe asthma), intravenous cortisol in large doses, e.g., 0.5–2 g, may be used acutely and repeated at 2- to 4-hour intervals according to the patient's response. The goals of therapy are to produce a satisfactory clinical response with minimal corticosteroid dosage.

Topical hydrocortisone (0.5–1%) is used in a variety of bases for the treatment of a wide variety of noninfectious skin and ocular disorders.

Special Dosage Situations

In children, chronic steroid administration produces early closure of epiphyses, leading to stunted growth. For this reason, use small doses and schedule treatment for alternate days rather than daily if possible. Care is advised in treating patients with osteoporosis, personality disorders, or tuberculosis. Thyrotoxicosis shortens the half-life of cortisol, while cirrhosis and uremia prolong it [1, 2].

Therapeutic Concentrations

Physiological concentration ranges from 5–25 μg/dl, diurnal variation producing the highest plasma level in the morning and the lowest level around midnight. Response is generally more important than plasma level, except in Addison's disease when checking dosage adequacy and compliance is possible.

Adverse Reactions

Serious catabolic effects, suppression of the pituitary-adrenal axis, and iatrogenic Cushing's syndrome are the main problems that result from prolonged or excessive corticosteroid use. Injudicious use may lead to worsening of skin, ocular, or systemic infections. Tuberculosis and herpes ophthalmicus are especially important in this respect. Candidiasis may develop, especially in patients with immunosuppression and in those patients receiving antibiotics. Mood is generally improved, but some patients become pathologically euphoric or dysphoric. Gastrointestinal ulceration and perforation are disputed effects of steroids. Pseudotumor cerebri ("benign intracranial hypertension") and acute addisonian crisis may occur on rapid discontinuation of steroid therapy.

Interactions

Drugs with enzyme-inducing activity such as phenobarbital, phenytoin, and rifampin may increase cortisol metabolism to a variable and probably unimportant extent.

The increased production and urinary excretion of 6β-hydroxy-cortisol after the administration of some drugs and chemicals are recognized as signs of enzyme induction.

References

1. Bacon, G. E., and Kenny, F. M.   Prolonged serum half-life of cortisol in renal failure: *John Hopkins Med. J.* 132:127–131, 1973.
2. Peterson, R. E.   Metabolism of adrenocorticoids in man. *Ann. N.Y. Acad. Sci.* 82:846–853, 1959.
3. Peterson, R. E.   The miscible pool and turnover rate of adrenocortical steroids in man. *Recent Prog. Horm. Res.* 15:231–261, 1959.
4. Sandberg, A. A., and Slaunwhite, W. R.   Transcortin, a corticosteroid-binding plasma protein. *J. Clin. Invest.* 37:928, 1958.

CROMOLYN SODIUM
(Disodium Cromoglycate)

An agent used in the prophylaxis of asthma, allergic rhinitis, and vernal conjunctivitis. Probably acts by stabilizing the mast cell membrane, thus inhibiting the release of the pharmacological mediators of anaphylaxis such as histamine and slow-reacting substance of anaphylaxis (SRS-A) in response to an antibody challenge [4]. In asthma, cromolyn has been shown to inhibit both immediate and late antigen-induced bronchospasm. Indicated in the management of allergic, exercise-induced, and intrinsic asthma. The success rate may be higher in patients with allergy demonstrated by skin testing [2], intermittent attacks [6], and sputum eosinophilia than in patients who do not fulfill these criteria [1]. However, all patients who require regular treatment of asthma should probably be given a trial dosage of cromolyn for at least 4–6 weeks. Cromolyn frequently must be administered with other medications but may be used to decrease steroid dosage in asthma and antihistamine dosage in allergic rhinitis. In allergic rhinitis, it is most useful in seasonal rhinitis and of less value in perennial rhinitis and nasal polyps. Commercially available in combination with isoproterenol for those individuals who develop bronchial irritation with cromolyn alone. Under investigation in the oral treatment of ulcerative colitis.

Absorption

When inhaled, about 50–80% of the dose is deposited in the mouth and pharynx and subsequently swallowed. Intestinal absorption is poor [1%]. The portion of the dose that reaches the lung appears to be totally absorbed. t_{max}: 15–20 minutes [3].

Distribution

V_d: unknown. Protein binding: unknown. Probably no transfer to fetus.

Elimination

Plasma $t_{\frac{1}{2}}$: 4 minutes. $t_{\frac{1}{2}}$ in lung: 0.6–0.9 hours. Excreted unchanged in urine (50%) and bile (50%) [3].

Dosage Schedule

20–40 mg (1–2 capsules) 4 times daily by *Spinhaler** for both adults and children. Dose may be reduced to twice daily in maintenance therapy. In rhinitis, use either micronized powder of 1% or 2% solution, 10 mg every 4–6 hours.

Special Dosage Situations

Useful as prophylactic only. Of *no value* in aborting acute attack of asthma. No known contraindications.

Therapeutic Concentrations

Not relevant, since cromolyn appears to act locally on the bronchial mucosa.

Adverse Reactions

Bronchial irritation and bad aftertaste. Severe bronchoconstriction has been reported in a sensitive individual [5]. Rare effects include pulmonary eosinophilia, anaphylaxis, skin eruptions, urticaria, and angioneurotic edema [7].

Interactions

None known.

Reviews

Brogden, R. N., Speight, T. M., et al. Sodium cromoglycate (cromolyn sodium). I. A review of its mode of action, pharmacology, therapeutic efficacy, and use. *Drugs* 7:164–282, 1974.

Brogden, R. N., Speight, T. M., et al. Sodium cromoglycate (cromolyn sodium). II. Allergic rhinitis and other conditions. *Drugs* 7:283–296, 1974.

---

*Spinhaler is the brand name of a device manufactured in the United Kingdom by Fisons, Ltd.

References

1. Altounyan, R. E. C. Developments in the treatment of asthma with disodium cromoglycate (Lomudal). *Acta Allergol.* [Kbh.] 30 (Suppl. 12):65–86, 1975.
2. Brompton Hospital/Medical Research Council Collaborative Trial. Long-term study of disodium cromoglycate in treatment of severe extrinsic or intrinsic bronchial asthma in adults. *Br. Med. J.* 4:383–388, 1972.
3. Cox, J. S. G. Review of chemistry, pharmacology, toxicity, metabolism, specific side-effects, anti-allergic properties *in vitro* and *in vivo* of disodium cromoglycate. In J. Pepys and A. W. Frankland (Eds.), *Disodium Cromoglycate in Allergic Airways Disease.* London: Butterworth, 1970. Pp. 13–25.
4. Orr, T. S. C., Pollard, M. C., et al. Mode of action of disodium cromoglycate, studies on immediate type hypersensitivity reactions using "double sensitization" with two antigenically distinct rat reagins. *Clin. Exp. Immunol.* 7:745–757, 1970.
5. Paterson, I. C., Grant, I. W. B., et al. Severe bronchoconstriction provoked by sodium cromoglycate. *Br. Med. J.* 4:916, 1976.
6. Press, P. Remarques sur les indications thérapeutiques du cromoglycate de sodium. *Schweiz. Med. Wochenschr.* 101: 934–940, 1971.
7. Sheffer, A. L., Rocklin, R. E., et al. Immunologic components of hypersensitivity reactions to cromolyn sodium. *N. Engl. J. Med.* 293:1220–1224, 1975.

CYCLOPHOSPHAMIDE

Relatively stable, nonvesicant nitrogen mustard used alone and in many combinations in the treatment of a wide variety of malignant diseases. Inactive until metabolized by the liver; the drug acts at least in part by forming covalent linkages with various groups, e.g., phosphate and hydroxyl, that are associated with the cell nucleus and DNA, thus exerting most damage on cells that are dividing rapidly. Cellular and biochemical effects are therefore widespread, involving cell destruction, teratogenicity, carcinogenicity, and many derangements of cell nutrition. Best results have been demonstrated in solid lymphoreticular tumors, cancer of the breast, bronchus, and ovary, Wegener's granulomatosis, and in acute lymphoblastic leukemia of childhood. Also extensively studied in an immunosuppressive role with steroids in the control of the allergic disturbances associated with conditions such as organ transplants, systemic lupus erythematosus, rheumatoid arthritis, and minimal change nephrotic syndrome in children.

Absorption

Apparently complete but little available information.

Distribution

V_d: 0.4–0.6 L/kg [1, 6]. Protein binding of cyclophosphamide: 10–20%. Protein binding of alkylating metabolites: 50–60% [1].

Elimination

$t_{\frac{1}{2}}$: 4–8 hours [1, 5]. Cyclophosphamide is oxidized by the hepatic mixed-function oxidases to 4-hydroxycyclophosphamide and aldophosphamide, both of which are active. The latter is further oxidized by the nonmicrosomal enzyme aldehyde oxidase to carboxyphosphamide, which is inactive. The degradation products of aldophosphamide, phosphoramide mustard, and acrolein are also toxic [2]. Excreted mainly in urine, approximately 10% as cyclophosphamide and 16–40% as alkylating metabolites [1, 5]. The $t_{\frac{1}{2}}$ of the total metabolites appears to be shorter than that of cyclophosphamide [1].

Dosage Schedule

Treatment should be instituted only as part of an overall plan for cancer treatment or immunosuppression in an institution in which such procedures are common. Many regimens involve single, intermittent, or continuous dosage, usually orally or intravenously, but doses are occasionally instilled directly into the chest or abdomen. Chronic oral maintenance dosage is usually about 2 mg/kg daily.

Special Dosage Situations

The attempt to cure cancer or other life-threatening disorders such as systemic lupus erythematosus overrides all other concerns. Clearly detrimental to women during pregnancy; breast-feeding should be discontinued. In patients with gross renal failure the half-lives of cyclophosphamide and its metabolites are prolonged [6], and thus suitable adjustments must be made. Severe toxicity has been reported in uremia in association with high plasma levels [1].

Therapeutic Concentrations

Since cyclophosphamide is inactive, its plasma concentration is relevant only as a source of metabolites. No available data on therapeutic concentrations of alkylating metabolites. Effect of the drug is usually monitored by improvement in disease and symptoms or signs of dangerous adverse effects, e.g., dysuria, hematuria, and white cell count approaching 3000/cu mm.

Adverse Reactions

Alopecia is common and marked, but hair growth usually recovers between treatments. Nausea, vomiting, diarrhea, oral ulceration, and hepatotoxicity; depression of bone marrow; menstrual irregularities; male sterility because of impaired spermatogenesis; interstitial pulmonary fibrosis; hemorrhagic cystitis (even carcinoma of the bladder has been reported); inappropriate antidiuretic hormone secretion with large doses; and depression of immunity, with resulting opportunistic infections, especially by varicella and fungi.

Interactions

Attention has focused on possible induction and inhibition of the cytochromes P-450 system. Phenobarbital increases metabolism twofold or threefold but produces little effect on metabolite levels [4]. Prednisone acutely reduces metabolism but accelerates biotransformation after chronic use [3], apparently without major clinical effect. Allopurinol prolongs cyclophosphamide half-life [1]. Inducing or depressing metabolism appears to have little effect on the product of time and concentration of alkylating metabolites [1].

Review

Torkelson, A. R., LaBudde, J. A., et al. The metabolic fate of cyclophosphamide. *Drug Metab. Rev.* 3:131–165, 1974.

References

1. Bagley, C. M., Bostick, F. W., et al. Clinical pharmacology of cyclophosphamide. *Cancer Res.* 33:226–233, 1973.
2. Connors, T. A., Cox, P. J., et al. Some studies of the active intermediates formed in the microsomal metabolism of cyclophosphamide and isophosphamide. *Biochem. Pharmacol.* 23:115–129, 1974.
3. Faber, O. K., Mouridsen, H. T., et al. The biotransformation of cyclophosphamide in man: Influence of prednisone. *Acta Pharmacol. Toxicol.* 35:195–200, 1974.
4. Jao, J. Y., Jusko, W. J., et al. Phenobarbital effects on cyclophosphamide pharmacokinetics in man. *Cancer Res.* 32:2761–2764, 1972.
5. Mouridsen, H. T., Faber, O., et al. The metabolism of cyclophosphamide. *Cancer* 37:665–670, 1976.
6. Mouridsen, H. T., and Jacobsen, E. Pharmacokinetics of cyclophosphamide in renal failure. *Acta. Pharmacol. Toxicol.* 36:409–414, 1975.

DIAZEPAM

A benzodiazepine, used as an hypnotic and in the treatment of anxiety, alcoholic withdrawal, and status epilepticus. Has the advantage of a very wide therapeutic index.

Absorption

Oral bioavailability: about 75%. t_{max}: 1 hour after oral administration [6]; 1–2 hours after intramuscular injection. Plasma levels of the drug fluctuate considerably during the 10 hours following parenteral dosing, and an enterohepatic recirculation has been suggested [1]. However, recirculation is not clearly proven.

Distribution

V_d: 1.1 L/kg. Protein binding: 98% [6]. Diazepam and its metabolite, N-desmethyldiazepam, appear in the fetal circulation in plasma concentrations of about 40% of maternal plasma levels. However, in the first 2 hours after administration, fetal levels may be considerably higher than this figure [4].

1–4% of diazepam and 3–4% of the metabolite plasma concentrations [5] appear in CSF; this amount equals the unbound fraction in plasma.

Elimination

$t_{\frac{1}{2}}$ in adults: 1–3 days [6]. $t_{\frac{1}{2}}$ in children: 18 hours, but longer half-lives have been recorded in neonates [7]. Partially metabolized by demethylation to the active metabolite N-desmethyldiazepam and by hydroxylation to the active metabolites oxazepam and tenazepam. N-desmethyldiazepam is also metabolized to oxazepam in plasma. All these metabolites undergo glucuronidation and appear in the urine. The major metabolite in plasma is N-desmethyldiazepam, while in urine it is oxazepam [6, 8].

Dosage Schedule

Nighttime sedative: 2–5 mg, increased weekly until desired effect achieved. Status epilepticus: 0.1–0.35 mg/kg intravenously. Anxiety: 5–10 mg/day. Alcoholic withdrawal: adjust dose against degree of agitation and tremulousness and respiratory status.

Special Dosage Situations

For status epilepticus in children, dosage is the same as that for adults. For anxiety in children, 0.12–0.8 mg/kg/day. No teratogenicity is reported, but the fetus may require assisted ventilation if diazepam is given to the mother around the time of delivery. Diazepam and its metabolite, N-desmethyldiazepam, are transferred to breast milk and may produce somnolence in the baby [3].

Dosage should be reduced for elderly patients [6]; $t_{\frac{1}{2}}$ is related to age and is prolonged to 90 hours as age approaches 80 years. In cirrhosis, the $t_{\frac{1}{2}}$ is doubled and the V_d is increased to 1.5 L/kg, even in the absence of gross biochemical abnormalities. In acute hepatitis, the $t_{\frac{1}{2}}$ is increased to 2–4 days [6]. No dosage change required in renal failure.

Therapeutic Concentrations

Epileptic seizures are suppressed when the plasma level of diazepam exceeds 600 ng/ml [2].

Adverse Reactions

Psychological dependence. Apnea and hypotension, which are rare but serious, generally follow parenteral dose. Confusion, drowsiness, ataxia, menstrual irregularities, and, rarely, agranulocytosis.

Interactions

Additive effects with other sedatives and tranquilizers (including alcohol).

References

1. Baird, E. S., and Hailey, D. M.   Plasma levels of diazepam and its major metabolite following intramuscular administration. *Br. J. Anaesth.* 45:546–548, 1973.

2. Booker, H. E., and Celesia, G. G. Serum concentrations of diazepam in subjects with epilepsy. *Arch. Neurol.* 19:191–194, 1973.
3. Cole, A. P., and Hailey, D. M. Diazepam and active metabolite in breast milk and their transfer to the neonate. *Arch. Dis. Child.* 50:741–742, 1975.
4. Erkkola, R., Kanto, J., et al. Diazepam in early human pregnancy. *Acta Obstet. Gynecol. Scand.* 53:135–138, 1974.
5. Kanto, J., Kangas, L., et al. Cerebrospinal-fluid concentrations of diazepam and its metabolites in man. *Acta Pharmacol. Toxicol.* [Kbh]. 36:328–334, 1975.
6. Klotz, U., Avant, G. R., et al. The effects of age and liver disease on the disposition and elimination of diazepam in adult man. *J. Clin. Invest.* 55:347–359, 1975.
7. Morselli, P. L., Principi, N., et al. Diazepam elimination in premature and full-term infants and children. *J. Perinatal Med.* 1:133–141, 1973.
8. Schwartz, M. A., Koechlin, B. A., et al. Metabolism of diazepam in rat, dog, and man. *J. Pharmacol. Exp. Ther.* 149:423–435, 1965.

DIAZOXIDE

A nondiuretic thiazide, the major indications of which are hypertensive emergencies, refractory hypertension, and chronic hypoglycemia, especially hypoglycemia caused by insulinoma, glycogen storage disease, and infantile hypoglycemia. Diazoxide exerts its antihypertensive effect directly on vascular smooth muscle [6] and its hyperglycemic effect by direct inhibition of insulin release from the beta cell [2].

Absorption

Oral bioavailability: 100% [7]. t_{max}: no available data.

Distribution

V_d: 0.2 L/kg [9]. Protein binding in adults: 90– 95% [10]. Protein binding in children: 85–90% [10]. Binding decreased in renal failure [5]. Crosses placenta [4].

Elimination

$t_{\frac{1}{2}}$ in adults: 20–40 hours [10]. $t_{\frac{1}{2}}$ in children: 10–24 hours [10]. 55–60% metabolized by sulfate conjugation of alcohol metabolite and production of carboxylic acid metabolite.

Metabolites are not active pharmacologically and have approximately the same $t_{\frac{1}{2}}$ as the parent drug. Elimination is by glomerular filtration. There appears to be significant tubular reabsorption of the parent drug [1].

Dosage Schedule

Intravenous: 150–300 mg by rapid injection (less than 30 seconds); repeat as needed. Peak effect occurs 2–5 minutes after injection. Because of the high protein binding of the drug [11], it has been suggested that the full dosage of the drug should be used at one administration to achieve an effect, but this topic is controversial. The patient should be recumbent during intravenous administration.

Oral, in hypertension: 200–1000 mg/day in 2 or 3 divided doses. Oral, in hypoglycemia: 150–450 mg/day in 2 or 3 divided doses.

Not used intramuscularly.

Special Dosage Situations

Because of the high incidence of hyperglycemia in the dosage used for hypertension, this drug should be used only in severe disease that has proved refractory to more conventional medication. Avoid chronic use in young patients with hypertension, diabetics, and in patients with chronic renal failure in whom nonketotic hyperglycemic coma may occur [3]. Safe for use in preeclampsia. Recommended dose for hypoglycemia and hypertension in children is 5 mg/kg/day.

Therapeutic Concentrations

No available data.

Adverse Reactions

Glucose intolerance, edema, hypertrichosis, and hyperuricemia are main side-effects. Hypotension is accompanied by tachycardia.

Interactions

Displaces warfarin from albumin-binding sites [10]. Antagonizes the action of sulfonylureas and increases the hyperglycemic effect of thiazide diuretics. Decreases plasma levels of phenytoin in man, possibly because of increased metabolism [8]. Sulfonylureas may be useful in antagonizing hyperglycemic effect of diazoxide.

References

1. Dayton, P. G., Pruitt, A. W., et al.   Metabolism and disposition of diazoxide. A mini-review. *Drug Metab. Dispos.* 3:226–229, 1975.
2. Fajans, S. S., Floyd, J. C., Jr., et al.   Further studies on diazoxide suppression of insulin release from abnormal and normal islet tissue in man. *Ann. N.Y. Acad. Sci.* 150:261–279, 1968.
3. Lancaster-Smith, M., Leigh, N. I., et al.   Death following non-ketotic hyperglycemic coma during diazoxide therapy and peritoneal dialysis. *Postgrad. Med. J.* 50:175–177, 1974.
4. Milner, R. D. G., and Chouksey, S. L.   Effects of fetal exposure to diazoxide in man. *Arch. Dis. Child.* 47:537–543, 1972.
5. Pearson, R. M., and Breckenridge, A. M.   Renal function, protein binding, and pharmacological response to diazoxide. *Br. J. Clin. Pharmacol.* 3:169–175, 1976.
6. Powell, W. J., Green, R. M., et al.   Action of diazoxide on skeletal muscle vascular resistance. *Circ. Res.* 28:167–178, 1971.
7. Pruitt, A. W., Dayton, P. G., et al.   Disposition of diazoxide in children. *Clin. Pharmacol. Ther.* 14:73–82, 1972.

8. Roe, T., Podosin, R., et al. Effect of diazoxide on diphenylhydantoin metabolism. *Clin. Res.* 23:143A, 1975.
9. Sadee, W. E., Segal, J., et al. Diazoxide urine and plasma levels in humans by stable-isotope dilution-mass fragmentography. *J. Pharmacokinet. Biopharm.* 1:295–305, 1973.
10. Sellers, E. M., and Koch-Weser, J. Influence of intravenous injection rate on protein binding and vascular activity of diazoxide. *Ann. N.Y. Acad. Sci.* 226:319–332, 1973.
11. Sellers, E. M., and Koch-Weser, J. Protein binding and vascular activity of diazoxide. *N. Engl. J. Med.* 281:1141–1145, 1969.

DIETHYLCARBAMAZINE

An antihelminthic agent derived from piperazine; effective against *Wuchereria bancrofti, Brugia malayi, Loa loa, Ascaris lumbricoides,* and *Onchocerca volvulus.* Indicated in the management of filariasis, loiasis, tropical pulmonary eosinophilia, onchocerciasis, and *Ascaris* infestations. Has also been used in filariasis eradication programs [4]. May be used as a provocative test in onchocerciasis and filariasis, in which diseases it may replace night blood collections [6].

Its mechanism of action is not clear, but it is known to be rapidly active in vivo and inactive in vitro. For this reason, it has been postulated that the drug enhances host defense mechanisms [3]. Administration of the drug is accompanied within 30–45 minutes by the appearance of microfilariae in peripheral blood, urine, and sputum [2]. However, it is known to affect only the microfilariae, leaving the parent worms intact.

Despite the drug's widespread use for 30 years, very little is known about its pharmacological properties.

Absorption
Oral bioavailability: unknown. Approximately 20% appears in urine after an oral dose. t_{max}: 3 hours [5]. No available data about first-pass metabolism or biliary excretion.

Distribution
No available data.

Elimination
$t_{\frac{1}{2}}$: about 12 hours [5]. No available information about metabolism.

Dosage Schedule
Filariasis, onchocerciasis, and loiasis: 2 mg/kg t.i.d. for 3–4 weeks. Filariasis prophylaxis: 2 mg/kg t.i.d. for 3–5 days. Tropical eosinophilia and *Ascaris* infestation: 5 mg/kg t.i.d. for 7 days. Resistant *Ascaris:* 6–10 mg/kg t.i.d. for 10 days; repeat if necessary.

In onchocerciasis involving the eye, a 3% topical solution is available that temporarily clears microfilariae from the cornea and anterior chamber [1].

Special Dosage Situations

Use carefully in debilitated patients and in patients with severe filarial and onchocercal infections. No available data about its use in patients with hepatic or renal failure and in the elderly. Adult dosage may be given to children.

Therapeutic Concentrations

No available information.

Adverse Reactions

Hypersensitivity reactions, probably due to destruction of micro-filariae. In onchocerciasis, this reaction may be manifested as pruritus, edema of the skin, and conjunctiva and urticaria (Mazzotti reaction). Anterior uveitis may also occur with the use of eyedrops [1]. Pulmonary edema and cardiovascular collapse may occur rarely but only in those patients with heavy infestations. Other general side-effects include general malaise and gastrointestinal disturbances. In filariasis, nodular swellings and leukocytosis may occur [7].

Interactions

No available information.

References

1. Anderson, J., and Fuglsang, H.   Topical diethylcarbamazine in ocular onchocerciasis. *Trans. R. Soc. Trop. Med. Hyg.* 67:710–717, 1973.
2. Fazen, L. E., Anderson R. I., et al.   Clinical and laboratory changes consequent to diethylcarbamazine in patients with onchocerciasis. *Am. J. Trop. Med. Hyg.* 25:250–256, 1976.
3. Gibson, D. W., Connor, D. H., et al.   Onchocercal dermatitis: Ultrastructural studies of microfilariae and host tissues, before and after treatment with diethylcarbamazine (Hetrazan). *Am. J. Trop. Med. Hyg.* 25:74–87, 1976.
4. Kessel, J. F., Siliga, N., et al.   Periodic mass treatment with diethylcarbamazine for the control of filariasis in American Samoa. *Bull. WHO* 43:817–825, 1970.
5. Lubran, M.   Determination of Hetrazan in biological fluids. *Br. J. Pharmacol.* 5:210–216, 1950.
6. Rajapakse, Y. S.   Diethylcarbamazine provocation of the microfilariae of Wuchereria bancrofti. *J. Trop. Med. Hyg.* 77: 182–184, 1974.
7. Santiago-Stevenson, D., Oliver-Gonzalez, J., et al.   Treatment of filariasis bancrofti with 1-diethylcarbamyl-4-methylpiperazine hydrochloride ("Hetrazan"). *J.A.M.A.* 135:708–712, 1947.

DIETHYLSTILBESTROL (DES)

A synthetic estrogen that is active when administered orally, unlike equine estrogens. Used in the suppression of lactation, the control of menopausal symptoms, and as a postcoital contraceptive ("morning-after pill"). Occasionally used in the management of acne vulgaris. Widely used in the treatment of disseminated breast carcinoma in postmenopausal and castrated subjects for whom curative surgery and radiotherapy are not feasible (remission rate 30–40%). Also used in the management of inoperable carcinoma of the prostate. The mechanism of action for its role in the therapy of cancer remains speculative.

Absorption
No available data.

Distribution
V_d: unknown. Protein binding: unknown. Crosses placenta (see Adverse Reactions).

Elimination
Less than 5% recovered in urine [7, 11]. No other available studies of its elimination in humans. In rats, entire elimination is via bile, and there is significant enterohepatic recirculation [4]. This recirculation is presumed to occur also in humans.

Dosage Schedule
Suppression of lactation: 5 mg t.i.d. for 3 days, beginning within 12 hours of delivery; then reduce to 10 mg for 1 day and 5 mg for 2 days. May be repeated if breast engorgement occurs. (Bromocriptine may soon supersede DES for this condition.)

Suppression of menopausal symptoms: 0.2–0.5 mg/day long-term. May be given continuously or on a schedule of 6 days out of 7 or 25 days out of 30. The latter regimen appears to be most physiological.

Carcinoma of the breast: 10–25 mg/day, but this dosage may be varied to suit the individual, depending on occurrence of side-effects and patient's response. Continue until remission occurs.

Carcinoma of the prostate: 1–3 mg/day long-term.

Morning-after pill: 25 mg b.i.d. for 5 days, beginning within 72 hours of coitus. Failure rate is less than 1/1000, but failure may have serious consequences (see Adverse Reactions).

Special Dosage Situations
Absolutely contraindicated in pregnant women. Use cautiously in patients with atheromatous disease.

Therapeutic Concentrations
No available data. In carcinoma of the prostate, adequacy of therapy may be checked by estimation of the serum testosterone level [8, 9], which should be lowered into the female range (10–50 ng/dl), or the serum acid phosphatase level.

Adverse Reactions
Increased incidence of cardiovascular deaths from congestive heart failure, myocardial infarction, arteriosclerotic heart disease,

pulmonary embolism, and cerebrovascular accident. This enhanced atherogenesis is generally not evident at doses of less than 1 mg/day [2].

Carcinogenesis manifested by vaginal adenomatosis is common in young women whose mothers were exposed to DES during the first 18 weeks of pregnancy (DES was previously used to prevent threatened abortion). Administration of DES may lead to adenocarcinoma or squamous metaplasia of the vagina [1, 3, 5, 6]. There is an increased incidence of endometrial carcinoma in postmenopausal women who are taking estrogens [10].

Alterations in laboratory measurements, i.e., suppression of pituitary, adrenal, and ovarian function tests. Elevation of Bromsulphalein (BSP) retention, serum calcium, triglycerides, thyroxine (T_4) and protein-bound iodine (PBI), thyroid-binding globulin (free thyroxine index unchanged), gamma globulins, growth hormone, clotting Factors I and VIII, and serum glutamic-oxaloacetic transaminase (SGOT) levels. Decrease in serum cholesterol, glucose, and triiodothyronine (T_3) resin values.

Interactions

None known.

Review

Notter, K. L., and Fish, C. R.   Diethylstilbestrol usage: Its interesting past, important present, and questionable future. *Med. Clin. North Am.* 58:793–810, 1974.

References

1. Bibbo, M., Maysoon, A. M., et al.   Follow-up study of male and female offspring of DES-treated mothers. *J. Reprod. Med.* 15:29–32, 1975.
2. Byar, D. P.   The Veterans Administration cooperative urological research group's studies of cancer of the prostate. *Cancer* 32:1126–1130, 1973.
3. Fetherston, W. C.   Squamous neoplasia of vagina related to DES syndrome. *Am. J. Obstet. Gynecol.* 122:176–181, 1975.
4. Hanahau, D. J., and Daskalakis, E. G.   The metabolic pattern of C^{14}-diethylstilbestrol. *Endocrinology* 53:163–170, 1953.
5. Herbst, A. L., Ulfelder, H., et al.   Adenocarcinoma of the vagina. Association of maternal stilbestrol therapy with tumor appearance in young women. *N. Engl. J. Med.* 284:878–881, 1971.
6. Herbst, A. L., Poskanzer, D. C., et al.   Prenatal exposure to stilbestrol. A prospective comparison of exposed female offspring with unexposed controls. *N. Engl. J. Med.* 292:334–339, 1975.
7. Jellinck, P. H.   The excretion of synthetic oestrogens. *Biochem. J.* 58:262–265, 1954.
8. Robinson, M. R. G., and Thomas, B. S.   Effect of hormonal therapy on plasma testosterone levels in prostatic carcinoma. *Br. Med. J.* 4:391–394, 1971.
9. Shearer, R. J., and Hendry, W. F.   Plasma testosterone: An

accurate monitor of hormone treatment in prostatic cancer. *Br. J. Urol.* 45:668–677, 1973.

10. Smith, D. C., and Prentice, R. Association of exogenous estrogen and endometrial carcinoma. *N. Engl. J. Med.* 293:1164–1170, 1975.

11. Tompsett, S. L. Note on the detection of hexoestrol, stilbestrol, dienestrol, and the *p*-hydroxy metabolites of phenobarbitone and phenytoin in urine. *J. Pharm. Pharmacol.* 16: 207–208, 1964.

DIGITOXIN

A cardiac glycoside derived from foxglove; molecule consists of the pharmacologically active aglycone digitoxigenin and three molecules of the sugar digitoxose. Differs structurally from digoxin by absence of hydroxyl group at 12 position on aglycone, which accounts for the lesser polarity of digitoxin and its decreased propensity for bioavailability problems. Primary actions include increase in force of myocardial contraction, increased electrical excitability of the heart, and decreased atrioventricular (A-V) conduction. Shortens atrial refractory period (except when vagus blocked with atropine), increases A-V and ventricular refractory periods, and increases automaticity at ventricular ectopic pacemaker sites. Primary uses are the treatment of heart failure and the control of ventricular rate in patients with atrial fibrillation and atrial flutter.

Absorption

Oral absorption: 90–100%. Oral t_{max}: 1–3 hours [2]. Onset of action: 0.5–2 hours [2]. Peak effect: 4–6 hours [2].

Distribution

V_d: about 0.5 L/kg [8]. Protein binding: 95–97%. Cardiac levels: approximately 7 times plasma levels. Fetal plasma levels: equal to maternal levels.

Elimination

$t_{\frac{1}{2}}$: 4–6 days [2]. Extensive hepatic metabolism to predominantly inactive metabolites. 75% is excreted in urine and 25% in stools: 8% is converted to digoxin [3], which is increased in renal failure. There is enterohepatic recirculation of digitoxin [1].

Dosage Schedule

Loading dose: 0.25–1.0 mg, approximately 10 μg/kg [2]. Maintenance dose: 0.05–0.2 mg/day, approximately 1.5 μg/kg/day; give once daily. IM route is not recommended, because it is painful and absorption is erratic.

Special Dosage Situations

Loading dose is 0.045 mg/kg for children over 4 weeks and 0.022 mg/kg for infants under 4 weeks; maintenance dose is one-tenth of loading dose. No special precautions are indicated in women during pregnancy or lactation, in the elderly, or in patients with renal [9] or hepatic failure.

Therapeutic Concentrations

15–25 ng/ml [4].

Adverse Reactions

Low margin of safety. Hypokalemia often aggravates toxicity. Anorexia, nausea, and vomiting; extrasystoles, bigeminy, A-V block, sinus arrhythmia, paroxysmal atrial tachycardia, ventricular tachycardia, atrial fibrillation, and ventricular fibrillation; and headache, fatigue, malaise, drowsiness, confusion, and blurred vision. In children, toxicity is manifested by depression of the sinus node and rarely by ectopic beats. Stop digitoxin for appropriate number of half-lives if toxic. Add potassium if necessary. Phenytoin, lidocaine, or propranolol is useful if ventricular arrhythmia is present.

Interactions

Phenobarbital [5] and possibly phenylbutazone [6] and phenytoin [6] can cause reduction in plasma levels by inducing metabolism, but the exact effect is not known. Unbound fraction is increased twofold or threefold during hemodialysis, probably because of concomitant heparin administration [7]. Cholestyramine reduces half-life of digitoxin by about 50% [1].

References

1. Caldwell, J. H., Bush, C. A., et al.   Interruption of the enterohepatic circulation of digitoxin by cholestyramine. *J. Clin. Invest.* 50:2638–2644, 1971.
2. Lukas, D. S.   Some aspects of the distribution and disposition of digitoxin in man. *Ann. N.Y. Acad. Sci.* 179:338–361, 1971.
3. Marcus, F. I.   Digitalis pharmacokinetics and metabolism. *Am. J. Med.* 58:452–459, 1975.
4. Smith, T. W., and Haber, E.   The clinical value of serum digitalis glycoside concentrations in the evaluation of drug toxicity. *Ann. N.Y. Acad. Sci.* 179:322–337, 1971.
5. Solomon, H. M., and Abrams, W. B.   Interactions between digitoxin and other drugs in man. *Am. Heart J.* 83:277–280, 1972.
6. Solomon, H. M., Reich, S., et al.   Interactions between digitoxin and other drugs *in vitro* and *in vivo*. *Ann. N.Y. Acad. Sci.* 179:362–369, 1971.
7. Storstein, L., and Janssen, H.   Studies on digitalis. VI. The effect of heparin on serum protein binding of digitoxin and digoxin. *Clin. Pharmacol. Ther.* 20:15–23, 1976.
8. Vöhringer, H. F., and Rietbrock, N.   Metabolism and excretion of digitoxin in man. *Clin. Pharmacol. Ther.* 16:796–806, 1974.
9. Vöhringer, H. F., Rietbrock, N., et al.   Disposition of digitoxin in renal failure. *Clin. Pharmacol. Ther.* 19:387–395, 1976.

DIGOXIN

A cardiac glycoside derived from foxglove; molecule consists of the pharmacologically active aglycone digoxigenin and three molecules of the sugar digitoxose. Primary actions include increase in force of myocardial contraction, increased electrical excitability of the heart, and decreased atrioventricular (A-V) conduction. Shortens atrial refractory period (except when vagus blocked with atropine), increases A-V and ventricular refractory periods, and increases automaticity at ventricular ectopic pacemaker sites. Primary uses are the treatment of heart failure and the control of ventricular rate in patients with atrial fibrillation and atrial flutter.

Absorption

Bioavailability problems exist, depending on preparation [15]. Availability of tablets: 50–93%; mean 65% [11]. Availability of elixir: 70–100%; mean 80% [11]. t_{max} of tablets: 0.75–2 hours [15]. t_{max} of elixir: 0.5–1 hour [11]. Onset of action of IV preparation: 15–30 minutes [6]. IM route is not recommended because absorption is no faster than the oral route and it may be erratic. The injection is often painful.

Distribution

V_d: 6–10 L/kg [13]; greater in infants [7]. Protein binding: about 25% [8]. Cardiac levels of digoxin are about 70 times that of plasma levels in adults [3] and 140 times that of plasma levels in infants [7]. Fetal plasma levels equal maternal plasma levels [19].

Elimination

$t_{\frac{1}{2}}$: 33–51 hours [17]. Excreted by glomerular filtration and some by tubular secretion; 25% eliminated by nonrenal mechanism [13]. $t_{\frac{1}{2}}$ in anuria: 2.5–6 days [4]. About 30% undergoes enterohepatic recirculation in 24 hours [2].

Dosage Schedule

Loading dose: 10–15 μg/kg in 2 or 3 divided doses in 24 hours. Maintenance dose: 3–5 μg/kg/day (for tablets of good availability).

Special Dosage Situations

In children adjust dosage according to the following guidelines [21]:

	Oral Maintenance (μg/kg/day)
Premature or newborn	10–12.5
1 month–1 year	20–25
1 year–2 years	16–20
2–12 years	10–15

In patients with renal failure, adjust dose according to creatinine clearance. If creatinine clearance is 50–100 ml/min, give 75% of estimated dose. If creatinine clearance is 25–50 ml/min, give 60%

of estimated dose. If creatinine clearance is less than 25 ml/min, give 30% of estimated dose [17] (see also Table 1, p. 30). Reduce dose in elderly according to renal function. No special precautions necessary in women during pregnancy or lactation or in patients with hepatic failure [18]. Thyrotoxic patients may need larger doses because of increased elimination; myxedematous patients may need smaller doses because of decreased elimination [5]. Mucosal disease that is associated with intestinal malabsorption may lead to decreased absorption [10]. Reduce estimated dose in obese individuals because of lower lean body mass relative to total weight. Contraindicated in heart failure caused by constrictive pericarditis (when tachycardia is compensatory) and subaortic hypertrophic cardiomyopathy (idiopathic hypertrophic subaortic stenosis, IHSS).

Therapeutic Concentrations

0.8–2 ng/ml [1]; may be higher in infants [7].

Adverse Reactions

Low margin of safety. Hypokalemia and possibly hypomagnesemia [20] often aggravate toxicity. Anorexia, nausea, and vomiting; extrasystoles, bigeminy, A-V block, sinus arrhythmia, paroxysmal atrial tachycardia, ventricular tachycardia, atrial fibrillation, and ventricular fibrillation; and headache, fatigue, malaise, drowsiness, confusion, and blurred vision. In children, toxicity is manifested by depression of the sinus node and rarely by ectopic beats. Stop digoxin for appropriate number of half-lives if the drug has toxic effects. Add potassium if necessary. Phenytoin, lidocaine, or propranolol is useful if ventricular arrhythmia is present. Charcoal may be used to absorb drug in gastrointestinal tract in patients with overdosage [9].

Interactions

Cholestyramine, neomycin [14], sulfasalazine [12], metoclopramide [16], magnesium trisilicate (and other antacids to a lesser extent), kaolin, and pectin (Kaopectate) may reduce absorption; these drugs should be administered at least 6 hours before or after administration of digoxin. Propantheline may increase absorption [16].

References

1. Butler, V. P., and Lindenbaum, J.   Serum digitalis measurements in the assessment of digitalis resistance and sensitivity. *Am. J. Med.* 58:460–469, 1975.

2. Caldwell, J. H., and Cline, C. T.   Biliary excretion of digoxin in man. *Clin. Pharmacol. Ther.* 19:410–415, 1976.

3. Coltart, H., Howard, M., et al.   Myocardial and skeletal muscle concentrations of digoxin in patients on long-term therapy. *Br. Med. J.* 2:318–319, 1972.

4. Doherty, J. E., Flanigan, W. J., et al.   Studies with tritiated digoxin in anephric human subjects. *Circulation* 35:298–303, 1967.

5. Doherty, J. E., and Perkins, W. H.   Digoxin metabolism in

hypo- and hyperthyroidism: Studies with tritiated digoxin in thyroid disease. *Ann. Intern. Med.* 64:489–507, 1966.

6. Forester, W., Lewis, R. P., et al. The onset and magnitude of the contractile response to commonly used digitalis glycosides in normal subjects. *Circulation* 49:517–521, 1974.

7. Gorodischer, R., Jusko, W. J., et al. Tissue and erythrocyte distribution of digoxin in infants. *Clin. Pharmacol. Ther.* 19:256–263, 1976.

8. Gorodischer, R., Krasner, J., et al. Serum protein binding of digoxin in newborn infants. *Res. Commun. Chem. Pathol. Pharmacol.* 9:387–390, 1974.

9. Härtel, G., Manninen, V., et al. Treatment of digoxin intoxication. *Lancet* 2:158, 1973.

10. Heizer, W. D., Smith, J. W., et al. Absorption of digoxin in patients with malabsorption syndromes. *N. Engl. J. Med.* 285:257–259, 1971.

11. Huffman, D. H., Manion, C. V., et al. Absorption of digoxin from different oral preparations in normal subjects during steady state. *Clin. Pharmacol. Ther.* 16:310–317, 1974.

12. Juhl, R. P., Summers, R. W., et al. Effect of sulfasalazine on digoxin bioavailability. *Clin. Pharmacol. Ther.* 20:387–394, 1976.

13. Koup, J. R., Greenblatt, D. J., et al. Pharmacokinetics of digoxin in normal subjects after intravenous bolus and infusion doses. *J. Pharmacokin. Biopharm.* 3:181–192, 1975.

14. Lindenbaum, J., Maulitz, R. M., et al. Impairment of digoxin absorption by neomycin. *Clin. Res.* 20:410, 1972.

15. Lindenbaum, J., Mellow, M. H., et al. Variation in biologic availability of digoxin from four preparations. *N. Engl. J. Med.* 285:1344–1347, 1971.

16. Manninen, V., Melin, J., et al. Altered absorption of digoxin in patients given propantheline and metoclopramide. *Lancet* 1:398–400, 1973.

17. Marcus, F. I. Digitalis pharmacokinetics and metabolism. *Am. J. Med.* 58:452–459, 1975.

18. Marcus, F. I., and Kapadia, G. G. The metabolism of tritiated digoxin in cirrhotic patients. *Gastroenterology* 47:517–524, 1964.

19. Rogers, M. C., Willerson, J. T., et al. Serum digoxin concentrations in the human fetus, neonate, and infant. *N. Engl. J. Med.* 287:1010–1013, 1972.

20. Seller, R. H., Cangiano, J., et al. Digitalis toxicity and hypomagnesemia. *Am. Heart J.* 79:57–68, 1970.

21. Soyka, L. F. Clinical pharmacology of digoxin. *Pediatr. Clin. North Am.* 19:241–256, 1972.

DIPHENHYDRAMINE

A competitive histamine H_1 antagonist that possesses anticholinergic, antitussive, antiemetic, and sedative properties. Indicated for symptomatic relief in a variety of allergic conditions, including hay fever, allergic rhinitis, urticaria, angioedema, and atopic and contact dermatitis. Also used in the management of motion sickness, nausea and vomiting, parkinsonism, and acute drug-induced extrapyramidal syndromes. Does not antagonize histamine-induced gastric acid secretion (H_2 effect).

Absorption

Systemic bioavailability of oral dose: about 50% [1]. t_{max}: 2–4 hours [1, 3].

Distribution

V_d: 3–4 L/kg. Protein binding: 98–99% [1]. Blood-plasma ratio: 0.82 [1].

Elimination

$t_{\frac{1}{2}}$: 4–10 hours [3]. Less than 4% of dose excreted unchanged in urine [1]. The remainder is excreted in urine as a primary and secondary amine (the result of N-desmethylation) and diphenyl-methoxyacetic acid, a carboxylic acid that is partly free and partly conjugated [2, 3].

Dosage Schedule

25–50 mg orally as required. May be repeated at 6- to 8-hour intervals. 10–50 mg parenterally by IV or IM route, as required.

Special Dosage Situations

No specific information about use in the elderly and in patients with renal or hepatic disease. No evidence of adverse effects when used in women during pregnancy or lactation, but the drug should be used cautiously in these situations. Avoid use, if possible, in patients with glaucoma and prostatism.

Therapeutic Concentrations

Monitor patient's clinical response and attempt to avoid adverse effects.

Adverse Reactions

Side-effects are mainly related to anticholinergic and sedative properties: dryness of mouth, nose, and throat, nasal stuffiness, blurring of vision, urinary retention, and constipation; and drowsiness, restlessness, confusion, convulsions, and coma. Sleepiness is associated with plasma concentration above 70 ng/ml [1].

In serious overdose, treatment with a cholinesterase inhibitor with central activity (physostigmine) may be necessary, in addition to the usual supportive measures.

Interactions

Avoid concurrent use of other drugs with anticholinergic, sympathomimetic, or sedative effects. Further deterioration of motor activity and increased sedation occur with alcohol [4]. Monoamine oxidase inhibitors (MAOI) should be discontinued for at least 48 hours. A precipitate forms when diphenhydramine is mixed in vitro with the radiopaque dye meglumine iodipamide (Cholografin) [5]. Allergic reactions to this agent during IV cholangiography should be treated by injection of the antihistamine at a separate site.

References

1. Albert, K. S., Hallmark, M. R., et al. Pharmacokinetics of diphenhydramine in man. *J. Pharmacokinet. Biopharm.* 3:159–170, 1975.
2. Chang, T., Okerholm, R. A., et al. Identification of diphenhydramine (Benadryl®) metabolites in human subjects. *Res. Commun. Chem. Path. Pharmacol.* 9:391–404, 1974.
3. Glazko, A. J., Dill, W. A., et al. Metabolic disposition of diphenhydramine. *Clin. Pharmacol. Ther.* 16:1066–1076, 1974.
4. Linnoila, M. Effects of antihistamines, chlormezanone, and alcohol on psychomotor skills related to driving. *Eur. J. Clin. Pharmacol.* 5:247–254, 1973.
5. Stevens, J. S. Incompatibility of diphenhydramine hydrochloride (Benadryl®) with meglumine iodipamide (Cholografin®). *Radiology* 117:224–225, 1975.

DOPAMINE

A naturally occurring catecholamine that acts as a CNS transmitter. Known to be depleted in Parkinson's disease [10]. Increases cardiac output and decreases peripheral resistance without altering heart rate or blood pressure [5]. Has a specific action on the renal artery, causing vasodilation that is not blocked by alpha- and beta-adrenergic blocking agents, thus suggesting a specific receptor [1]. IV infusion produces an increase in renal plasma flow, inulin clearance, and sodium excretion [8]. Because of these properties, dopamine is indicated in the management of congestive heart failure [8] and shock of any etiology [4, 6, 9], especially if shock is associated with prerenal failure. Probably also useful as a renal vasodilator in the management of malignant hypertension that is associated with progressive renal failure, hepatorenal syndrome, or drug overdose when the drug is cleared by the kidney.

Absorption

Given only by IV route.

Distribution

V_d: probably very large but no exact data available. Protein binding: unknown.

Elimination

$t_{\frac{1}{2}}$: 1–2 minutes. 75% metabolized by monoamine oxidase to 3-methoxytyramine, 3-methoxy-4-hydroxyphenylacetic acid, 3,4-dihydroxyphenylacetic acid, 3-methoxy-4-hydroxyphenylethanol, and 3,4-dihydroxyphenylethanol, as well as their respective conjugates, all of which are inactive. 25% metabolized to norepinephrine (noradrenaline) [2].

Dosage Schedule

Generally, 1–10 μg/kg/hr is given by IV infusion, although doses up to 50 μg/kg/hr have been used. Never dilute in an alkaline solution, such as sodium bicarbonate, for example, because the drug tends to deteriorate in this kind of solution [3]. For shock with severe vasoconstriction, dopamine may be successfully combined with isoproterenol, phenoxybenzamine, or phentolamine. Should never be given to patients with intravascular volume depletion; keep central venous pressure at 14–18 cm water at all times.

Special Dosage Situations

Use cautiously in patients with angina and peripheral vascular disease (see Adverse Reactions). Probably safe for use in women during pregnancy. Use carefully with cyclopropane and halogenated hydrocarbon anesthetics, since there is a theoretical possibility of potentiation, resulting in arrhythmias. Increased dosage required in patients with cirrhosis [7]. No dosage change required in patients with renal failure.

Therapeutic Concentrations

Titrate dose against blood pressure.

Adverse Reactions

Angina and vasoconstriction, which may lead to gangrene in patients with peripheral vascular disease. Ectopic beats, nausea, vomiting, tachycardia, dyspnea, hypotension, and headache. Less common reactions are aberrant cardiac conduction, bradycardia, widening of QRS complex, azotemia, and piloerection. Hypertension may occur rarely; if it does, the infusion must be suspended.

Important: Subcutaneous infiltration leads to necrosis and sloughing of the tissues. Counteract this adverse effect with subcutaneous infiltration of 10–15 mg of phentolamine as soon as possible.

Interactions

Pressor action counteracted by phenoxybenzamine. Monoamine oxidase inhibitors (MAOI) prolong effects, and dose should be decreased to one-tenth in the presence of these agents. May also provoke hypertensive reaction when given with MAOI.

Review

Goldberg, L. I.   Cardiovascular and renal actions of dopamine: Potential clinical applications. *Pharmacol. Rev.* 24(1):1–29, 1972.

References

1. Breckenridge, A., Orme, M., et al.   The effect of dopamine on renal blood flow in man. *Eur. J. Clin. Pharmacol.* 3:131–136, 1971.
2. Goodall, McC., and Alton, H.   Metabolism of 3-hydroxytyramine (dopamine) in human subjects. *Biochem. Pharmacol.* 17:905–914, 1968.
3. Gardella, L. A., Zaroslinski, J. F., et al.   Intropin (dopamine hydrochloride) intravenous admixture compatibility. Part 1. Stability with common intravenous fluids. *Am. J. Hosp. Pharm.* 32:575–578, 1975.
4. Holzer, J., Karliner, J. S., et al.   Effectiveness of dopamine

in patients with cardiogenic shock. *Am. J. Cardiol.* 32:79–84, 1973.

5. Horwitz, D., Fox, S. M., et al.   Effects of dopamine in man. *Circ. Res.* 10:237–243, 1962.

6. MacCannell, K. L., McNay, J. L., et al.   Dopamine in the treatment of hypotension and shock. *N. Engl. J. Med.* 275:1389–1398, 1966.

7. MacGaffey, K., and Jick, H.   Studies on the mechanism of sodium diuresis following dopamine. *Clin. Res.* 13:311, 1965.

8. McDonald, R. H., Goldberg, L. I., et al.   Effect of dopamine in man: Augmentation of sodium excretion, glomerular filtration rate, and renal plasma flow. *J. Clin. Invest.* 43:1116–1124, 1964.

9. Rosenblum, R., and Frieden, J.   Intravenous dopamine in the treatment of myocardial dysfunction after open-heart surgery. *Am. Heart. J.* 83:743–748, 1972.

10. Sandler, M.   Catecholamine synthesis and metabolism in man: Clinical implications (with special reference to parkinsonism). *Hand. Exp. Pharmacol.* 33:845–899, 1972.

ERGOTAMINE

An amino acid alkaloid; derivative of lysergic acid. Product of the fungus *Claviceps purpurea,* which grows on rye and other grains. Ergotamine causes peripheral vasoconstriction, and in high doses, acts as a beta-adrenergic blocking agent. Used in the treatment of the migraine syndrome. Administered parenterally as dihydroergotamine mesylate or as ergotamine tartrate. Oral preparations of ergotamine tartrate are often combined with caffeine. Best results are achieved if the drug is given during the prodromal phase of migraine or very soon after the onset of the headache.

Absorption

Incomplete. Absolute systemic bioavailability: unknown. However, the rate and possibly the extent of absorption are enhanced by the simultaneous administration of caffeine [7]. t_{max}: 2–4 hours [7]. 16% of a dose is absorbed by the buccal route [8].

Distribution

V_d: unknown. Protein binding: unknown. No available data on distribution to the human fetus. Drug in breast milk may produce toxicity in the child (see Special Dosage Situations).

Elimination

$t_{\frac{1}{2}}$: 34 hours [4]. Approximately 4% of a dose is eliminated in the urine unchanged [4, 7]; metabolic fate of the remainder is not known.

Dosage Schedule

Orally: 1–2 mg ergotamine tartrate with caffeine initially, followed by 1 mg every 30 minutes if necessary, until a maximum of

6 mg has been taken. No more than 6 mg should be taken in 24 hours and no more than 10 mg in 1 week. Sublingually: same as oral dosage schedule. Parenterally: 0.25–0.5 mg of ergotamine tartrate initially, repeated once if necessary (total dose over a 24-hour period should not exceed 1.0 mg), or 1–2 mg of dihydroergotamine mesylate. Rectal suppositories: 2 mg, with a maximum of 3 suppositories daily or 6 suppositories in any one week.

Special Dosage Situations

Children: no available data. Pregnancy: contraindicated because of the oxytocic action of ergotamine. Lactation: contraindicated because the baby may develop vomiting, diarrhea, cardiovascular instability, and convulsions.

Contraindicated in patients with liver disease, renal disease, coronary artery disease, or peripheral vascular insufficiency. Avoid in patients with sepsis, which appears to increase the vasoconstrictive complications of ergotamine.

Therapeutic Concentrations

Not established.

Adverse Reactions

Nausea and vomiting, numbness and tingling of the fingers and toes, and chronic headache may develop in habitual users taking 1–2 mg/day [6]. In susceptible individuals or in patients who have ergotamine poisoning, coronary, peripheral, and retinal artery insufficiency may occur [2, 5]. Chronic ergotamine poisoning is also associated with arterial intimal lesions and thrombosis. Treat acute poisoning with infusion of phenoxybenzamine, 100 mg in 500 ml 5% dextrose in water over 5 hours [3], or with sodium nitroprusside infusion, starting at 50 μg/min and adjusting the rate of infusion in relation to patient's response and side-effects.

Interactions

In one patient propranolol and Cafergot given together produced severe peripheral vasoconstriction, which was not evident when Cafergot was given alone [1].

References

1. Baurucker, J. E.   Drug interaction—propranolol and Cafergot. *N. Engl. J. Med.* 288:916–917, 1973.
2. Gupta, D. R., and Strobos, R. J.   Bilateral papillitis associated with Cafergot® therapy. *Neurology* 22:793–797, 1972.
3. Hessov, I., Kromann-Anderson, C., et al.   Peripheral arterial insufficiency during ergotamine treatment. *Dan. Med. Bull.* 19:236–244, 1972.
4. Meier, J., and Schrier, E.   Human plasma levels of some anti-migraine drugs. *Headache* 16:96–104, 1976.
5. Pearce, J.   Hazards of ergotamine tartrate. *Lancet* 1:834–835, 1976.
6. Rose, F. C., and Wilkinson, M.   Ergotamine tartrate overdose. *Lancet* 1:525, 1976.

7. Schmidt, R., and Fanchamps, A.   Effect of caffeine on intestinal absorption of ergotamine in man. *Eur. J. Clin. Pharmacol.* 7:213–216, 1974.

8. Sutherland, J. M., Hooper, W. D., et al.   Buccal absorption of ergotamine. *J. Neurol. Neurosurg. Psychiatry* 37:1116–1120, 1974.

ERYTHROMYCIN

A basic, water- and acid-unstable bacteriostatic macrolide antibiotic. Active against most gram-positive cocci, including penicillin-resistant staphylococci. Also active against gram-negative diplococci, *Hemophilus*, and *Bordetella pertussis* and effective in *Mycoplasma* infections. Resistance develops easily. Mechanism of action is inhibition of protein synthesis by binding to the 50 S ribosome subunit.

Absorption
Oral bioavailability: unknown. Although erythromycin estolate is absorbed more completely than the salts, it is not recommended because of risk of liver toxicity [4]. The bioavailability of the salts is reduced by concomitant food. t_{max}: 1–4 hours.

Distribution
V_d: about 0.6 L/kg. Protein binding: 70–90% [1]. Diffuses readily intracellularly. Concentration in CSF is about 10% of the serum concentration and is only a little higher in meningeal inflammation [2, 3]. The concentration in breast milk is about 50%, and in fetal circulation it is about 10% of the concentration in the maternal serum [3].

Elimination
$t_{\frac{1}{2}}$: 1.5–2 hours [2, 5]. About 30% is excreted unchanged in the bile [6, 7]. About 15% is excreted in the urine [2]. The rest is metabolized to unknown metabolites.

Dosage Schedule
Oral (erythromycin stearate or succinate): 0.5–1 g every 6 hours, preferably at least 1 hour before meals. IM: not recommended because of severe pain. IV (erythromycin lactobionate): up to 1 g every 6 hours. The powder is initially dissolved in at least 30 ml of sterile water (not saline or dextrose) and then added to an intravenous solution with saline or dextrose for infusion over at least 30 minutes.

Special Dosage Situations
Children (oral): 30–50 mg/kg/day in 4 divided doses. No adjustments in patients with kidney failure, in elderly, or in women during pregnancy or lactation. Avoid use in patients with severe hepatic failure.

Therapeutic Concentrations
0.5–3.0 μg/ml.

Adverse Reactions

Allergy accompanied by fever, eosinophilia, and rash is rare. Cholestatic hepatitis is seen only when the estolate-ester form of the drug is administered [7]. Local irritation is common: gastrointestinal reactions are epigastric pain, vomiting, and diarrhea; the IM reaction is severe muscle pain; and the IV reaction is thrombophlebitis. Superinfection, especially with *Candida,* is a risk. Drug not removed by hemodialysis.

Interactions

Avoid concomitant treatment with chloramphenicol, lincomycin, and clindamycin, since no additional benefit can be obtained because of a similar mechanism of action. Physical incompatibility with chloramphenicol has also been reported.

Review

Griffith, R. S., and Black, H. R.   Erythromycin. *Med. Clin. North Am.* 54:1199–1215, 1970.

References

1. Gordon, R. C., Regamey, C., et al.   Serum protein binding of erythromycin, lincomycin, and clindamycin. *J. Pharm. Sci.* 62:1074–1077, 1973.
2. Griffith, R. S., Johnstone, D. M., et al.   The distribution and excretion of erythromycin following intravenous injection. *Antibiot. Annu.* 496–499, 1953–54.
3. Heilman, F. R., Herrell, W. E., et al.   Some laboratory and clinical observations on a new antibiotic, erythromycin (Ilotycin). *Proc. Staff Meet. Mayo Clin.* 27:285–304, 1952.
4. Hepatotoxicity of erythromycin (editorial).   *J. Infect. Dis.* 119:300–306, 1969.
5. Kunin, C. M., and Finland, M.   Persistence of antibiotics in blood of patients with acute renal failure. III. Penicillin, streptomycin, erythromycin, and kanamycin. *J. Clin. Invest.* 38:1509–1519, 1959.
6. Takimura, Y., and Lopez-Belio, M. Excretion of erythromycin through the biliary tract. *Antibiot. Med.* 1:561-566, 1955.
7. Twiss, J. R., Berger, W. V., et al.   The biliary excretion of erythromycin (Ilotycin). *Surg. Gynecol. Obstet.* 102:355–357, 1956.

ETHAMBUTOL

A water-soluble compound with a tuberculostatic effect. Only the active *d*-form is used. Mechanism of action unknown. 75% of the strains of human *Mycobacterium tuberculosis* are sensitive to 1 μg/ml, including several strains resistant to streptomycin. To avoid bacterial resistance, always use in combination with other antituberculous drugs.

Absorption

Oral bioavailability: about 80%, unchanged by food. t_{max}: 2–4 hours [3, 4].

Distribution

V_d: unknown. Protein binding: about 40% [2]. No passage through normal meninges. In meningitis: 20–50% of serum concentration in CSF [5]. No available information about concentration in breast milk or in fetal circulation.

Elimination

$t_{\frac{1}{2}}$: 3–4 hours [1, 3]. 50–80% excreted unchanged, most probably by glomerular filtration. 10% metabolized to the inactive dicarboxylic acid derivative.

Dosage Schedule

Only used orally. 15–25 mg/kg in 1 daily dose.

Special Dosage Situations

No specific information is available about dosage for children or for women during pregnancy or lactation. In the elderly and in patients with renal failure, reduce dosage according to Table 1, page 30. No dosage adjustment necessary for patients with hepatic failure. No contraindications to use, but use cautiously in patients with hyperuricemia.

Therapeutic Concentrations

Peak serum level 2–4 hours after oral administration: 2–5 μg/ml. Predose serum level: below 1 μg/ml.

Adverse Reactions

Optic neuritis, which produces a defect in visual acuity, especially for green, is the most important side-effect. This side-effect occurs more frequently if the daily dose is above 25 mg/kg or the peak serum concentration is above 5 μg/ml. Recovery is usually complete after discontinuation of the drug. Other rare side-effects are dermatitis, peripheral neuritis, hyperuricemia, and leucopenia. Drug is easily eliminated by hemodialysis [1].

Interactions

None reported.

Reviews

Place, V. A., and Thomas, J. P. Clinical pharmacology of ethambutol. *Am. Rev. Resp. Dis.* 87:901–904, 1963.
Place, V. A., and Black, H. (Eds.). New antituberculous agents: Laboratory and clinical studies. *Ann. N.Y. Acad. Sci.* 135:683–939, 1966.
Pyle, M. M. Ethambutol and viomycin. *Med. Clin. North Am.* 54:1317–1327, 1970.

References

1. Dume, T., Wagner, C., et al. Zur Pharmakokinetik von Ethambutol bei Gesunden und Patienten mit terminaler Niereninsuffizienz. *Dtsch. Med. Wochenschr.* 96:1430–1434, 1971.
2. Gundert-Remy, U., Klett, M., et al. Concentration of ethambutol in cerebrospinal fluid in man as a function of the non-protein bound drug fraction in serum. *Eur. J. Clin. Pharmacol.* 6:133–136, 1973.
3. Peets, E. A., Sweeney, W. M., et al. The absorption, excretion, and metabolic fate of ethambutol in man. *Am. Rev. Resp. Dis.* 91:51–58, 1965.
4. Place, A. V., Peets, E. A., et al. Metabolic and special studies of ethambutol in normal volunteers and tuberculous patients. *Ann. N.Y. Acad. Sci.* 135:775–795, 1966.
5. Place, V. A., Pyle, M. M., et al. Ethambutol in tuberculous meningitis. *Am. Rev. Resp. Dis.* 99:783–785, 1969.

ETHOSUXIMIDE

A succinimide derivative; the drug of choice in the treatment of petit mal or absence seizures but ineffective in other forms of epilepsy. Mode of action not understood.

Absorption

Oral bioavailability: 100%. t_{max}: 3–7 hours with the capsule form of the drug and less with the syrup form [1].

Distribution

V_d: not known. Protein binding: none [6]. CSF level equals plasma level [6]. No available information about human placental transfer or concentration in breast milk.

Elimination

$t_{\frac{1}{2}}$ in adults: 60 hours [6]. $t_{\frac{1}{2}}$ in children: 30 hours [6]. 80% metabolized by hydroxylation and ethylation [3, 5]. Metabolites and parent drug appear in urine.

Dosage Schedule

20 mg/kg/day in a single daily dose [4]. No available information about adequate loading doses.

Special Dosage Situations

No available information about use in patients with renal or hepatic disease.

Therapeutic Concentrations

40–80 μg/ml [6]. A level of 60 μg/ml is usually achieved with a dose of 20 mg/kg/day, although considerable individual variation exists.

Interactions

Increases plasma phenytoin levels [2].

Adverse Reactions

Anorexia, nausea, vomiting, tiredness, headaches, and unsteadiness; rarely, a syndrome similar to systemic lupus erythematosus (SLE), leukopenia, or pancytopenia may occur.

Review

Eadie, M. J., and Tyrer, J. H. *Anticonvulsant Therapy.* Edinburgh and London: Churchill/Livingstone, 1974. Pp. 113–117.

References

1. Buchanan, R. A., Fernandez, L., et al. Absorption and elimination of ethosuximide in children. *J. Clin. Pharmacol.* 9:393–398, 1969.
2. Frantzen, E., Hansen, J. M., et al. Phenytoin (Dilantin) intoxication. *Acta Neurol. Scand.* 43:440–446, 1967.
3. Horning, M. G., Stratton, C., et al. Metabolism of 2-ethyl-2-methylsuccinimide (ethosuximide) in the rat and human. *Drug Metab. Disp.* 1:569–576, 1973.
4. Penry, J. K., Porter, R. J., et al. Ethosuximide. Relation of Plasma Levels to Clinical Control. In D. M. Woodbury, J. K. Penry, and R. P. Schmidt (Eds.), *Antiepileptic Drugs.* New York: Raven Press, 1972. Pp. 431–441.
5. Preste, P. G., Westerman, C. E., et al. Identification of 2-ethyl-2-methyl-3 hydroxysuccinimide as a major metabolite of ethosuximide in humans. *J. Pharm. Sci.* 63:467–469, 1974.
6. Sherwin, A. L., and Robb, J. P. Ethosuximide. Relation of Plasma Levels to Clinical Control. In D. M. Woodbury, J. K. Penry, and R. P. Schmidt (Eds.), *Antiepileptic Drugs.* New York: Raven Press, 1972. Pp. 443–448.

FUROSEMIDE
(Frusemide)

An anthranilic acid diuretic that acts by inhibiting sodium and chloride reabsorption in the ascending loop of Henle and perhaps in the proximal and distal convoluted tubules. Indicated in the management of all types of edema, including edema caused by advanced renal failure, and in ascites caused by cirrhosis. Also indicated in the management of acute hypercalcemia. Unlike the thiazide diuretics, it has little place in the chronic therapy of hypertension because of its tendency to cause pronounced hypokalemia. Administration accompanied by elevation of plasma renin activity. Used as an indicator of plasma renin hypersecretion.

Absorption

Oral bioavailability: 50–60% [4]. Oral t_{max}: 1 hour. Intramuscular t_{max}: 30 minutes [2]. Maximum diuresis occurs 1–3 hours after oral administration and 30–90 minutes after IV injection. Diuretic action is generally complete in about 6 hours if the patient has normal renal function.

Distribution

V_d: 0.1 L/kg [3]. Protein binding: 95–99% [1]. Binding reduced by 9–14% in acute renal failure [1].

Elimination

$t_\frac{1}{2}$: 30–70 minutes [2, 3]. 90% is eliminated in urine unchanged, both by glomerular filtration and by proximal tubular secretion. The remainder is excreted into the bile [3].

Dosage Schedule

Orally: 40–120 mg/day in 1 or 2 doses. In an emergency, drug may be given by IV route in a dose of 20–120 mg and repeated as required. Therapeutic regimen should be initiated with small doses and adjusted upward to meet the needs of the individual patient.

Special Dosage Situations

Larger doses (e.g., up to 1000 mg/day) have been given in renal failure ($t_\frac{1}{2}$: 80 minutes in anephric patients. V_d: 0.2 L/kg) [3]. Dehydration is more likely to occur in the elderly. There is no contraindication to use in women during pregnancy. Children: 1–2 mg/kg initially, may be increased if necessary.

Therapeutic Concentrations

It is usual simply to monitor the patient's response, but plasma levels of 0.2–0.3 μg/ml are associated with diuresis [6].

Adverse Reactions

Hyponatremia, hypokalemia, and hypomagnesemia; and hypovolemia, which may cause syncope. Also hyperglycemia, hyperuricemia, pancreatitis, and hyperosmolar coma. Plasma levels in excess of 50 μg/ml are likely to cause tinnitus and hypoacusis. Bone marrow depression, exfoliative dermatitis, and erythema multiforme occur rarely. Occasionally, gastrointestinal distress may occur.

Interactions

Increased ototoxicity in combination with aminoglycosides; increased nephrotoxicity in association with cephaloridine. These interactions are more likely to occur in patients with renal failure. Hypokalemia may increase effect of curare and the risk of digitalis and other cardiac glycoside toxicity. Furosemide's hypotensive and natriuretic effects are antagonized by indomethacin [5].

Review

Kennedy, A. C., de Wardener, H. E., et al. (Eds.).   Symposium on Lasix. *Scott. Med. J.* 19(Suppl. 1):1–64, 1974.

References

1. Andreasen, F., and Jakobsen, P. Determination of furosemide in blood plasma and its binding to proteins in normal plasma and in plasma from patients with acute renal failure. *Acta. Pharmacol. Toxicol.* 55:49–57, 1974.
2. Calesnick, B., Christensen, J. A., et al. Absorption and excretion of furosemide-S^{35} in human subjects. *Proc. Soc. Exp. Biol. Med.* 123:17–22, 1966.
3. Cutler, R. E., Forrey, A. W., et al. Pharmacokinetics of furosemide in normal subjects and functionally anephric patients. *Clin. Pharmacol. Ther.* 15:588–596, 1974.
4. Kelly, M. R., Cutler, R. E., et al. Pharmacokinetics of orally administered furosemide. *Clin. Pharmacol. Ther.* 15:178–186, 1974.
5. Patak, R. V., Mookerjee, B. K., et al. Antagonism of the effects of furosemide by indomethacin in normal and hypertensive man. *Prostaglandins* 10:649–659, 1975.
6. Rupp, W. Pharmacokinetics and pharmacodynamics of Lasix. *Scott. Med. J.* 19(Suppl. 1):5–13, 1974.

GLIBENCLAMIDE

A potent short-acting "second generation" sulfonylurea that mediates hypoglycemic action, at least initially, through stimulation of pancreatic insulin release (beta-cytotropic activity). Used in the management of patients with adult-onset nonketotic diabetes with functional islet tissue, in whom weight control and carbohydrate restriction have been unsuccessful in controlling hyperglycemia. Comparable in effect to glibornuride [3], glipizide [1], and tolbutamide [2].

Absorption

Completely absorbed by oral route [1]. Systemic bioavailability: unknown. t_{max}: 2 hours.

Distribution

V_d: 0.1 L/kg [1]. Protein binding: 90–95%.

Elimination

$t_{\frac{1}{2}}$: 4–8 hours [1]. Elimination in feces and urine about equal. No parent drug in urine [1]; 4–6% in feces; remainder is in the form of unidentified metabolites [1].

Dosage Schedule

5 mg daily as a single oral dose with breakfast. Dosage may be increased at weekly intervals by 2.5–5 mg to a maximum of 15 mg.

Special Dosage Situations

Glibenclamide is contraindicated in juvenile diabetes mellitus, in patients with ketoacidosis, or in those patients who have undergone pancreatectomy. Care is advised for use in the elderly and in patients with renal or hepatic disease. During stressful periods, such as infection, operation, or trauma, transfer to insulin therapy may be advisable.

Therapeutic Concentrations

It is usual to monitor the blood glucose response. This procedure is especially important during acute illness and after dosage adjustments.

Adverse Reactions

Gastrointestinal disturbances such as nausea and vomiting, skin rash, occasional leukopenia and thrombocytopenia, and transient disturbance of hepatic function. Hypoglycemia is a serious potential problem with all sulfonylureas, especially if dietary intake is reduced or if an overdose is taken. Children may be at greater risk of prolonged, marked hypoglycemic effects than adults are [4].

Interactions

Little available information. Chloramphenicol, dicumarol, phenylbutazone, propranolol, and salicylates may enhance glibenclamide's hypoglycemic effect, while corticosteroids, thiazides, and phenytoin may antagonize this effect.

References

1. Fuccella, L. M., Tamassia, V., et al.   Metabolism and kinetics of the hypoglycemic agent glipizide in man—comparison with glibenclamide. *J. Clin. Pharmacol.* 13:68–75, 1973.
2. Heine, P., Kewitz, H., et al.   Dose-response relationships of tolbutamide and glibenclamide in diabetes mellitus. *Eur. J. Clin. Pharmacol.* 7:321–330, 1974.
3. Logie, A. W., and Stowers, J. M.   Clinical trial of glibornuride in diabetes. *Br. Med. J.* 3:514–515, 1975.
4. Sillence, D. O., and Court, J. M.   Glibenclamide-induced hypoglycemia. *Br. Med. J.* 3:490–491, 1975.

GOLD

Originally tried unsuccessfully as an antituberculous agent. Inhibits lysosomal hydroxylases, suppresses anaphylactic release of histamine, prostaglandin release in vitro, and cellular immunity. Used in the treatment of early active rheumatoid arthritis that progresses despite adequate salicylate therapy, bed rest, and physical treatment. May be of value in the management of pemphigus [11].

Absorption

Administered intramuscularly, usually as gold sodium thiomalate, because oral preparations are erratically absorbed. t_{max}: 4–6 hours [10]. A thiosulfate preparation for intravenous administration is also available. Crysotherapy with a new oral preparation may be more rewarding, although in one study plasma gold levels in patients who took the drug orally were one-third to one-half less than levels produced by IM dosage [2].

Distribution

V_d: 0.1 L/kg [4]. Protein binding: 95% [10]. Synovial fluid concentration is half that found in plasma [3], and arthritic joints have been found to contain twice the amount of the drug found in normal joints [8]. Binding of gold to connective tissue has been demonstrated [6]. The concentration of gold in breast milk seems to be of the same order as that in plasma [1].

Elimination

Aurothiomalate is excreted unchanged. The distribution phase has a half-life of about 10 hours and lasts for about 40 hours. The elimination half-life is about 6 days [7].

The distribution and elimination phases are longer with gold sodium thioglucose, which is a longer acting preparation, the half-life being about 10 days [12]. Renal excretion accounts for about 70% of the elimination [5]. About 40% of a dose remains unexcreted after 2 months, suggesting a "deep" compartment caused by extensive binding [4].

Dosage Schedule

Usually given as IM gold sodium thiomalate, which contains 50% gold. The usual regimen is to give 10 mg in the first week, 25 mg in the second and third weeks, and 50 mg weekly thereafter to a total dose of 750 mg. If remission occurs, continue to give 50 mg at 2-week intervals for 4 doses, then at 3-week intervals for 4 doses, and then every month for 1 year. For pemphigus the dose is 25 mg at 2-month intervals [11].

Special Dosage Situations

There is no definitive information about the use of gold in children and in women during pregnancy. Gold is contraindicated in patients with renal and hepatic disease. It should be given cautiously to the elderly because of reduction in renal function.

Therapeutic Concentrations

3 μg/ml has been suggested [9].

Adverse Reactions

The majority of adverse reactions usually occur earlier and more frequently in patients with chronic disease. 25–50% of patients have some adverse reactions. The incidence of reactions seems unrelated to the plasma level [9, 12]. Skin reactions vary from erythema to exfoliative dermatitis. Other side-effects are glossitis, pharyngitis, tracheitis, gastritis, and colitis; chrysiasis (a gray-blue pigmentation, especially on the exposed areas); vaginitis; thrombocytopenia; and leucopenia, agranulocytosis, and aplastic anemia, which may occur several months after the cessation of therapy. Trace proteinuria occurs in 50% of patients. Heavy albuminuria and hematuria occur in 1–3% of patients; the site of damage is usually the proximal tubule. Nephrotic syndrome, which is reversible, may also occur. Encephalitis, peripheral neuropathy, and hepatitis rarely occur. Before administration of each dose, check the patient's skin, urine, and blood count. For severe reactions, glucocorticoids, dimercaprol, or penicillamine may be used.

Interactions
May potentiate myelotoxic potential of antimalarials, immuno-suppressives, and phenylbutazones.

References
1. Blau, S. P.   Metabolism of gold during lactation. *Arthritis Rheum.* 16:777–778, 1973.
2. Finkelstein, A. E., Walz, D. T., et al.   Auranofin. New oral gold compound for treatment of rheumatoid arthritis. *Ann. Rheum. Dis.* 35:251–257, 1976.
3. Gerber, R. C., Paulus, H. E., et al.   Kinetics of aurothioma-late in serum and synovial fluid. *Arthritis Rheum.* 15:625–629, 1972.
4. Gerber, R. C., Paulus, H. E., et al.   Gold kinetics following aurothiomalate therapy: Use of a whole body radiation counter. *J. Lab. Clin. Med.* 83:778–789, 1974.
5. Gottlieb, N. L., Smith, P. M., et al.   Gold excretion correlated with clinical course during chrysotherapy in rheumatoid arthritis. *Arthritis Rheum.* 15:582–592, 1972.
6. Grahame, R., Billings, R., et al.   Tissue gold levels after chrysotherapy. *Ann. Rheum. Dis.* 33:536–539, 1974.
7. Harth, M.   Serum gold levels during chrysotherapy with relation to urinary and fecal excretion. *Clin. Pharmacol. Ther.* 15:354–360, 1974.
8. Lawrence, J. S.   Studies with radioactive gold. *Ann. Rheum. Dis.* 20:341–351, 1961.
9. Lorber, A., Atkins, C. J., et al.   Monitoring serum gold values to improve chrysotherapy in rheumatiod arthritis. *Ann. Rheum. Dis.* 32:133–139, 1973.
10. Mascarenhas, B. R., Granda, J. L., et al.   Gold metabolism in patients with rheumatoid arthritis treated with gold compounds—reinvestigated. *Arthritis Rheum.* 15:391–402, 1972.
11. Penneys, N. S., Eaglstein, W. H., et al. Gold sodium thio-malate treatment of pemphigus. *Arch. Dermatol.* 108:56–60, 1973.
12. Rubinstein, H. M., and Dietz, A. A.   Serum Gold. II. Levels in rheumatoid arthritis. *Ann. Rheum. Dis.* 32:128–132, 1973.

GRISEOFULVIN

A water-insoluble, fungistatic antibiotic with activity against most strains of *Microsporum, Epidermophyton,* and *Trichophyton.* Ineffective against bacteria and all other fungi, including *Actinomycetes* and *Nocardia.* Mechanism of action is uncertain, but the drug probably binds to sterols in fungus wall, damaging the integrity of the wall.

Griseofulvin is bound to keratin in cells of the host's epidermis, making the cells resistant to fungal infestation. Indicated in severe mycotic infections caused by susceptible organisms. Of special value in hair and nail infections. A few studies have shown a beneficial effect of griseofulvin in patients with Raynaud's phenomenon [7].

Absorption
Oral bioavailability of the micronized formulation: 40–70% [6]. Oral bioavailability of new preparation that contains ultramicronized particles: 75–90% [1]. A fatty meal enhances absorption. t_{max}: 2–4 hours.

Distribution
V_d: 1–2 L/kg [6]. Protein binding: unknown. No available information about distribution to breast milk, across placenta, or to CNS.

Elimination
$t_{\frac{1}{2}}$: 10–24 hours [4, 6]. Less than 1% is excreted unchanged. About 60% is excreted in urine as 6-desmethylgriseofulvin, partly as the glucuronidated compound [2, 4]. 4-desmethylgriseofulvin and several minor, unidentified metabolites have also been detected in the urine [6].

Dosage Schedule
500 mg 1–2 times daily of micronized preparations. Treatment should be continued at least 3 months for skin infections and for 6 and 12 months for infections in fingernails and toenails, respectively, i.e., the time for complete epithelial regeneration.

Special Dosage Situations
Children: 10 mg/kg daily in 2–3 divided doses. No available information about use in the elderly, in women during lactation, or in patients with renal or hepatic disease. Contraindicated in pregnancy because of possible teratogenicity.

Adverse Reactions
Headache, peripheral neuritis, blurred vision, and mental confusion. Nausea, heartburn, and diarrhea. Blood dyscrasias, hepatotoxicity, and proteinuria without renal insufficiency. Photosensitivity and serum sickness. May precipitate acute attacks of porphyria in disposed individuals. Gynecomastia has been reported in children. Griseofulvin is embryotoxic and teratotoxic in rats and should not be given to pregnant women. Long-term feeding of griseofulvin to mice has produced hepatic carcinomas.

Interactions
Phenobarbital decreases the bioavailability of griseofulvin [5]. Griseofulvin antagonizes the effects of warfarin, possibly by enzyme induction [3].

Review

Lin, C., and Symchowicz, S.   Absorption, distribution, metabolism, and excretion of griseofulvin in man and animals. *Drug Metab. Rev.* 6:75–95, 1975.

References

1. Barrett, W. E., and Hanigan, J. J.   The bioavailability of griseofulvin PEG ultramicrosize (Gris-Peg) tablets in man under steady-state conditions. *Curr. Ther. Res.* 18:491–500, 1975.
2. Bates, T. R., and Sequeira, J. A.   Bioavailability of micronized griseofulvin from corn oil-in-water emulsion, aqueous suspension, and commercial tablet dosage forms in humans. *J. Pharm. Sci.* 64:793–797, 1975.
3. Cullen, S. I., and Catalano, P. M.   Griseofulvin—warfarin antagonism. *J.A.M.A.* 199:582–583, 1967.
4. Lin, C., Masat, J., et al.   Absorption, metabolism, and excretion of ^{14}C-griseofulvin in man. *J. Pharm. Sci.* 187:415–422, 1973.
5. Riegelman, S., Rowland, M., et al.   Griseofulvin—phenobarbital interaction in man. *J.A.M.A.* 213:426–431, 1970.
6. Rowland, M., Riegelman, S., et al.   Absorption kinetics of griseofulvin in man. *J. Pharm. Sci.* 57:984–989, 1969.
7. Sabri, S., Higgins, R. F., et al.   A double blind clinical trial of griseofulvin in patients with Raynaud's phenomenon. *Postgrad. Med. J.* 49:641–643, 1973.

GUANETHIDINE

An antihypertensive, postganglionic adrenergic blocking agent. Actively transported into peripheral nerve endings, where it is bound to norepinephrine storage sites and displaces norepinephrine from nerve endings. Guanethidine may then be released by nerve stimulation and may act either by persistent nerve stimulation or as a "false neurotransmitter" [4]. Guanethidine causes an initial pressor response that is followed by a decrease in blood pressure. This decrease is caused partly by diminished venous return secondary to a decrease in venous tone and partly by a direct depression of cardiac output. Guanethidine is indicated for the management of all forms of hypertension, *except* pheochromocytoma.

Absorption

50–80% absorbed, but systemic availability probably much less because of first-pass metabolism. t_{max}: 3 hours [2].

Distribution

V_d: unknown. Protein binding: unknown.

Elimination

$t_{\frac{1}{2}}$: 43 hours. 40% metabolized. Major metabolites are guanethidine-N-oxide, 2-(6-carboxyhexylamino)ethylguanidine, and (6-carboxyhexyl)2-iminoimidazolidine. Parent drug and metabolites appear in urine; biliary excretion is insignificant. Excretion is by both glomerular filtration and tubular secretion. Elimination curve is triexponential, suggesting slowly released "deep" tissue store [1].

Dosage Schedule

No fixed dose; adjust against blood pressure level. Usual starting dose is 10 mg daily, which may be increased slowly to 400 mg/day. Because of the long $t_{\frac{1}{2}}$, the drug needs to be given only once daily, and maximum action will not occur for at least 1 week. In emergencies, the following loading regimen has been recommended:

Day 1	80 mg	25 mg	35 mg
Day 2	40 mg	50 mg	75 mg
Day 3	90 mg	110 mg	125 mg
Day 4	150 mg	150 mg	150 mg

This type of regimen may produce early results, which would otherwise not occur for 3–4 days [5].

Special Dosage Situations

Avoid use in patients with cardiac and cerebrovascular disease because of postural hypotensive effect (see Adverse Reactions). Dose may need to be decreased in patients with renal failure because of lengthened $t_{\frac{1}{2}}$. Avoid use in males because of poor compliance caused by high incidence of failure of ejaculation.

Therapeutic Concentrations

Not relevant, since plasma levels do not correlate well with antihypertensive effect. Levels greater than 8 ng/ml are associated with adrenergic blockade [6].

Adverse Reactions

Failure of ejaculation, postural and exercise hypotension, dry mouth, and diarrhea.

Interactions

Uptake of guanethidine into nerve endings is blocked by tricyclic antidepressants, cocaine, and amphetamine. Functional denervation leads to a hypersensitive response to infused ephedrine and epinephrine [3, 4].

Review

Lukas, G. Metabolism and biochemical pharmacology of guanethidine and related compounds. *Drug Metab. Rev.* 2:101–116, 1974.

References

1. McMartin, C. The separation detection of metabolites of guanethidine. *Pharmacology* 18:238–243, 1969.

2. McMartin, C., Rondel, M. B., et al.   The fate of guanethidine in two hypertensive patients. *Clin. Pharmacol. Ther.* 11:423–431, 1970.
3. Mitchell, J. R., and Oates, J. A.   Guanethidine and related agents. I. Mechanism of the selective blockade of adrenergic neurons and its antagonism by drugs. *J. Pharmacol. Exp. Ther.* 172:100–107, 1970.
4. Mitchell, J. R., Arias, L., et al.   Antagonism of the antihypertensive action of guanethidine sulfate by desipramine hydrochloride. *J.A.M.A.* 202:973–976, 1967.
5. Shand, D. G., Nies, A. S., et al.   A loading-maintenance regimen for more rapid initiation of the effect of guanethidine. *Clin. Pharmacol. Ther.* 18:139–144, 1975.
6. Walter, I. E., Khandelwal, J., et al.   The relationship of plasma guanethidine levels to adrenergic blockade. *Clin. Pharmacol. Ther.* 18:571–580, 1975.

HALOPERIDOL

Major tranquilizer of the butyrophenone family. Acts by forming a monomolecular film on membranes in the CNS that bear γ-aminobutyric acid (GABA) and dopamine. In this way, haloperidol is thought to inhibit specific areas in the extrapyramidal system, unlike chlorpromazine, which exerts a more global effect. Has also been shown to elevate serum prolactin levels.

Indicated in the management of schizophrenia; the best response is found in patients with acute manic symptoms, paranoia, and social withdrawal. Also indicated in the manic phase of manic-depressive psychosis, aggressive behavior in emotionally disturbed children, Gilles de la Tourette's disease [5], and delirium tremens. Effective antiemetic agent [4]. Possibly of value in treatment of stuttering and of persistent hiccups. Of no value in psychotic depression or in the management of neuroses.

Absorption
Systemic bioavailability: unknown. t_{max}: 3–6 hours [2].

Distribution
V_d: 20–30 L/kg [1]. Protein binding: unknown. Possibly crosses placenta.

Elimination
Distribution phase: about 30 minutes. $t_{\frac{1}{2}}$: 12–22 hours [1]. Metabolism: no data.

Dosage Schedule
Adjust clinically to patient's needs. Dosage range is generally 0.5–30 mg daily, although doses of 1000 mg/day have been used without adverse effects. Incidence of side-effects increases sharply with dosages that exceed 30 mg/day. Dosage of 5 mg/day is generally adequate in the psychoses of old age. Antiemetic dose is 1 mg given parenterally.

Special Dosage Situations
No available information. Possibly contraindicated in pregnancy.

Therapeutic Concentrations
No available information.

Adverse Reactions
Parkinsonism, dystonias, and akathisia are the most frequent side-effects, especially with dosages exceeding 30 mg/day. Agitation and tremor occur, generally with doses greater than 100 mg/day. Less common reactions are hypotension, tachycardia, fever, vomiting, hepatic impairment, stupor, catalepsy, confusion, and urticaria. Parkinsonism and other extrapyramidal syndromes (acute dystonia and akathisia) generally respond to the usual antiparkinsonian medications. May cause limb malformations when administered in the first trimester of pregnancy [3].

Interactions
Response diminished by administration of benztropine and other anticholinergic antiparkinsonian drugs. Possibly serious irreversible brain damage with lithium.

Review
Ban, T. A.   Haloperidol and the butyrophenones. *Psychosomatics* 14:286–297, 1973.

References
1. Forsman, A., Mortensson, E., et al.   A gas chromatographic model for determining haloperidol. A sensitive procedure for studying serum concentration and pharmacokinetics of haloperidol in patients. *Naunyn-Schmiedeberg's Arch. Pharmacol.* 286:113–124, 1974.
2. Johnson, P. C., Charalampous, K. D., et al.   Absorption and excretion of tritiated haloperidol in man (a preliminary report). *Int. J. Neuropsychiatry* 3(Suppl. 1):S24–S25, 1967.
3. Kopelman, A. E., McCullar, F. W., et al.   Limb malformations following maternal use of haloperidol. *J.A.M.A.* 231:62–64, 1975.
4. Robbins, E. L., and Nagel, J. D.   Haloperidol parenterally for treatment of vomiting and nausea from gastrointestinal disorders in a group of geriatric patients: Double-blind, placebo-controlled study. *J. Am. Geriat. Soc.* 23:38–41, 1975.
5. Shapiro, A. K., Shapiro, E., et al.   Treatment of Tourette's syndrome with haloperidol, review of 34 cases. *Arch. Gen. Psychiatry* 28:92–97, 1973.

HEPARIN

A sulfated mucopolysaccharide, which is a strong acid that carries electronegative charge at physiological pH. Binds strongly to many proteins, which is the basis of its anticoagulant action. Clinically the mechanism of action is thought to be the activation of antithrombin III (At III) with inhibition of the activation of Factor X and the rest of the clotting cascade. Indicated for prophylaxis and management of deep venous thrombosis, pulmonary thromboembolic disease, and disseminated intravascular coagulation.

Absorption
Not used orally because of poor bioavailability. Effective, although absorbed erratically when given subcutaneously. IM use should be avoided because of high risk of hematoma.

Distribution
V_d: 0.05–0.2 L/kg [1, 3]. Protein binding: 95% [7].

Elimination
$t_{\frac{1}{2}}$: usually about 60–90 minutes [1, 2, 3, 7]. However, a wide variation in $t_{\frac{1}{2}}$ (45–355 minutes) has been described in patients undergoing open-heart surgery [2]. Lower concentrations may be cleared more rapidly, suggesting that dose-dependent metabolism exists. Metabolism has not been well defined; apparently metabolized by liver heparinase, with 20% excreted unchanged in urine [6].

Dosage Schedule
Heparin is a complex molecule of uncertain molecular weight, and therefore it is prescribed in units rather than milligrams. 1 mg = 80–120 units USP. The regimen is empirical: common dosages have been 30,000–40,000 units over 24 hours via constant infusion or 5000–10,000 units every 4–6 hours by intermittent IV injections. Attempts have been made to individualize regimens based on the anticoagulant effect desired in relation to the patient's weight, blood volume, and renal function [2, 7]. The regimen of 70 units/kg IV, followed after 90 minutes by 400 units/kg/24 hours by infusion [3], is satisfactory, although interindividual variations in effect are quite large. In disseminated intravascular coagulation, smaller doses are needed, e.g., 500–1000 units/hr IV. In prophylaxis of postoperative deep venous thrombosis, subcutaneous heparin may be given, 5000 units b.i.d. or t.i.d., commencing 2 hours before the operation and continuing for 7 days afterward [5]. Use of this drug in a large multicenter trial has clearly shown that this regimen reduces the postoperative death rate from pulmonary embolism [4].

Special Dosage Situations
Hepatic failure: care should be taken, since a tendency toward bleeding already exists in this condition. Renal failure: $t_{\frac{1}{2}}$ of heparin is prolonged by approximately 25%, but no major adjustment is necessary [7]. Pulmonary embolism: heparin clearance is enhanced [3], although the mechanism is not fully understood.

Therapeutic Concentrations
Not measured directly. Clotting time of whole blood should be twice that of normal clotting time.

Adverse Reactions

Overdose causes hemorrhage—beware of "silent" retroperitoneal bleeding, gastrointestinal bleeding, or intracranial hemorrhage. To stop the hemorrhaging, it is usually only necessary to discontinue heparin. If an antidote is needed, protamine can be given in a dose of 1 mg/100 units heparin. Because protamine is a positively charged basic protein that not only has its own anticoagulant effect but also acts for a longer time than heparin, care must be taken not to use so much protamine that the patient will receive an overdose. A practical dose may be calculated by seeing how much protamine is required to coagulate a sample of the patient's blood and then giving about 60% of the calculated dose.

Heparin suppresses aldosterone secretion and causes potassium retention in days to weeks. When given chronically, heparin may cause osteoporosis or alopecia.

Interactions

Increased risk of bleeding with drugs that inhibit platelet aggregation, e.g., aspirin, dipyridamole, phenylbutazone, and indomethacin. Basic drugs such as antihistamines, phenothiazines, quinine, quinidine, and tetracycline will form a precipitate in injection fluids if mixed with heparin.

Special Notes

High concentrations of heparin prolong prothrombin time. If patient is concurrently receiving warfarin, the effect of this anticoagulant should be measured at least 6 hours after previous dose of heparin. To help prevent the catastrophe of a dangerously large dose of heparin being inadvertently infused too rapidly, only enough heparin for a 6- to 8-hour period should be added to the infusion bottle [2].

Review

Sherry, S.   Low-dose heparin for the prophylaxis of pulmonary embolism. *Am. Rev. Respir. Dis.* 114:661–6, 1976.

References

1. Estes, J. W.   The kinetics of heparin. *Ann. N.Y. Acad. Sci.* 179:187–204, 1971.
2. Goodman, T., Todd, M. E., et al.   Laboratory observations and clinical implications of monitoring the effect of heparin by bioassay. *Surg. Gynecol. Obstet.* 142:673–685, 1976.
3. Hirsh, J., van Aken, W. G., et al.   Heparin kinetics in venous thrombosis and pulmonary embolism. *Circulation* 53:691–695, 1976.
4. International Multicentre Trial.   Prevention of fatal postoperative pulmonary embolism by low doses of heparin. *Lancet* 2:45–51, 1975.
5. Nicolaides, A. N., Dupont, P. A., et al.   Small doses of subcutaneous sodium heparin in preventing deep venous thrombosis after major surgery. *Lancet* 2:890–893, 1972.
6. Olsson, P., Lagergren, H., et al.   The elimination from

plasma of intravenous heparin: An experimental study on dogs and humans. *Acta Med. Scand.* 173:619–630, 1963.
7. Perry, P. J., Herron, G. R., et al.   Heparin half-life in normal and impaired renal function. *Clin. Pharmacol. Ther.* 16:514–519, 1974.

HYDRALAZINE

A phthalazine derivative that exerts hypotensive activity through direct relaxation of vascular smooth muscle.

Absorption

80% absorbed after oral dose, but first-pass absorption through the gut wall and liver substantially reduces systemic availability. In fast acetylators, about 22% of the oral dose appears in plasma; in slow acetylators, this figure rises to about 38%. t_{max}: 2–4 hours [4].

Distribution

V_d: 0.3–0.7 L/kg. This amount is unchanged by the acetylator status of the patient [4]. Protein binding: about 87% [1].

Elimination

$t_{\frac{1}{2}}$: 2–8 hours for fast acetylators [4]. $t_{\frac{1}{2}}$: 2–6 hours for slow acetylators [4]. Acetylation appears relatively unimportant after the first-pass effect. There is extensive hydroxylation and other unidentified processes in addition to acetylation, and thus only 1.5–3% is excreted unchanged in urine. Spontaneous degradation to phthalazine occurs in vitro in plasma at 37° C and is also thought to occur in vivo. From a plasma concentration of 0.42 μg/ml, degradation was a zero-order process at the rate of 0.07 μg/ml/hr [4]. Degradation may continue in the urinary bladder.

Dosage Schedule

Starting dose is 10–20 mg twice daily, with the dose being increased rapidly according to the patient's response. To avoid toxicity, dosage should be limited in slow acetylators to 200 mg daily in 2–4 divided doses. In combination with propranolol and a thiazide diuretic, doses of 2.4 mg/kg (for slow acetylators) and 3.7 mg/kg (for fast acetylators) are usually satisfactory [4]. Dosage once or twice daily may be adequate [2].

Special Dosage Situations

Use with caution in slow acetylators. Relative contraindications include angina pectoris and mitral valve disease, since exacerbation of chest pain and increased pulmonary hypertension, respectively, may occur. In renal failure higher levels and longer $t_{\frac{1}{2}}$ are reported [4], suggesting greater renal elimination as unchanged drug than indicated. No available information about use in pregnant women or in children.

Therapeutic Concentrations

Dosage is usually adjusted to blood pressure response, within the dose limits indicated. Therapeutic response is usually associated with plasma levels of 0.5–1.5 μg/ml [5].

Adverse Reactions

Side-effects, of which there is a relatively high incidence, include flushing, tachycardia, headache, dizziness, tremors, and muscle cramps; gastrointestinal symptoms such as nausea, vomiting, and diarrhea; nasal congestion, lacrimation, urinary retention, and paralytic ileus; and angina pectoris in susceptible individuals, arrhythmias, and myocardial infarction. Hypersensitivity reactions include fever, urticaria, rash, polyneuritis, anemia, and pancytopenia (structural relationship with sulfas). The SLE (systemic lupus erythematosus) syndrome, a serious and notable toxic effect that is characterized by fever, malaise, chest and joint pains, and various serological disorders, occurs more frequently in slow acetylators than in fast acetylators [3]. This effect may require steroid therapy. Tolerance to minor side-effects may develop. A supportive measure in hydralazine overdose is expansion of the fluid volume; epinephrine (adrenaline), which may aggravate tachycardia, should be avoided.

Interactions

None reported.

Special Note

Beta-blocking drugs offer a useful drug combination by preventing reflex tachycardia and problems associated with it.

References

1. Lesser, J. M., Israili, Z. H., et al.   Metabolism and disposition of hydralazine-^{14}C in man and dog. *Drug Metab. Disp.* 2:352–360, 1974.
2. O'Malley, K., Segal, J. L., et al.   Duration of hydralazine action in hypertension. *Clin. Pharmacol. Ther.* 18:581–586, 1975.
3. Perry, H. M.   Late toxicity to hydralazine resembling systemic lupus erythematosus or rheumatoid arthritis. *Am. J. Med.* 54:58–72, 1973.
4. Reidenberg, M. M., Drayer, D., et al.   Hydralazine elimination in man. *Clin. Pharmacol. Ther.* 14:970–977, 1973.
5. Zacest, R., and Koch-Weser, J.   Relation of hydralazine plasma concentration to dosage and hypotensive action. *Clin. Pharmacol. Ther.* 13:420–425, 1972.

IBUPROFEN

Phenylalkanoic acid, a nonsteroidal anti-inflammatory agent, with analgesic and antipyretic properties, Approximately 2–4 times as potent as aspirin in improving symptoms and signs of inflammation in rheumatoid arthritis but not as potent as indomethacin or phenylbutazone. Efficacy equal to that of aspirin. Mechanism of action is not known; however, formation of prostaglandins is inhibited, and lysosomal membranes are stabilized in vitro [1]. Indicated in the symptomatic management of rheumatoid arthritis and osteoarthritis.

Absorption

Only used orally. Systemic bioavailability: unknown. t_{max}: 30–90 minutes [2]. Absorption delayed when the drug is taken after a meal.

Distribution

V_d: unknown. Protein binding: 99% [5]. Distribution to other tissues: no available data.

Elimination

$t_{\frac{1}{2}}$: 2 hours [4]. Completely metabolized by hydroxylation [4]. Conjugated and unconjugated metabolites appear in the urine [5].

Dosage Schedule

600–1200 mg/day in 3–4 divided doses. Occasionally, doses up to 2400 mg/day may be required, but with doses as large as this, a higher incidence of gastrointestinal intolerance occurs.

Special Dosage Situations

Although incidence of peptic ulcer is said to be less with ibuprofen than with aspirin in equipotent doses, use cautiously in patients with a history of this disease. No available data about administration of this drug to the elderly or to patients with renal or hepatic disease. Children: 10–20 mg/kg/day in 3–4 divided doses.

Therapeutic Concentrations

Plasma levels have not been shown to correlate well with clinical effect.

Adverse Reactions

Gastrointestinal upsets. Occult gastrointestinal bleeding may occur when 900–1200 mg/day of ibuprofen is given. This is similar to the bleeding that might occur from 3.6 g/day of aspirin [3] but half the amount of bleeding that might occur from 4.8 g/day of calcium aspirin [6]. Headache, dizziness, anxiety, elevation of serum glutamic-oxalocetic transaminase and alkaline phosphatase levels, and the formation of serum uric acid. Rash, leukopenia, and toxic amblyopia have been reported.

Interactions

None known.

References

1. Adams, S. S., Bough, R. G., et al.   Some aspects of the pharmacology, metabolism, and toxicology of ibuprofen. *Rheumatol. Phys. Med.* 10(Suppl. 1):9–14, 1970.
2. Adams, S. S., Cliffe, E. E., et al.   Some biological properties of 2-(4-isobutylphenyl)-propionic acid. *J. Pharm. Sci.* 56:1686, 1967.
3. Brooks, C. D., Schmid, F. R., et al.   Ibuprofen and aspirin in

the treatment of rheumatoid arthritis. *Rheumatol. Phys. Med.* 10(Suppl. 1):48–63, 1970.

4. Kaiser, D. G., and Vangiessen, G. J. GLC determination of ibuprofen (+)-2-(*p*-isobutylphenyl) propionic acid in plasma. *J. Pharm. Sci.* 63:219–221, 1974.
5. Mills, R. F., Adams, S. S., et al. The metabolism of ibuprofen. *Xenobiotica* 3:589–598, 1973.
6. Thompson, M., and Anderson, M. Studies of gastrointestinal blood loss during ibuprofen therapy. *Rheumatol. Phys. Med.* 10(Suppl. 1):104–107, 1970.

IMIPRAMINE (and Desipramine)

Original dibenzazepine derivative used in the treatment of endogenous depression. Produces sedation and anticholinergic effects in normal people. Tricyclic antidepressants, unlike their close chemical relatives the phenothiazines, do not calm agitated psychotic patients but are indicated in the treatment of endogenous depression. Mode of action remains uncertain but may be related to inhibition of synaptic re-uptake of brain norepinephrine and 5-hydroxytryptamine, with increased concentrations of these transmitters in the synaptic cleft [10]. Other indications include the treatment of enuresis and of hyperactive, aggressive behavior in minimally brain-damaged children.

Absorption

Complete. Systemic bioavailability: 29%–77%; large variation in systemic bioavailability because of hepatic first-pass metabolism [7]. t_{max}: 30–60 minutes [5].

Distribution

V_d: 10–20 L/kg [7]. Protein binding: 95% [2]. There appears to be considerable distribution into many regions of the brain [3].

Elimination

Distribution phase: 3–8 hours [7]. Elimination $t_{\frac{1}{2}}$: 8–16 hours [7]. Metabolic processes include N-demethylation to desmethylimipramine (desipramine), which is active and plays an important therapeutic role, N-oxidation, and aliphatic and aromatic hydroxylation. Variable degrees of conjugation follow hydroxylation. Proportions of parent drug and metabolites found in urine are 1–4% for imipramine and desipramine, 40–60% for conjugated metabolites, 15–35% for nonconjugated metabolites, and the remaining percentage for nonextractable polar metabolites [4, 6].

The following absorption, distribution, and elimination figures apply for desipramine: t_{max}: 2–8 hours. V_d: 28–60 L/kg [1]. Protein binding: 90% [2]. $t_{\frac{1}{2}}$: 10–26 hours [1].

Dosage Schedule

25 mg 2–4 times daily in the first 2 weeks of treatment. If response is inadequate after 2 weeks, the dose may be increased at

weekly intervals by 25–50 mg daily to a maximum of 300 mg/day. Tolerance to minor side-effects may develop if increases in dosage are gradual.

Special Dosage Situations

Patients who have recently received monoamine oxidase inhibitors (MAOI) should not receive imipramine within a 2-week period of stopping therapy with MAOI. In children, the dose is usually 1–2.5 mg/kg daily for enuresis and up to 5 mg/kg/day for behavioral disturbance. A dose of 5 mg/kg/day should not be exceeded. ECG monitoring may be of value [9]. All tricyclic antidepressants should be used with care in the elderly and in patients with known cardiovascular disease. Urinary retention may be potentiated in elderly patients and in patients with prostatic obstruction. No special problems in women during pregnancy or lactation have been described.

Therapeutic Concentrations

Plasma concentrations of imipramine greater than 45 ng/ml and of desipramine greater than 75 ng/ml are necessary for a satisfactory clinical response [8]. Therapeutic response is limited by adverse reactions. Worsening of depression does not occur at high plasma concentrations, in contrast to the effect observed with high concentrations of nortriptyline [8].

Adverse Reactions

Anticholinergic effects are most common. These include dry mouth, blurred vision, constipation, urinary retention, and tachycardia. Weakness, fatigue, tremulousness, sweating, and parkinsonism may occur. Cardiovascular effects include ST-segment and T-wave changes on ECG, postural hypotension, arrhythmias, conduction defects, precipitation of heart failure, and possibly acute myocardial infarction.

Acute toxicity is characterized by high fever, hypotension or hypertension, cardiac arrhythmias, convulsions, and coma. The average acute lethal dose is 30 mg/kg. Treatment is generally symptomatic. The long duration of action is a problem, and therefore observation with ECG monitoring may be necessary for up to 72 hours after an overdose. Lidocaine or propranolol may be used to suppress ectopic arrhythmias. Specific treatment is available in the form of the centrally acting cholinesterase inhibitor physostigmine in a dose of 1–3 mg given by slow IV injection. This dose may be repeated every 30–60 minutes if necessary.

Interactions

MAOI and imipramine together may produce severe hypertension, hyperpyrexia, and convulsions.

Both imipramine and desipramine inhibit the antihypertensive effect of guanethidine and similar compounds, e.g., bethanidine and debrisoquine, by prevention of their uptake into nerve endings. Alpha-methyldopa is not affected.

Barbiturates may increase imipramine metabolism, by induction of mixed-function oxidase enzymes. Phenothiazines may decrease imipramine metabolism by enzyme inhibition.

Directly acting sympathomimetics, e.g., epinephrine and isoproterenol, should be used with care, since their effects may be enhanced. Indirectly acting sympathomimetics may have reduced activity.

The sympathomimetic effects of tricyclic antidepressants and thyroid hormone may be additive.

Other drugs with anticholinergic activity may in theory have additive effects with tricyclic antidepressants.

References

1. Alexanderson, B. Pharmacokinetics of nortriptyline in man after single and multiple oral doses: The predictability of steady state plasma concentrations from single dose plasma level data. *Eur. J. Clin. Pharmacol.* 5:1–10, 1972.
2. Borgå, O., Azarnoff, D. L., et al. Plasma protein binding of tricyclic antidepressants in man. *Biochem. Pharmacol.* 18:2135–2143, 1969.
3. Christiansen, J., and Gram, L. F. Imipramine and its metabolites in human brain. *J. Pharm. Pharmacol.* 25:604–608, 1973.
4. Christiansen, J., Gram, L. F., et al. Imipramine metabolism in man. A study of urinary metabolites after administration of radioactive imipramine. *Psychopharmacologia* 11:255–264, 1967.
5. Dencker, H., Dencker, S. J., et al. Intestinal absorption, demethylation, and enterohepatic circulation of imipramine. *Clin. Pharmacol. Ther.* 19:584–586, 1976.
6. Gram, L. F. Metabolism of tricyclic antidepressants. A review. *Dan. Med. Bull.* 21:218–231, 1974.
7. Gram, L. F., and Christiansen, J. First-pass metabolism of imipramine in man. *Clin. Pharmacol. Ther.* 17:555–563, 1975.
8. Gram, L. F., Reisby, N., et al. Plasma levels and antidepressant effect of imipramine. *Clin. Pharmacol. Ther.* 19:318–324, 1976.
9. Hayes, T. A., Panitch, M. L., et al. Imipramine dosage in children: A comment on imipramine and electrocardiographic abnormalities in hyperactive children. *Am. J. Psychiatry* 132:546–547, 1975.
10. Schildkraut, J. J., and Kety, S. S. Biogenic amines and emotion. *Science* 156:21–30, 1967.

INDOMETHACIN

An antipyretic analgesic with anti-inflammatory activity. Acts by inhibition of prostaglandin E_1 [4]. Major indications are rheumatoid arthritis, osteoarthritis, ankylosing spondylitis, psoriatic arthritis, pseudogout, and acute gouty arthritis.

Absorption

Systemic bioavailability: 90–100% orally and rectally [1, 6]. t_{max}: 1–2 hours [1]. Suppository acts like a delayed-release preparation [1].

Distribution

V_d: 0.3–1.6 L/kg [1]. Protein binding: 90% [5]. No available data about distribution to breast milk or across placenta.

Elimination

$t_{\frac{1}{2}}$: 3–11 hours [1]. About 80% metabolized by O-demethylation, N-deacylation, and glucuronidation to inactive metabolites excreted in bile and urine [3]. 10–20% is excreted unchanged in urine by both glomerular filtration and tubular secretion. About 50% of an IV dose undergoes enterohepatic circulation [6].

Dosage Schedule

Usual analgesic dose is 50–150 mg/day in 3 divided doses. A 100-mg suppository may be taken in evening to reduce morning stiffness. In acute gout, 200–400 mg/day for 2–3 days may be used. The drug should be taken after meals to lessen chance of gastric distress.

Special Dosage Situations

Use cautiously in patients with gastric or duodenal ulcer or psychiatric disorders. No available information about use in children or in women during pregnancy or lactation.

Therapeutic Concentrations

0.5–3 μg/ml, although it is usual to simply measure effect and adjust dosage accordingly. Side-effects become very common at levels above 6 μg/ml [1].

Adverse Reactions

High incidence of side-effects. Untoward symptoms appear in approximately 35–50% of patients on usual therapeutic doses [2]. Anorexia, nausea, dyspepsia, peptic ulcer, acute pancreatitis, and hepatitis; frontal throbbing headache, dizziness, light-headedness, mental confusion, depression, psychosis, hallucination, blurred vision, visual disturbance, and hearing disturbance; and neutropenia and aplastic anemia.

Interactions

Probenecid inhibits the tubular secretion of indomethacin [7]. Indomethacin reduces platelet adhesion and should be used with caution with anticoagulants and other drugs with this property. Increases incidence of peptic ulcer when given with other ulcerogenic drugs. Decreases hypotensive and natriuretic effect of furosemide.

References

1.   Alvan, G., Orme, M., et al.   Pharmacokinetics of indomethacin. *Clin. Pharmacol. Ther.* 18:364–373, 1975.

2. Boardman, P. L., and Hart, F. D.   Side effects of indomethacin. *Ann. Rheum. Dis.* 26:127–132, 1967.
3. Duggan, D. E., and Hogans, A. F.   The metabolism of indomethacin in man. *J. Pharmacol. Exp. Ther.* 181:563–575, 1972.
4. Ferreira, S. H., and Vane, J. R.   New aspects of the mode of action of nonsteroid anti-inflammatory drugs. *Ann. Rev. Pharmacol.* 14:57–73, 1974.
5. Hvidberg, E., Lausen, H. H., et al.   Indomethacin: Plasma concentrations and protein binding in man. *Eur. J. Clin. Pharmacol.* 4:119–124, 1972.
6. Kwan, K. E., Breault, G. O., et al.   Kinetics of indomethacin absorption, elimination, and enterohepatic circulation in man. *J. Pharmacokin. Biopharm.* 4:255–280, 1976.
7. Skeith, M. D., Simkin, P. A., et al.   The renal excretion of indomethacin and its inhibition by probenecid. *Clin. Pharmacol. Ther.* 9:89–93, 1968.

INSULIN

A polypeptide consisting of 51 amino acids arranged in 2 chains (A and B), joined together by 2 disulfide linkages. Porcine and bovine insulin differ by 1 and 3 amino acids, respectively, from human insulin, but their activity is practically the same. Synthesized and stored in the beta cells of pancreatic islets as proinsulin (86 amino acids). Secreted as insulin after a variety of stimuli: glucose, amino acids, and fatty acids; gastrointestinal hormones such as pancreozymin, gastrin, secretin, amd glucagon; and cholinergic and beta-adrenergic stimulation, alpha-adrenergic blockade, and sulfonylureas. The secretion is inhibited by alpha-adrenergic stimulating drugs and beta-adrenergic blocking drugs, diazoxide, phenytoin, and somatostatin. The secretory response is mediated through cyclic adenosine monophosphate (cAMP). The normal daily insulin production is about 40 units. The potency of the US Reference Standard is of the order of 25 units per milligram.

The primary action of insulin is to increase the transport of glucose from the extracellular fluid to muscle and fat cells, subsequently increasing the synthesis of glycogen, triglycerides, and peptides. The cellular uptake of potassium is also enhanced. The mobilization of fatty acids and gluconeogenesis is inhibited. The action of insulin appears to be independent of cAMP.

Insulin is indicated in the treatment of juvenile diabetes mellitus and in maturity-onset diabetes that cannot be treated satisfactorily with diet alone or with diet in combination with oral hypoglycemic agents.

Absorption

Not absorbed orally because of complete hydrolysis to amino acids in the gastrointestinal tract. Parenteral t_{max} is unknown, but it is probably close to the time of peak action. About 50% of the insulin secreted is inactivated in the liver during the first passage, a physiological first-pass effect.

Distribution
V_d: about 0.6 L/kg. Protein binding: 1–10%.

Elimination
$t_{\frac{1}{2}}$ (alpha): about 10 minutes. $t_{\frac{1}{2}}$ (beta): 90–120 minutes. However, there is much disagreement about these figures, depending on methodology [2, 3, 4]. Inactivated in the liver and kidneys. In severe renal failure, the half-life is prolonged to more than 3–4 hours [2]. Failing liver function affects the half-life less, since normal kidneys seem capable of increasing their metabolic capacity. Insulin is excreted by glomerular filtration, but little insulin is lost in the urine because of back-diffusion in the renal tubules. Urinary excretion of insulin is about 5 units daily [1].

Dosage Schedule
Insulins are classified by the following guidelines, according to duration of action after subcutaneous injection:

		Onset (hr)	Peak (hr)	Duration (hr)
Rapid	Crystalline insulin (regular insulin)	0.5	1–2	4–8
	Single peak purified insulin	0.5	1–2	4–8
	Semilente insulin	1	3–4	8–16
Interme- diate	NPH insulin (isophane insulin)	2	8–10	16–24
	Lente insulin	2	8–10	16–24
	Globin insulin	2	6–8	16–24
Delayed	Ultralente insulin	6	18–24	24–36
	Protamine zinc insulin	6	18–24	24–36

Note the difference in concentration of preparation: 40, 80, or 100 units/ml. Regular insulin can be mixed with all other insulins except protamine zinc insulin. Semilente, lente, and ultralente insulins may be mixed with each other but not with other insulins. Only regular insulin can be given IV. The dose is highly variable and must be adjusted individually. Usually, the initial dose is 16–20 units of intermediate-acting insulin given in the morning. If the dose has to be increased above 40 units per 24 hours, it is usual to give two-thirds of the dose in the morning and one-third in the evening. To match a high morning caloric intake, 20–50% of the morning dose can be given as rapidly acting insulin.

Special Dosage Situations
Ketoacidotic diabetic coma: correction of fluid depletion is essential. The current recommended regimen is intravenous infusion or frequent small IV or IM doses (5–10 unit/hr crystalline insulin) in conjunction with very careful monitoring of glucose, acid-base, and electrolyte status.

Hyperosmolar nonketotic coma: replace fluids. Small amounts of insulin usually restore euglycemia.

Renal disease: the need for insulin often reduced, probably because of reduced renal insulin inactivation.

Children, elderly, and patients with hepatic disease: no special dosage adjustments.

Pregnancy: increased demand for insulin in last 2–4 months of pregnancy.

Surgery: in the morning before the operation, about 50% of the total daily dose is given as a delayed action preparation. During the operation a glucose drip with rapid-acting insulin (24 units/L 5% dextrose solution) or dextrose solution by itself may be administered.

Therapeutic Concentrations

The plasma concentration of immunoreactive insulin (IRI) of fasting normal persons is 10–20 μU/ml. After a large glucose load, the concentration may increase to about 100 μU/ml.

Adverse Reactions

Most common side-effect is hypoglycemia from overdosage. Main symptoms and signs are sweating, weakness, tachycardia, hunger, "inner" trembling and later confusion, slurred speech, convulsions, and coma. The immediately effective treatment is 10–25 g glucose IV. If the patient is completely awake, glucose can be given orally. 1 mg of glucagon by the IM route is an alternative treatment; glucagon may be given by relatives of the patient after explanation by the physician of the appropriate procedure.

Other side-effects are insulin resistance, defined as the requirement of more than 200 units/day, and lipodystrophy, with localized atrophy and the formation of fibrous nodules. Allergic reactions such as urticaria and angioedema are rare.

Interactions

Increased risk of hypoglycemia, with concomitant treatment with beta blockers or salicylates.

Reviews

Nabarro, J. D. N. (Ed.). Symposium. Insulin metabolism. *Postgrad. Med. J.* 49(Suppl. 7):931–963, 1973.

Rubenstein, A. H., and Spitz, I. Role of the kidney in insulin metabolism and excretion. *Diabetes* 17:161–169, 1968.

References

1. Chamberlain, M. J., and Stimmler, L. The renal handling of insulin. *J. Clin. Invest.* 46:911–919, 1967.
2. O'Brien, J. P., and Sharpe, A. R. The influence of renal disease on the insulin I[131] disappearance curve in man. *Metabolism* 16:76–83, 1967.
3. Ørskov, H., and Christensen, N. J. Plasma disappearance rate of injected human insulin in juvenile diabetic, maturity-onset diabetic, and nondiabetic subjects. *Diabetes* 18:653–659, 1969.

4. Stimler, L., Mashiter, K., et al.   Insulin disappearance after intravenous injection and its effect on blood glucose in diabetic and non-diabetic children and adults. *Clin. Sci.* 42:337–344, 1972.

ISONIAZID

Chemically related to the monoamine oxidase inhibitor (MAOI) iproniazid, isoniazid is effective as a primary antituberculous chemotherapeutic agent; the mechanism of action is unknown. No MAOI effect. Active against most strains of mycobacteria, but resistance develops easily if used alone. No cross-resistance to other antituberculous drugs. Indicated in all forms of tuberculosis (given in a combination regimen) and the drug of choice for chemoprophylaxis (given alone).

Absorption
Oral biovailability: 90%. t_{max}: 1–2 hours.

Distribution
V_d: about 0.6 L/kg [4]. Protein binding: 50% [14]. The concentration in CSF is about 20% of the serum concentration [5], which is similar to the concentration in pleural fluid and breast milk [2].

Elimination
$t_{\frac{1}{2}}$: 0.7–2 hours in fast acetylators and 2–4 hours in slow acetylators. This effect is due to a genetically determined bimodal difference of the enzyme acetyl transferase in the population [10, 13]. Slow acetylators are recessive homozygous; fast acetylators are heterozygous or dominant homozygous. The distribution in the population between fast and slow acetylators is independent of sex but highly variable between different ethnic groups. A low prevalence of slow acetylators is found among most Orientals (10–20%), whereas 50–60% of whites and blacks are slow acetylators [6, 7]. Among diabetics there seems to be a slightly higher prevalence of rapid acetylators than in the general population [10]. Slow or rapid acetylation may be determined by measuring the plasma concentration of isoniazid 6 hours after an oral dose of 4 mg/kg. Slow acetylators have a serum concentration above 0.8 μg/ml; rapid acetylators have a concentration below 0.8 μg/ml [6]. Alternatively, measurements of sulfamethazine (sulphadimidine) elimination from serum or urine can be used to determine if a patient has slow or fast acetylation [8]. 10–40% of isoniazid is excreted unchanged; about 50% is acetylated by the liver; and the remainder is hydrolyzed to isonicotinic and isonicotinuric acids, which are all excreted by the renal route [4, 5]. Slow acetylators excrete a relatively higher fraction of unchanged isoniazid than fast acetylators [11, 13].

Dosage Schedule
5 mg/kg up to a maximum of 300 mg daily, given in a single dose or in divided doses. Acetylation status does not seem to affect therapeutic success.

Special Dosage Situations

Children: 10–15 mg/kg/day; in tuberculous meningitis up to 30 mg/kg/day, in 2–3 divided doses. Renal disease: no dosage adjustments; the $t_{\frac{1}{2}}$ and the rate of acetylation seem to be almost normal [3, 12]. Hepatic disease: use isoniazid with great caution and in reduced doses because of delayed elimination. $t_{\frac{1}{2}}$ in advanced liver failure is 5–7 hours [1]. Pregnancy and lactation: dosage unchanged.

Prophylaxis with isoniazid is not recommended in patients over the age of 35 years who have a positive tuberculin conversion, because of an increased risk of hepatotoxicity.

Therapeutic Concentrations

Not established. Minimum tuberculostatic concentration is about 0.5 μg/ml.

Adverse Reactions

Dose-related side-effects are dermatitis, neuritis (often including the optic nerve), convulsions, mental disturbances (such as euphoria, loss of memory, or psychosis), dizziness, ataxia, and paresthesiae. Pyridoxine 50–100 mg daily reduces or abolishes all of these side-effects. Hepatocellular toxicity seems to be more frequent in fast acetylators than in slow acetylators, presumably because of the formation of the toxic metabolite acetylhydrazine [11].

Allergic reactions are fever, skin rashes, bone marrow depression, vasculitis, and systemic lupus erythematosus, which are all rare. Isoniazid is not eliminated by dialysis.

Interactions

In slow acetylators isoniazid may inhibit the metabolism of phenytoin [9]. Para-aminosalicylic acid inhibits acetylation and prolongs the half-life in both rapid and slow acetylators, but the clinical significance is uncertain [14].

References

1. Acocella, G., Bonollo, L., et al.   Kinetics of rifampicin and isoniazid administered alone and in combination to normal subjects and patients with liver disease. *Gut* 13:47–53, 1972.
2. Barclay, W. R., Ebert, R. H., et al.   Distribution and excretion of radioactive isoniazid in tuberculous patients. *J.A.M.A.* 151:1384–1388, 1953.
3. Bowersox, D. W., Winterbrauer, R. H., et al.   Isoniazid dosage in patients with renal failure. *N. Engl. J. Med.* 289:84–87, 1973.
4. Boxenbaum, H. G., and Riegelman, S.   Pharmacokinetics of isoniazid and some metabolites in man. *J. Pharmacokin. Biopharm.* 4:287–325, 1976.
5. DesPrez, R., and Boon, I. U.   Metabolism of C^{14}-isoniazid in humans. *Am. Rev. Resp. Dis.* 84:42–51, 1961.
6. Dufour, A. P., Knight, R. A., et al.   Genetics of isoniazid metabolism in Caucasian, Negro, and Japanese populations. *Science* 145:391, 1964.

7. Evans, D. A. P.   Genetic variations in the acetylation of isoniazid and other drugs. *Ann. N.Y. Acad. Sci.* 151:723–733, 1968.

8. Evans, D. A. P.   An improved and simplified method of detecting the acetylator phenotype. *J. Med. Genet.* 6:405–407, 1969.

9. Kutt, H., Brennan, R., et al.   Diphenylhydantoin intoxication. A complication of isoniazid therapy. *Am. Rev. Resp. Dis.* 101:377–383, 1970.

10. Mattila, M. J., and Tiitinen, H.   The rate of isoniazid inactivation in a Finnish diabetic and non-diabetic patients. *Ann. Med. Exp. Biol. Fenn.* 45:423–427, 1967.

11. Mitchell, J. R., Thorgeirsson, U. P., et al.   Increased incidence of isoniazid hepatitis in rapid acetylators: Possible relation to hydrazine metabolites. *Clin. Pharmacol Ther.* 18:70–79, 1976.

12. Reidenberg, M. M., and Shear, L.   Elimination of isoniazid in patients with impaired renal function. *Am. Rev. Resp. Dis.* 108:1426–1428, 1973.

13. Tiitinen, H.   Isoniazid and ethionamide serum levels and inactivation in Finnish subjects. *Scand. J. Resp. Dis.* 50:110–124, 1969.

14. Tiitinen, H.   Modification by para-aminosalicylic acid and sulfamethazine of the isoniazid inactivation in man. *Scand. J. Resp. Dis.* 50:281–290, 1969.

ISOPROTERENOL
(Isoprenaline)

Isopropylnorepinephrine, a potent synthetic sympathomimetic amine with nonselective beta-adrenoceptor agonist activity; used as a bronchodilator, a cardiac stimulant, and occasionally to enhance atrioventricular (A-V) conduction. Pharmacological actions include an increase in cardiac inotropic and chronotropic activities; a reduction of peripheral vascular resistance, with additional vasodilation of renal and mesenteric arteries; an increase in cardiac output; and a slight increase in systolic pressure but a reduction in mean arterial pressure. Excitability and conductivity of cardiac tissues are greatly increased. Relaxation of smooth muscle accompanies a nonspecific reduction in histamine release after allergic stimulus. There is relaxation of the pregnant uterus. The main metabolic effect of the drug in man is the release of free fatty acids.

Absorption
Oral absorption is almost complete, but there is extensive first-pass metabolism, probably by sulfation in the intestine. Oral t_{max}: 80 minutes [2]. Inhalation t_{max}: 10 minutes [1]. Most of the drug given by inhaler is in fact swallowed [3].

Distribution
V_d: about 0.5 L/kg [1]. Protein binding: unknown.

Elimination

$t_{\frac{1}{2}}$: 2½ hours [2]. The metabolic pattern of drug given by the IV route differs markedly from that given orally or by spray. After IV dosage, 66% of drug is excreted unchanged, the remainder is excreted as free and conjugated 3-*O*-methyl metabolite [2]. After oral dosage 6–16% of drug is excreted unchanged, 3–11% of the dose is excreted as mainly conjugated 3-*O*-methyl isoproterenol, and 80%, or the majority, as sulfuric acid conjugated isoproterenol [2]. 3-*O*-methyl isoproterenol is a very weak beta-adrenergic antagonist formed by the action of catechol-*O*-methyl transferase (COMT).

Dosage Schedule

Reversible airway disease: 20 μg by aerosol produces a maximum response [5]. However, most commercial aerosols contain much more than 20 μg of the drug. Total daily dosage should not exceed 900 μg–1000 μg, and patients should be strongly advised to seek medical attention if asthmatic symptoms are not readily relieved.

Shock: infusion at a rate of 1–10 μg/min dilates the vascular bed and improves the peripheral circulation, resulting in diminution of anaerobic metabolism. Generally, the blood pressure decreases. Dopamine is usually preferred to isoproterenol as an inotropic agent, since tachycardia and arrhythmias are less likely to occur and renal artery dilation is greater.

Heart block: sublingual and sustained-release preparations are available, but absorption of these preparations is erratic and side-effects are often troublesome. In this situation, a cardiac pacemaker is usually the treatment of choice.

Special Dosage Situations

There is no available specific information about renal or hepatic disease. No contraindication to use of bronchodilating doses in women during pregnancy. Angina pectoris may be precipitated in patients with ischemic heart disease.

Therapeutic Concentrations

No available data.

Adverse Reactions

Tachycardia, arrhythmias, palpitations, headache, flushing, tremor, apprehension, and dizziness.

An epidemic of deaths among young asthmatics in certain countries appears to have been related to an excessive use of concentrated solutions of isoproterenol (10 mg/ml) [4]. Other factors contributing to these deaths which are under debate include anoxemia; the Freons used as propellants; refractoriness to the effect of isoproterenol, followed by vasodilation and cardiovascular collapse; and sensitization, producing serious cardiac arrhythmias.

Toxicity may be controlled by careful IV administration of a beta-blocking drug such as propranolol, noting that this drug may aggravate airway obstruction in individuals with pulmonary disease.

Interactions

Possibility of toxicity is increased when given concurrently with other directly or indirectly acting sympathomimetics, theophylline, and thyroid replacement.

References

1. Blackwell, E. W., Briant, R. H., et al.   Metabolism of isoprenaline after aerosol and direct intrabronchial administration in man and dog. Br. J. Pharmacol. 50:587–591, 1974.
2. Conolly, M. E., Davies, D. S., et al.   Metabolism of isoprenaline in dog and man. Br. J. Pharmacol. 46:458–472, 1972.
3. Paterson, J. W., Conolly, M. E., et al.   Isoprenaline resistance and the use of pressurised aerosols in asthma. Lancet 2:426–429, 1968.
4. Stolley, P. D.   Asthma mortality. Why the United States was spared an epidemic of deaths due to asthma. Am. Rev. Resp. Dis. 105:883–890, 1972.
5. Williams, M. H., Jr., and Kane, C.   Dose response of patients with asthma to inhaled isoproterenol. Am. Rev. Resp. Dis. 111:321–324, 1975.

LEVODOPA

3-4-Dihydroxyphenylalanine; indicated in the management of Parkinson's disease that is idiopathic, postencephalitic, or caused by manganese toxicity. Especially valuable in the relief of muscle stiffness and akinesia but less valuable in the control of tremor. Of no value in the treatment of arteriosclerotic Parkinson's syndrome or the extrapyramidal syndrome associated with phenothiazine usage. Also indicated in the management of hepatic coma and may have value as a provocative agent in predicting the onset of Huntington's chorea. Has been used as a test of pituitary function because of its ability to raise blood levels of growth hormone (GH) [3] and thyrotrophic hormone (TRH) [4] and to lower levels of prolactin [5].

Acts by being metabolized by dopa decarboxylase to dopamine, replacing this CNS neurotransmitter that is deficient in Parkinson's disease. Metabolism occurs throughout the body as well as in the brain. The blood-brain barrier is impervious to dopamine but not to levodopa. This metabolism may be blocked peripherally but not centrally by dopa decarboxylase inhibitors (e.g., benzserazide and alpha-methyldopahydrazine), thus allowing more levodopa to cross the blood-brain barrier. The inhibition of peripheral metabolism also decreases the peripheral side-effects of dopamine.

Absorption

Orally, 20–30% absorbed from the stomach and duodenum by active transport. Degradation in the bowel is increased and absorption decreased by delayed gastric emptying time, decreased stomach pH, and prolonged intestinal transit time [1]. t_{max}: 0.5–4 hours. Absorption is not only highly variable between individuals but also in the same individual at different times. A first-pass effect exists [7] and may be saturable if drug is delivered rapidly to the duodenum, e.g., by the concurrent administration of metoclopramide [6].

Distribution

V_d: unknown. Protein binding: unknown. Widely distributed to tissues, where it is metabolized rather than stored. This phenomenon also appears to apply to the brain, where it does not enter storage granules in presynaptic nerve endings.

Elimination

$t_{\frac{1}{2}}$: 3 hours. Completely metabolized, the major metabolites being phenylcarboxylic acid and 3-*O*-methyldopa. Metabolism is inhibited 70–80% by dopa decarboxylase inhibitors and the $t_{\frac{1}{2}}$ is prolonged to 15 hours [2].

Dosage Schedule

0.5–8 g orally once daily. Initial regimen should be small doses, e.g., 250 mg 1–4 times daily after meals. This regimen may be increased by 250–1000 mg/day every 2–3 days, thus allowing the patient to develop tolerance to the side-effects. Multiple small doses have a more uniform effect than single large doses. The induction period may be shortened and the dose diminished by at least 50% by the concurrent use of a decarboxylase inhibitor, e.g., alpha-methyldopahydrazine (carbidopa), in a dose of 100 mg/day. Note that carbidopa is available only as a combination tablet with levodopa. Therefore, both levodopa and levodopa plus carbidopa may need to be given in certain dosage requirements of levodopa.

Long-term dosage often requires frequent readjustment because of sudden loss of muscular control or development of side-effects. The reasons for these fluctuations are not clear.

Special Dosage Situations

Care should be taken in administering levodopa to patients with episodic cardiac arrhythmias, previous mental illness, hemolytic anemia, gastrointestinal bleeding, and renal, hepatic, and gouty disease. Contraindicated in malignant melanoma.

Therapeutic Concentrations

Not known.

Adverse Reactions

"On-off effect," i.e., rapid fluctuation between freedom from side-effects and full-blown Parkinsonism, due to inadequate medication and paralysis due to excessive blood levels. Side-effects, such as gastrointestinal upsets, generally occur early, but tolerance usually develops and can be avoided with carbidopa. Orthostatic hypotension, ventricular premature contractions, and ventricular tachycardia are diminished with carbidopa. Anxiety, insomnia, and acute toxic delirium also occur. Involuntary movements sometimes occur after therapy has been established and may be exacerbated by carbidopa. Transient pancytopenia, development of a positive Coombs' test, and elevations of serum alkaline phosphatase and serum glutamic-oxaloacetic transaminase, blood urea nitrogen, and uric acid may occur. Occasionally, clinical gout may ensue. Levodopa also appears to enhance the recurrence of malignant melanoma, although the evidence for this effect is not conclusive.

Interactions

Monoamine oxidase inhibitors (MAOI), pyridoxine, papaverine, phenothiazines, and other major tranquilizers interfere with levodopa's effect; pyridoxine (vitamin B_6) is present in many vitamin preparations sold over the counter. Levodopa causes false positive results in tests for urinary glucose and ketones.

Reviews

Pelton, E. W., III, and Chase, T. N.   L-Dopa and the treatment of extrapyramidal disease. *Acta Pharmacol. Toxicol.* 13:253–304, 1975.

Yahr, M. D.   Levodopa. *Ann. Int. Med.* 83:677–682, 1975.

References

1. Bianchine, J. R., Calimlim, L. R., et al.   Metabolism and absorption of 1-3, 4 dihydroxyphenylalanine in patients with Parkinson's disease. *Ann. N.Y. Acad. Sci.* 179:126–140, 1971.
2. Bianchine, J. R., Messiha, F. S., et al.   Peripheral aromatic L-amino acids decarboxylase inhibitor in Parkinsonism. II. Effect on metabolism of L-2-^{14}C-dopa. *Clin. Pharmacol. Ther.* 13:584–594, 1972.
3. Boyd, A. E., Lebovitz, H. E., et al.   Stimulation of human growth hormone secretion by L-dopa. *N. Engl. J. Med.* 283:1425–1429, 1970.
4. Burrow, G. N., Spaulding, S. W., et al.   The effect of L-dopa on the hypothalamic-pituitary-thyroid axis. *Adv. Neurol.* 5:489–493, 1974.
5. Frantz, A. G., and Shuh, H. K.   L-Dopa and the control of prolactin secretion. *Adv. Neurol.* 5:447–455, 1974.
6. Mearick, P. T., Wade, D. N., et al.   Metoclopramide, gastric emptying and L-dopa absorption. *Aust. N.Z. J. Med.* 4:144–148, 1974.
7. Peaston, M. J. T., and Bianchine, J. R.   Metabolic studies and clinical observations during L-dopa treatment of Parkinson's disease. *Br. Med. J.* 1:400–403, 1970.

LIDOCAINE
(Lignocaine)

A member of the procaine family of local anesthetics; is a weak base. Indicated for therapy of ventricular ectopic arrhythmias in addition to its common use as a local anesthetic.

Absorption
Orally, less than 15% systemically bioavailable due to high clearance by liver [4]. IV route most satisfactory for antiarrhythmic therapy.

Distribution
V_d: 1.6 L/kg [6]. Protein binding: 60% [9]. Distributed within minutes to heart, lungs, and liver; later stored in adipose tissue and muscle [1].

Elimination
$t_\frac{1}{2}$ in adults: 90 minutes. About 70% metabolized by the liver; major metabolites are 4-hydroxy-2,6-dimethylalanine, mono-ethylglycinexylidide (MEGX), and glycinexylidide (GX) [5]. MEGX and GX have some antiarrhythmic activity and are probably responsible for the CNS effects of lidocaine. $t_\frac{1}{2}$ of GX: 10 hours [7]. Metabolites and small amounts of parent drug appear in urine, with greater amounts of parent drug appearing in alkaline urine [2].

Dosage Schedule
Loading dose of 1.5 mg/kg repeated after 20 minutes should yield plasma level above 2.0 μg/ml [3]. At the same time an intravenous infusion should be commenced, 25–30 μg/kg/min, to give plasma level in the therapeutic range. Without loading dose, infusion will take 4–5 hours to reach steady state in normal subjects.

Special Dosage Situations
Care is required in administering lidocaine to patients with cardiac failure (V_d reduced and $t_\frac{1}{2}$ increased to 10–12 hours) and those with hepatic failure ($t_\frac{1}{2}$ increased), since clearance of the drug is reduced in these conditions; loading dose should be used to achieve therapeutic levels and a lowered rate of infusion. Although drug is excreted by the kidneys, no toxic effects from accumulation of parent drug or metabolites in the blood have yet been demonstrated in patients with renal disease [8]. No known contraindications.

Therapeutic Concentrations
1–5 μg/ml.

Adverse Reactions
Hypotension, heart block, confusion, and seizures. Note that CNS effects, probably due to metabolites, occur most frequently at lidocaine plasma levels in excess of 9 μg/ml. Treatment is to stop administration of the drug.

Interactions
Propranolol $t_\frac{1}{2}$ prolonged by simultaneous administration of lidocaine, probably because of alteration of hepatic hemodynamics.

References

1. Benowitz, N., Forsyth, R. P., et al. Lidocaine disposition kinetics in monkey and man. 1. Prediction by a perfusion model. *Clin. Pharmacol. Ther.* 16:87–98, 1974.
2. Eriksson, E., and Granberg, P. Studies on the renal excretion of Citanest and Xylocaine. *Acta Anaesthesiol. Scand.* 16(Suppl. 1):79–85, 1965.
3. Greenblatt, D. J., Bolognini, V., et al. Pharmacokinetic approach to the clinical use of lidocaine intravenously. *J.A.M.A.* 236:273–277, 1976.
4. Gugler, R., Lain, P., et al. Effect of portocaval shunt on the disposition of drugs with or without first-pass effect. *J. Pharmacol. Exp. Ther.* 195:416–423, 1976.
5. Keenaghan, J. B., and Boyes, R. N. The tissue distribution metabolism and excretion of lidocaine in rats, guinea pigs, dogs, and man. *J. Pharmacol. Exp. Ther.* 180:454–463, 1972.
6. Rowland, M., Thomson, P. D., et al. Disposition kinetics of lidocaine in normal subjects. *Ann. N.Y. Acad. Sci.* 179:383–398, 1971.
7. Strong, J. M., Mayfield, D. S., et al. Pharmacological activity, metabolism, and pharmacokinetics of glycinexylidide. *Clin. Pharmacol. Ther.* 17:184–194, 1975.
8. Thomson, P. D., Melmon, K. L., et al. Lidocaine pharmacokinetics in advanced heart failure, liver disease, and renal failure in humans. *Ann. Intern. Med.* 78:499–503, 1973.
9. Tucker, G. T., Boyes, R. N., et al. Binding of anilide-type local anesthetics in human subjects. 1. Relationship between binding, physicochemical properties, and anesthetic activity. *Anesthesiology* 33:287–303, 1970.

LINCOMYCIN

Water-soluble, acid-stable antibiotic related to clindamycin. Bacteriostatic—in high concentrations bacteriocidal—by inhibition of bacterial protein synthesis. Active against most grampositive species, including penicillinase-producing staphylococci. Inactive against enterococci. Inactive against all gram-negative species except obligate anaerobes such as *Bacteroides*. Often cross-resistant with erythromycin.

Absorption

Oral bioavailability: about 40% [4, 5, 6]. Reduced by food [3]. Oral t_{max}: 2–4 hours. Intramuscular t_{max}: about 1 hour [5].

Distribution

V_d: about 0.35 L/kg [4]. Protein binding: 70% [2]. No passage through normal meninges; in meningitis, CSF concentration is about 40% of serum concentration [5]. Concentration in fetal circulation is 50% and in breast milk is 50–75% of the maternal serum concentration [5]. Penetrates into bone better than most antibiotics, producing a level of about 20% of the serum concentration [1].

Elimination

t$_{\frac{1}{2}}$: about 5 hours [4]. Mainly eliminated by the liver as unknown metabolites. 10–30% of parent drug excreted unchanged in the urine by glomerular filtration [6].

Dosage Schedule

Oral: 500 mg 6–8 hourly, at least 2 hours before meals. IM: 600 mg every 6–12 hours, by deep injection. IV: 600 mg dissolved in 250 ml of isotonic saline or glucose every 8–12 hours; infusion time at least 1 hour because of risk of cardiopulmonary arrest.

Special Dosage Situations

Children: oral dose is 20–60 mg/kg/day in 2 or 3 divided doses, and the IV dose is 10 mg/kg once or twice daily in a 200-ml solution. Renal failure: no dosage adjustment. Hepatic failure: half of usual dose may be satisfactory. No specific dose adjustment in elderly or in women during pregnancy or lactation. No contraindications to use except allergy to lincomycin and clindamycin.

Therapeutic Concentrations

2–10 μg/ml, depending on bacterial sensitivity.

Adverse Reactions

Especially with oral dosage, diarrhea (20%), pseudomembranous colitis (10% of cases may be fatal), glossitis, stomatitis; skin rashes, vaginitis, leucopenia, and thrombocytopenia. Cross-allergy with clindamycin. Drug not removed by dialysis.

Interactions

Lincomycin, chloramphenicol, and erythromycin mutually antagonize each other's antibiotic effect. Lincomycin potentiates neuromuscular blocking agents.

Review

Sanders, E. Lincomycin, fact, fancy, and future. *Med. Clin. North Am.* 54:1295–1303, 1970.

References

1. Davis, W. McL., and Balcom, J. H. Lincomycin studies of drug absorption and efficacy. *Oral Surg.* 27:688–696, 1969.
2. Gordon, R. C., Regamey, C., et al. Serum protein binding of erythromycin, lincomycin, and clindamycin. *J. Pharm. Sci.* 62:1074–1077, 1973.
3. Kaplan, K., Chew, W. H., et al. Microbiological, pharmacological, and clinical studies of lincomycin. *Am. J. Med. Sci.* 250:137–146, 1965.
4. Ma, P., Lim, M., et al. Human pharmacological studies of lincomycin, a new antibiotic for gram-positive organisms. *Antimicrob. Agents Chemother.* 183–188, 1963.
5. Medina, A., Fiske, N., et al. Absorption, diffusion, and

excretion of a new antibiotic, lincomycin. *Antimicrob. Agents Chemother.* 189–196, 1963.
6. Vavra, J. J., Sokolski, W. T., et al.   Absorption and excretion of lincomycin hydrochloride in human volunteers. *Antimicrob. Agents Chemother.* 176–182, 1963.

LITHIUM CARBONATE

The lithium ion has no known physiological role nor any psychotropic effect in normal people. Its close chemical relationship to sodium and potassium appears responsible for a variety of pharmacological actions in the brain, kidneys, thyroid gland, heart, and, to a lesser extent, other tissues. A probable mechanism for its action is replacement of intracellular potassium and extracellular sodium and also interference with magnesium involved in enzyme activity. Major indication for use of lithium is the prophylactic management of manic-depressive illness. May also be used in the treatment of acute manic (but not depressive) episodes of this illness. Its role in the treatment of thyrotoxicosis is being explored [5].

Absorption
t_{max}: 1–2 hours [6]. Absorption complete.

Distribution
V_d: 0.7 L/kg [6]. Protein binding: none. Salivary levels relate to plasma concentrations and are 2–3 times greater [6]. Erythrocyte concentrations are 5–40% of plasma concentrations. Red cell levels have been suggested as a means of assessing change in clinical condition and predicting toxicity [4]. Lithium is distributed readily to the fetus and to breast milk.

Elimination
Marked biphasic elimination. $t_{\frac{1}{2}}$: 4–6 hours for alpha distribution phase; $t_{\frac{1}{2}}$: 7–20 hours for beta elimination phase [1, 6]. Excretion in urine essentially complete, with minor amounts in sweat and feces. Renal clearance 20–30% of creatinine clearance; tubular reabsorption probably occurs [6].

Dosage Schedule
20–25 mg/kg/day orally in 2–4 divided doses. The plasma concentration 24 hours after a single 600-mg oral dose may help in determining long-term dosage requirements [3].

Special Dosage Situations
Avoid if possible in women during pregnancy; a higher than normal incidence of cardiovascular abnormalities has been reported in infants whose mothers take lithium during pregnancy [9]. Adjust dosage according to renal function in the elderly and in patients with known kidney disease. No special precautions for use in patients with liver disease.

Therapeutic Concentrations

0.8–1.4 mEq/L. The incidence of toxicity rises steeply with plasma concentrations above 2.0 mEq/L. Blood samples should be taken at least 10–15 hours after the previous dose to make sure that absorption and distribution are complete, e.g., in the morning after previous evening dose [1]. Initially, weekly measurements of plasma concentrations are advisable and, subsequently, after dosage adjustments. After stabilization, monthly measurements are usually satisfactory.

Adverse Reactions

Nausea, vomiting, diarrhea, abdominal cramps, tremor, sleepiness, coma, weight gain, electrocardiographic changes in S–T segment, renal and respiratory failure, and goiter. Nephrogenic diabetes insipidus may rarely develop.

Dialysis and the promotion of increased lithium excretion in urine by urea, acetazolamide, sodium bicarbonate, and theophylline may be used in the treatment of severe toxicity. Nevertheless, clinical improvement after overdose may take several days and probably relates to the slow removal of lithium from the brain.

Interactions

Single doses of furosemide, bendroflumethiazide, ethacrynic acid, ammonium chloride, and spironolactone produce no change in renal clearance, whereas sodium bicarbonate, acetazolamide, urea diuresis, and aminophylline increase clearance substantially [8]. Long-term thiazide therapy may, however, impair renal elimination of lithium [7]. Increased dietary sodium may lead to a gradual increase in lithium excretion [8].

A serious syndrome of irreversible brain damage has been reported in 4 patients who were given lithium and then received haloperidol for management of acute mania [2].

Reviews

Amdisen, A.   Monitoring of lithium treatment through determination of lithium concentration. *Dan. Med. Bull.* 22:277–291, 1975.

Gershon, S.   Lithium prophylaxis in recurrent affective disorders. *Compr. Psychiatry* 15:365–373, 1974.

Prien, R. F., and Caffey, E. M.   Lithium prophylaxis: A critical review. *Compr. Psychiatry* 15:357–363, 1974.

References

1. Amdisen, A.   Serum lithium estimations. *Br. Med. J.* 2:240, 1973.
2. Cohen, W. J., and Cohen, N. H.   Lithium carbonate, haloperidol, and irreversible brain damage. *J.A.M.A.* 230:1283–1287, 1974.
3. Cooper, T. B., Vergner, P.-E. E., et al.   The 24-hour serum lithium level as a prognosticator of dosage requirements. *Am. J. Psychiatry* 130:601–603, 1973.

4. Elizur, A., Shopsin, B., et al. Intra : Extracellular lithium ratios and clinical course in affective states. *Clin. Pharmacol. Ther.* 13:947–952, 1972.
5. Gerdes, H., Littmann, K. P., et al. Die Behandlung der Thyreotoxikose mit Lithium. *Dtsch. Med. Wochenschr.* 98:1551–1554, 1973.
6. Groth, U., Prellwitz, W., et al. Estimation of pharmacokinetic parameters of lithium from saliva and urine. *Clin. Pharmacol. Ther.* 16:490–498, 1974.
7. Petersen, V., Hvidt, S., et al. Effect of prolonged thiazide treatment on renal lithium clearance. *Br. Med. J.* 3:143–145, 1974.
8. Thomsen, K., and Schou, M. Renal lithium excretion in man. *Am. J. Physiol.* 215:823–827, 1968.
9. Weinstein, M. R., and Goldfield, M. D. Cardiovascular malformations with lithium use during pregnancy. *Am. J. Psychiatry* 132:529–531, 1975.

MEPERIDINE
(Pethidine)

A synthetic basic narcotic alkaloid that is one-tenth as potent as morphine as a parenteral analgesic. Used to counteract severe pain such as that which may occur in labor, terminal malignancy, myocardial infarction, biliary colic, and in the postoperative period. Also used in anesthetic premedication and in the management of acute pulmonary edema caused by left ventricular failure. Acts centrally at enkephalin receptors, producing analgesia, drowsiness, euphoria, and, in large doses, decreased sensitivity of the respiratory system to carbon dioxide and depression of the cough reflex. It may act peripherally to produce cardiovascular depression. As with all opiates, physical dependence and tolerance may develop readily.

Absorption
Systemic bioavailability: 50–60% [9]. t_{max}: 1–2 hours [3].

Distribution
V_d: about 4 L/kg; increases with increasing alcohol consumption. Protein binding: 65–75%; decreases with age and increasing alcohol intake [10]. Crosses placenta [13]. Appears in fetal circulation in concentrations equal to maternal blood levels.

Elimination
$t_{\frac{1}{2}}$: 2–4 hours [3]; dependent on urine pH. Extensively metabolized to inactive metabolites, meperedinic and normeperidinic acids, normeperidine, and meperidine-N-oxide, which are conjugated and appear in the urine [12]. About 6% appears as parent drug in alkaline urine, whereas as much as 28% appears in acid urine [1, 5]. In both cirrhosis and hepatitis, the $t_{\frac{1}{2}}$ is lengthened, the mean being 7–8 hours [8, 11]. There is no

change in $t_{\frac{1}{2}}$ in patients who develop tolerance to the drug [3]. In pregnant women, relatively more unchanged drug is excreted than in nonpregnant women [6]. Elderly subjects excrete less unchanged drug and more metabolite than younger subjects [12] but develop higher plasma levels for a given dose than younger people [4]. The reason for this phenomenon remains unclear.

Dosage Schedule

1.0–1.5 mg/kg, either orally or parenterally, repeated as required (usually every 4–6 hours).

Special Dosage Situations

Reduce dose in the elderly and in patients with hepatic and respiratory disease. Avoid in patients with chest trauma, undiagnosed acute abdominal pain, or head injury. Although meperidine is safe for use in labor [16], the neonate may have a resultant low Apgar score. This has been shown not to be detrimental to the child in the long run [2]. Contraindicated in myxedema, in which coma may be precipitated.

Therapeutic Concentrations

Widely variable, since the analgesic response is dependent on the tolerance of the individual. Peak plasma levels achieved by a given dose also vary widely but are of the order of 0.1 μg/ml for 50 mg of meperidine given by the IM route [17].

Adverse Reactions

Nausea, vomiting, gastric stasis, and constipation. In overdose, pinpoint pupils, coma, and cardiorespiratory depression occur; these adverse reactions may be counteracted with naloxone or doxapram [15]. In meperidine addicts, hallucinations, muscle twitching, and convulsions may develop with high dosage. The antidote of choice is naloxone, a pure opiate antagonist. This should be administered in a dose of 0.4–0.8 mg IV and may be repeated as necessary, since its half-life is much shorter than that of meperidine.

Interactions

Central depressant effect is additive with phenothiazines, tricyclic antidepressants, monoamine oxidase inhibitors (MAOI), and all sedatives and hypnotics. Analgesic effect is counteracted with nalorphine, levallorphan, naloxone, doxapram, and nikethamide [7]. Gastric emptying is delayed by meperidine, thus slowing absorption of paracetamol [14].

Special Note

Withdrawal from meperidine dependence may be carried out by using methadone. Sudden withdrawal without substitution of another drug may lead to symptoms as severe as those that accompany morphine withdrawal, reaching maximal intensity 8–12 hours after the last dose. Acute withdrawal symptoms may be treated with meperidine, with subsequent transfer to methadone.

References

1. Asatoor, A. M., London, D. R., et al. The excretion of pethidine and its derivatives. *Br. J. Pharmacol.* 20:285–298, 1963.
2. Buck, C., Gregg, R., et al. The effect of single prenatal and natal complications upon the development of children of mature birthweight. *Pediatrics* 43:942–954, 1969.
3. Burns, J. J., Berger, B. L., et al. The physiological disposition and fate of meperidine (Demerol) in man and a method for its estimation in plasma. *J. Pharmacol. Exp. Ther.* 114:289–298, 1955.
4. Chan, K., Kendall, M. J., et al. The effect of aging on plasma pethidine concentrations. *Br. J. Clin. Pharmacol.* 2:297–302, 1975.
5. Chan, K., Kendall, M. J., et al. Factors influencing the excretion and relative physiological availability of pethidine in man. *J. Pharmacol.* 27:235–241, 1975.
6. Crawford, J. S., and Rodulfsky, S. The placental transmission of pethidine. *Br. J. Anaesth.* 37:929–933, 1965.
7. Dundee, J. W., Gupta, P. D., et al. Modification of the analgesic action of pethidine and morphine by three opiate antagonists, a respiratory stimulant (doxapram), and an analeptic (nikethamide): A study using an experimental pain stimulus in man. *Br. J. Pharmacol.* 48:326P, 1973.
8. Klotz, U., McHorse, T. S., et al. The effect of cirrhosis on the disposition and elimination of meperidine in man. *Clin. Pharmacol. Ther.* 16:667–675, 1974.
9. Mather, L. E., and Tucker, G. T. Systemic availability of orally administered meperidine. *Clin. Pharmacol. Ther.* 20:535–540, 1976.
10. Mather, L. E., Tucker, G. T., et al. Meperidine kinetics in man. Intravenous injection in surgical patients and volunteers. *Clin. Pharmacol. Ther.* 17:21–30, 1975.
11. McHorse, T. S., Wilkinson, G. R., et al. Effect of acute viral hepatitis in man on the disposition and elimination of meperidine. *Gastroenterology* 68:775–780, 1975.
12. Mitchard, M., Kendall, M. J., et al. Pethidine-N-oxide: A metabolite in human urine. *J. Pharm. Pharmacol.* 24:915, 1972.
13. Moore, J., McNabb, T. G., et al. The placental transfer of pentazocine and pethidine. *Br. J. Anaesth.* 45(Suppl.):798–801, 1973.
14. Nimmo, W. S., Heading, R. C., et al. Inhibition of gastric emptying and drug absorption by narcotic analgesics. *Br. J. Clin. Pharmacol.* 2:509–513, 1975.
15. Ramamurthy, S., Steen, S. N., et al. Doxapram antagonism of meperidine-induced respiratory depression. *Anesth. Analg.* (Cleveland) 54:352–356, 1975.
16. Riffel, H. D., Nochimson, D. J., et al. Effects of meperidine and promethazine during labor. *Obstet. Gynecol.* 42:738–745, 1973.
17. Stambaugh, J. E., and Wainer, I. W. The bioavailability of meperidine. *J. Clin. Pharmacol.* 14:552–559, 1974.

METAPROTERENOL
(Orciprenaline)

A noncatechol (resorcinol) beta-adrenergic stimulant that is used in the treatment of reversible obstructive airway disease. Relatively selective beta-2-adrenergic stimulation, with little influence on heart rate, occurs at usual doses given orally, subcutaneously [4], or by inhalation spray. However, metaproterenol and isoproterenol if given IV produce comparable effects on both airway resistance and heart rate [5]. Its effect of reducing uterine contractions has led to its use in premature labor. Cellular action appears to be mediated by the stimulation of adenylcyclase, which increases the production of cyclic adenosine monophosphate (AMP) from adenosine triphosphate (ATP).

Absorption
Systemic bioavailability: unknown. t_{max}: unknown.

Distribution
V_d: unknown. Protein binding: unknown.

Elimination
$t_{\frac{1}{2}}$: about 6 hours. Metabolic pathway is uncertain. Catechol-O-methyl transferase (COMT) does not affect metaproterenol, which probably accounts for metaproterenol's $t_{\frac{1}{2}}$ being longer than the $t_{\frac{1}{2}}$ of the catechols [2, 3].

Dosage Schedule
Oral: 20 mg t.i.d. or q.i.d. Providing there is objective evidence of continued improvement in pulmonary function, dosage may be further increased within the limits of tolerance. Oral therapy is not useful in acute asthmatic attacks [6].

Inhalation: may be used prophylactically in a dose of 2 inhalations (1.5 mg) t.i.d. or q.i.d. In acute attacks, 2 inhalations may be repeated every 30 minutes to a maximum of 12 inhalations in 24 hours.

Special Dosage Situations
In children a good response with minimal toxicity has been observed with the following regimen [1]: 6–9 years old and under 27 kg body weight—10 mg (5 ml of syrup) q.i.d.; over 9 years old or over 27 kg body weight—20 mg (10 ml of syrup) q.i.d. Use with caution in the elderly and in patients with cardiovascular disease. No special precautions for women during pregnancy or lactation or in patients with renal or liver disease.

Therapeutic Concentrations
No available information. It is usual to monitor objectively the response in forced expiratory volume in 1 second (FEV_1), the FEV_1 percentage ($FEV_1\%$) of forced vital capacity (FVC), or peak flow rate (PFR).

Adverse Reactions

Tachycardia, palpitations, arrhythmias, flushing, headache, dizziness, and tremulousness; and angina in susceptible individuals. Careful use of a beta-blocking drug such as propranolol may be necessary in severe toxicity, although this drug may aggravate airway obstruction.

Interactions

Administer cautiously when indirectly acting or other directly acting sympathomimetic agents are being used concurrently and in patients with thyrotoxicosis. Theophylline and sympathomimetic amines administered together may increase chance of cardiac arrhythmia.

Review

Hurst, A.   Metaproterenol, a potent and safe bronchodilator. *Ann. Allergy* 31:460–466, 1973.

References

1. Brandon, M. L.   Long-term metaproterenol therapy in asthmatic children. *J.A.M.A.* 235:736–737, 1976.
2. Chervinsky, P., and Chervinsky, G.   Metaproterenol tablets: Their duration of effect by comparison with ephedrine. *Curr. Ther. Res.* 17:507–518, 1975.
3. Emirgil, C., Dwyer, K., et al.   Comparison of the duration of action and the cardiovascular effects of metaproterenol and an isoetharine-phenylephrine combination. *Curr. Ther. Res.* 19:371–378, 1976.
4. Koivikko, A.   A comparison of the effects of subcutaneous orciprenaline, salbutamol, and terbutaline in asthmatic children. *Ann. Clin. Res.* 6:99–104, 1974.
5. McEvoy, J. D. S., Vall-Spinosa, A., et al.   Assessment of orciprenaline and isoproterenol infusions in asthmatic patients. *Am. Rev. Resp. Dis.* 108:490–500, 1973.
6. Miller, M.   A comprehensive evaluation of metaproterenol, a new bronchodilator. *J. Clin. Pharmacol.* 7:34–40, 1967.

METHADONE

A synthetic opioid with pharmacological activities similar to morphine when given in equianalgesic doses. Analgesia is accompanied by sedation, euphoria, antitussive activity, respiratory depression, increase in smooth muscle tone, and peripheral vasodilation with postural hypotension. Indicated in the treatment of severe pain, in opiate abstinence syndrome, and in maintenance programs for morphine and heroin addicts [3].

Absorption

Oral absorption: essentially complete [1]. t_{max}: 4 hours [6, 7]. First-pass effect is indicated by diminished effect of oral doses compared with identical parenteral doses [2] and the enhanced excretion of major metabolite relative to parent drug after oral dosage [1].

Distribution

V_d: about 5 L/kg [7]. Protein binding: 84–87% [8], 70% binding to albumin and the remainder to globulin [8]. Concentrations in liver, lung, and kidneys greatly exceed those in blood [10]. Crosses placenta.

Elimination

$t_{\frac{1}{2}}$: 52 hours after single dose [11]; only 22 hours to 25 hours after chronic dosage [6, 11]. These mean values represent extensive interindividual differences. Hepatic N-desmethylation produces a major metabolite, mono-N-demethylmethadone (pyrrolidine), and pyrroline, a lesser metabolite of the latter, in addition to some less important hydroxylated and conjugated metabolites [1, 7, 11]. The major route of excretion appears to be in the bile, and an enterohepatic recirculation may exist. Since tubular reabsorption is pH-dependent, renal excretion is enhanced by acidifying the urine.

Dosage Schedule

5–10 mg IV repeated as necessary for relief of pain. 5–15 mg orally may be substituted if long-term outpatient use is required. Acute narcotic withdrawal or abstinence syndrome may be managed by prompt stabilization (by administering the drug of abuse if necessary), followed by gradual detoxification by stepwise withdrawal of methadone [12]. A practical program involves administration of 10 mg of methadone 4 times daily unless the patient is asleep. Higher doses are occasionally necessary for heroin substitution, but caution is advisable because most heroin addicts exaggerate their needs. When daily requirements are determined, a dose once daily is adequate and has advantages over divided doses [4]. A stepwise daily reduction of 5 mg of methadone is usually possible. The psychological effect on the addict may be diminished by apparently continuing the same dosage [1]. The addition of 10% by weight of naloxone to the methadone dose is safe if given orally, but it induces abstinence if injected parenterally [9]. This additive should prevent "street abuse" of methadone designed for clinical use.

Therapeutic Concentrations

No clear relationship between plasma concentrations and pharmacological effects [5]. Measuring plasma concentrations of methadone in patients on maintenance programs appears of little practical value, but it may identify patients with very low concentrations [5].

Special Dosage Situations

Patients with cirrhosis have diminished metabolism of methadone and reduced first-pass effect. Patients with renal or biliary calculi may require atropine or similar antispasmodic agents prophylactically. The elderly and patients with cardiovascular disease are especially prone to hypotensive syncope if they are ambulatory. Severe withdrawal has been described in a high percentage of babies of mothers on methadone programs [13].

Adverse Reactions

Identical to those of morphine. Depressed respiration, pinpoint pupils, and coma indicate acute overdose, and respiratory support is essential. Naloxone 5–10 μg/kg, given IV every 10–20 minutes if necessary (because of its much shorter duration of action), is a pure opiate antagonist without opiate (agonist) activity. Nausea, emesis, constipation, and hallucinations are usual problems when using therapeutic doses. Street abuse (IV methadone compares favorably with IV heroin) and addiction by patients are more serious problems; therefore, patients' requirements should be carefully controlled.

Interactions

Naloxone IV may provoke acute abstinence syndrome in addicts. Pentazocine has weak antagonist activity and may also produce withdrawal symptoms. Caution is advisable if other drugs that produce CNS depresssion, including alcohol, are to be taken concurrently, since additive effects have been described.

References

1. Änggård, E., Gunne, L. M., et al. Disposition of methadone in methadone maintenance. *Clin. Pharmacol. Ther.* 17:258–266, 1975.
2. Beaver, W. T., Wallenstein, S. L., et al. A clinical comparison of the analgesic effects of methadone and morphine administered intramuscularly and of orally and parenterally administered methadone. *Clin. Pharmacol. Ther.* 8:415–426, 1967.
3. Dole, V. P., and Nyswander, M. E. A medical treatment for diacetylmorphine (heroin) addiction. *J.A.M.A.* 193:646–650, 1965.
4. Goldstein, A. Blind comparison of once-daily and twice-daily dosage schedules in a methadone program. *Clin. Pharmacol. Ther.* 13:59–69, 1972.
5. Horns, W. H., Rado, M., et al. Plasma levels and symptom complaints in patients maintained on daily dosage of methadone hydrochloride. *Clin. Pharmacol. Ther.* 17:636–648, 1975.
6. Inturrisi, C. E., and Verebely, K. The levels of methadone in the plasma in methadone maintenance. *Clin. Pharmacol. Ther.* 13:633–635, 1972.
7. Inturrisi, C. E., and Verebely, K. Disposition of methadone in man after a single oral dose. *Clin. Pharmacol. Ther.* 13:923–929, 1972.
8. Olsen, G. D. Methadone binding to human plasma proteins. *Clin. Pharmacol. Ther.* 14:338–343, 1973.
9. Parwatikar, S. D., and Knowles, R. A. Methadone—naloxone in combination for the treatment of heroin addicts. *Clin. Pharmacol. Ther.* 14:941–948, 1973.

10. Robinson, A. E., and Williams, F. M. The distribution of methadone in man. *J. Pharm. Pharmacol.* 23:353–358, 1971.
11. Verebely, K., Volavka, J., et al. Methadone in man: Pharmacokinetic and excretion studies in acute and chronic treatment. *Clin. Pharmacol. Ther.* 18:180–190, 1975.
12. Wesson, D. R., and Smith, D. E. A conceptual approach to detoxification. *Psychedelic Drugs* 6:161–168, 1974.
13. Zelson, C., Lee, S. J., et al. Comparative effect of maternal intake of heroin and methadone. *N. Engl. J. Med.* 289:1216–1220, 1973.

METHYLDOPA

Antihypertensive agent, analogue of dihydroxyphenylalanine (dopa), a precursor of noradrenaline. Exact mechanism of action is not understood. Metabolized by dopa decarboxylase and dopamine-beta-hydroxylase to alpha-methyl dopamine [5] and alpha-methyl norepinephrine in both peripheral and central neurones, where it is stored in the same nerve ending granules that store other catecholamine granules (animal studies). It may act as a central "false transmitter" at alpha receptors [2] or as an inhibitor of catecholamine release by depletion of catecholamines [3]. Indicated in the management of all forms of hypertension *except* that due to pheochromocytoma.

Absorption
Oral bioavailability: variable. Metabolized to methyldopa-O-sulfate, probably in the gut wall (30–70%) [1]. t_{max}: 4 hours, parallels onset of antihypertensive response [4].

Distribution
V_d: 0.5 L/kg. Protein binding: 0–20%. Accumulated in nerve endings of brain and catecholaminergic peripheral nervous system.

Elimination
$t_{\frac{1}{2}}$: 2 hours. Cleared by glomerular filtration. 20–70% of parent drug appears in urine after oral dose, and as much as 90% after intravenous dose. Methyldopa-O-sulfate, the major metabolite, has a $t_{\frac{1}{2}}$ of 4 hours and probably has little or no antihypertensive activity [4]. However, it is cleared by the kidneys and therefore accumulates in the plasma in patients with renal failure. Under these circumstances, it may be pharmacologically active.

Note: Traditional pharmacokinetic parameters are not of much value, since the activity of methyldopa is related to its uptake and storage by nerve endings. Once stored, it is presumably not in equilibrium with the circulation (i.e., forms a "deep" compartment) and is subject to the same re-uptake as other catecholamines when released by the nerve endings.

Dosage Schedule
250 mg b.i.d. or t.i.d., increased by increments of 250–500 mg at daily intervals to a maximum of 3 g daily.

Special Dosage Situations

Renal failure: decreased dose may be required (see Elimination). Elderly: no special dosage adjustments. Pregnancy: no contraindications. Contraindicated in patients with depression, hepatitis, and hemolytic anemia; and if possible, avoid use in males because of high incidence of impotence.

Therapeutic Level

Plasma levels greater than 2 μg/ml are associated with a decrease in blood pressure [4]. However, the plasma level is relatively meaningless, since it does not necessarily reflect nerve ending stores of α-methyl norepinephrine and α-methyl dopamine.

Adverse Reactions

Drowsiness, depression, impotence, postural hypotension, drug fever, hepatitis, diarrhea, constipation, skin rash, positive Coombs' test (20%), Coombs' positive hemolytic anemia (0.02%), and galactorrhea.

Interactions

Competes with renal tubular reabsorption of amino acids, which may lead to aminoaciduria. Produces false increases of fluorometric measurements of urinary catecholamines; for this reason, beware of diagnosis of pheochromocytoma in patients taking methyldopa.

References

1. Conolly, M. E., Davies, D. S., et al.   Metabolism of isoprenaline in dog and man. *Br. J. Pharmacol.* 46:458–472, 1972.
2. Day, M. D., and Rand, M. D.   A hypothesis for the mode of action of α-methyldopa in relieving hypertension. *J. Pharm. Pharmacol.* 15:221–224, 1963.
3. Henning, M., and Van Zwieten, P. A.   Central hypotensive effect of α-methyldopa. *J. Pharm. Pharmacol.* 20:409–417, 1968.
4. Saavedra, J. A., Reid, J. L., et al.   Plasma concentrations of α-methyldopa and sulphate conjugate after oral administration of methyldopa and intravenous administration of methyldopa and methyldopa hydrochloride ethyl ester. *Eur. J. Clin. Pharmacol.* 8:381–386, 1975.
5. Waldmeier, P., Hedwall, P. R., et al.   On the role of α-methyl-dopamine in the antihypertensive effect of α-methyldopa. *Naunyn Schmiedeberg's Arch. Pharmacol.* 389:303–314, 1975.

METOCLOPRAMIDE

Methoxychlorprocainamide, although a derivative of procaine, is devoid of anesthetic or significant cardiovascular effects. Metoclopramide enhances peristalsis of the upper gastrointestinal tract, increases lower esophageal tone, and relaxes the pylorus. In addition, it exerts antiemetic activity, probably through a central effect on the medullary chemoreceptor [4] or possibly by central dopaminergic antagonism.

Increased upper gastrointestinal motility permits more rapid radiological examination of the small intestine by contrast media, with less exposure to radiation. Peroral jejunal biopsy may be performed more efficiently. The preoperative use of metoclopramide in accident victims and in pregnant women who must undergo emergency surgery after a recent meal helps prevent aspiration of stomach contents. Appears useful in management of persistent hiccups, esophageal reflux, and opiate- and digitalis-induced vomiting. No clear benefit in nystagmus, vertigo, sea-sickness, acute exacerbations of gastric or duodenal ulcer, or in the prevention of relapse of duodenal ulceration [2].

Absorption

Apparently complete, since therapeutic effects of an oral dose are comparable to those of an identical IV dose. t_{max}: 30–120 minutes.

Distribution

No available information.

Elimination

$t_{\frac{1}{2}}$: no available information. N-oxidation to monodealkylated and didealkylated derivatives has been described in vitro [1].

Dosage Schedule

A single parenteral dose of 10 mg is the usual dose given in preparation for investigative procedures.

Chronic oral treatment: 10–20 mg t.i.d.

Special Dosage Situations

No available information about use in the elderly, in women during pregnancy or lactation, or in patients with renal or hepatic disease. Children and young adults appear especially prone to develop extrapyramidal reactions, and thus the dosage should be limited to 0.5 mg/kg/day. Prolactin is released by metoclopramide and may adversely affect some breast cancers. Therefore women with this disease should probably not receive metoclopramide [7].

Therapeutic Concentrations

No available information.

Adverse Reactions

The most remarkable reactions are the extrapyramidal effects of akathisia (motor restlessness, jitteriness, and agitation); acute dystonia, which includes torticollis, oculogyric crisis, and opisthotonus (which may mimic tetanus); and parkinsonism. Women of all ages are affected more than men. Treatment with an IV anticholinergic agent such as biperiden, procyclidine, benztropine, or diphenhydramine is usually effective.

Drowsiness, lassitude, constipation, diarrhea, oral and periorbi-

tal edema, rashes, or galactorrhea may develop. A case of mul-
tifocal supraventricular cardiac arrhythmia has been reported [6].

Interactions

Avoid concurrent use of phenothiazines, since a higher incidence
of extrapyramidal effects occurs in combination with these drugs.
    The rate of absorption of some drugs such as acetaminophen,
ampicillin, tetracycline, L-dopa, and ethanol has been increased
with earlier and higher peak plasma concentrations, while digoxin may be absorbed less well because of enhanced gastrointestinal motility [2, 3, 5].

Review

Pinder, R. M., Brogden, R. N., et al.   Metoclopramide: A review
    of its pharmacological properties and clinical use. *Drugs*
    12:81–131, 1976.

References

1. Beckett, A. H., and Huizing, G.   *In vitro* metabolism of
    metoclopramide. *J. Pharm. Pharmacol.* 27(Suppl. 2):42P, 1975.
2. Gilliland, I., and Robinson, O. P. W., et al.   Metoclopramide.
    Postgrad. Med. J. 49(Suppl. 4):1–107, 1973.
3. Manninen, V., Apajalahti, A., et al.   Altered absorption of
    digoxin in patients given propantheline and metoclopramide.
    Lancet 1:398–400, 1973.
4. McNeilly, A. S., and Thorner, M. O.   Metoclopramide and
    prolactin. *Br. Med. J.* 2:729, 1974.
5. Nimmo, J., Heading, R. C., et al.   Pharmacological modifica-
    tion of gastric emptying: Effects of propantheline and meto-
    clopramide on paracetamol absorption. *Br. Med. J.* 1:587–
    589,1973.
6. Shalkai, M., Pinkhas, J., et al.   Metoclopramide and cardiac
    arrhythmia. *Br. Med. J.* 2:385, 1974.
7. Ward, H. W. C.   Metoclopramide and prolactin. *Br. Med. J.*
    3:169, 1974.

METRONIDAZOLE

A hydroxyethyl derivative of nitroimidazole. Highly effective in
the treatment of vaginal trichomoniasis, intestinal and hepatic
amebiasis, and giardiasis. Under investigation for the treatment
of cutaneous leishmaniasis [2], dracontiasis [4], Crohn's disease
[10], and infections with bacteroides [11] and other anaerobic
bacteria [8]. The mechanism of antimicrobial action is unknown.

Absorption

Oral bioavailability: 90–100% [7]. t_{max}: 1–2 hours [6].

Distribution

V_d: 0.6–0.7 L/kg [6]. Protein binding: 5–20% [6, 9]. Crosses
placenta. The concentration in CSF is probably equal to the concentration in serum [6].

Elimination

$t_{\frac{1}{2}}$: 8–14 hours [8, 9]. About 20% is excreted unchanged in the urine [8, 9]; the rest of the drug is predominantly metabolized by side-chain oxidation and subsequent glucuronidation, 1-(2-hydroxyethyl)-2-hydroxymethyl-5-nitroimidazole being the major metabolite [4].

Dosage Schedule

Trichomonas vaginalis: 250 mg orally 3 times daily for the same 10 days in both sexual partners. Retreatment can be initiated after 4 weeks if necessary. Vaginal pessaries may be used concurrently, but there is no evidence of a higher cure rate than with oral therapy alone. These regimens may be replaced by a single dose of 2 g to both sexual partners for the same period of time [1].

Amebiasis (intestinal infections and hepatic abscesses): 750 mg 3 times daily for 10 days.

Giardiasis: 250 mg 3 times daily for 10 days and repeated if necessary after 2 weeks for a further 10 days.

Special Dosage Situations

Children: 35–50 mg/kg in 3 divided daily doses (amebiasis). Liver disease: no available information about dosage adjustment. Renal failure: unchanged dose. Pregnancy: should be avoided in first trimester [5] and possibly during the remainder of pregnancy and during lactation because of reports of tumors in animals.

Therapeutic Concentrations

In cultures the antiprotozoal and antibacterial activity is 1–2.5 μg/ml.

Adverse Reactions

The reactions, which are few and reversible, are mild gastrointestinal symptoms such as metallic taste, stomatitis, oral candidiasis, nausea, diarrhea, proctitis, and epigastric pain. Headache, insomnia, and dizziness may occur. Mild leucopenia, ataxia, and confusion have been reported. Urine is often discolored (dark reddish-brown). There are reports of tumors in animals.

Interactions

Disulfiram-like reaction with alcohol, which should be avoided during treatment. Enhances anticoagulant effect of warfarin [3].

Review

Catterall, R. D. Trichomonal infections of the genital tract. *Med. Clin. North Am.* 56:1203–1209, 1972.

References

1. Dykers, J. R., Jr. Single dose metronidazole for trichomonas: Patient and consort. *N. Engl. J. Med.* 293:23–24, 1975.
2. Long, P. I. Cutaneous Leishmaniasis treated with metronidazole. *J.A.M.A.* 223:1378–1379, 1973.

3. O'Reilly, R. A.   The stereoselective interaction of warfarin and metronidazole in man. *N. Engl. J. Med.* 295:354–357, 1976.
4. Padonu, K. O.   A controlled trial of metronidazole in the treatment of dracontiasis in Nigeria. *Am. J. Trop. Med. Hyg.* 22:42–44, 1973.
5. Peterson, W. F., Stauch, J. E., et al.   Metronidazole in pregnancy. *Am. J. Obstet. Gynecol.* 94:343–353, 1966.
6. Ralph, E. D., Clarke, J. T., et al.   Pharmacokinetics of metronidazole as determined by bioassay. *Antimicrob. Agents Chemother.* 6:691–696, 1974.
7. Stambaugh, J. E., Leo, L. G., et al.   The isolation and identification of the urinary oxidative metabolites of metronidazole in man. *J. Pharmacol. Exp. Ther.* 161:373–381, 1968.
8. Tally, F. P., Sutter, V. L., et al.   Treatment of anaerobic infections with metronidazole. *Antimicrob. Agents Chemother.* 7:672–675, 1975.
9. Taylor, Jr., J. A., Migliardi, J. R., et al.   Tinidazole and metronidazole pharmacokinetics in man and mouse. *Antimicrob. Agents Chemother.* 267–270, 1969.
10. Ursing, B., and Kamme, C.   Metronidazole for Crohn's disease. *Lancet* 1:775–777, 1975.
11. Whelan, J. P. F., and Hale, J. H.   Bactericidal activity of metronidazole against *Bacteroides fragilis*. *J. Clin. Pathol.* 26:393–395, 1973.

MORPHINE

A narcotic alkaloid analgesic isolated from opium and acting directly on enkephalin receptors both centrally and peripherally in the bowel wall. Has analgesic effect mediated directly on CNS; also produces drowsiness, changes in mood, and mental clouding. Suppresses cough by a direct effect on the medullary center; causes respiratory depression by reducing responsiveness of the respiratory center to carbon dioxide and causes emesis by direct stimulation of the chemoreceptor trigger zone. Constipation is produced by direct action on bowel wall nerve plexuses; spasm of the spincter of Oddi may increase biliary tract pressure. Indicated for the relief of severe pain and the management of dyspnea that is caused by pulmonary edema in acute left ventricular failure.

Absorption
Systemic bioavailability: about 20% [2]. There is extensive first-pass metabolism. t_{max}: 10–20 minutes after oral, IM, and subcutaneous doses [2].

Distribution
V_d: 3–4 L/kg [2]. Protein binding: about 35%, mainly to albumin [3]. Crosses placenta, but no other information about distribution in man is available.

Elimination

t₄: 2–2½ hours [5]. Extensively metabolized; only 3–10% excreted unchanged in urine, 70% as glucuronide conjugate and about 5% as the *N*-demethylated active metabolite normorphine [2, 6]. About 10% is excreted in feces. After an oral dose, glucuronide conjugation probably occurs in the gut as well as in the liver [2].

Dosage Schedule

0.1–0.15 mg/kg parenterally, usually by the IM or IV route. The dose may be repeated as required for relief of pain. The equianalgesic oral dose is 4–5 times the parenteral dose.

Special Dosage Situations

Children: 0.05–0.15 mg/kg. Care must be exercised in using the drug in patients who have liver disease with jaundice because metabolism is reduced and the protein binding may be reduced to 22% with a consequent increase in the amount of free drug in plasma [4]. CNS effects may precipitate hepatic encephalopathy. Protein binding may be slightly reduced in renal failure [4]. If possible avoid use of drug in patients with diminished respiratory reserve. IV route is advisable in patients with poor peripheral circulation because absorption is often delayed. Morphine given 2–4 hours before parturition may produce respiratory depression in the neonate. No available specific information about use of the drug in elderly or in women during lactation.

Therapeutic Concentrations

It is usual to prescribe the dose according to patient's response. A plasma level of 0.05 μg/ml appears necessary for moderate analgesia [1].

Adverse Reactions

Nausea, vomiting, dizziness, mental changes, respiratory depression, epigastric discomfort, constipation, and biliary colic. Pinpoint pupils with coma strongly suggest narcotic overdose. 0.4–0.8 mg of naloxone IV or IM may be repeated while signs of acute overdosage persist, but the withdrawal syndrome may be provoked by giving this dosage to patients who are morphine addicts. Rapid development of tolerance and drug dependence are important limitations, and therefore the use of morphine should be carefully restricted to essential situations.

Interactions

Additive effects may occur with other centrally acting drugs, including the phenothiazines, monoamine oxidase inhibitors (MAOI), and tricyclic antidepressants.

Reviews

Boerner, U., Abbott, S., et al. The metabolism of morphine and heroin in man. *Drug Metab. Rev.* 4:39–73, 1975.
Snyder, S. H. Opiate receptors and internal opiates. *Sci. Am.* 236:44–56, 1977.

References

1. Berkowitz, B. A., Ngai, S. H., et al. The disposition of morphine in surgical patients. *Clin. Pharmacol. Ther.* 17:629–635, 1975.
2. Brunk, S. F., and Delle, M. Morphine metabolism in man. *Clin. Pharmacol. Ther.* 16:51–57, 1974.
3. Olsen, G. D. Morphine binding to human plasma proteins. *Clin. Pharmacol. Ther.* 17:31–35, 1975.
4. Olsen, G. D., Bennett, W. M., et al. Morphine and phenytoin binding to plasma proteins in renal and hepatic failure. *Clin. Pharmacol. Ther.* 17:677–684, 1975.
5. Stanski, D. R., Greenblatt, D. J., et al. Kinetics of high-dose intravenous morphine in cardiac surgery patients. *Clin. Pharmacol. Ther.* 19:752–756, 1976.
6. Yeh, S. Y. Urinary excretion of morphine and its metabolites in morphine-dependent subjects. *J. Pharmacol. Exp. Ther.* 192:201–210, 1975.

NALOXONE

N-allylnoroxymorphone, a synthetic congener of oxymorphone; a potent narcotic antagonist with no agonist effects. Used in the treatment of overdosage with narcotics and propoxyphene [8] and in the prophylaxis of narcotic abuse. Has been used in the treatment of diphenoxylate (Lomotil) poisoning in children [7]. Competes with morphine-like drugs for enkephalin receptor sites. Partial narcotic antagonists such as pentazocine are reversed only by naloxone.

Absorption

Systemic bioavailability: about 20% [2]. A high first-pass effect exists, probably because of hepatic metabolism [2]. t_{max}: 0.5–1 hour [2].

Distribution

V_d: 3 L/kg [4]. Protein binding: unknown. No available data about transfer to fetus or to breast milk.

Elimination

$t_{\frac{1}{2}}$: 1 hour [4]. Extensively inactivated by glucuronidation, N-dealkylation, and reduction [9].

Dosage Schedule

Not used orally in narcotic drug overdose because of high first-pass effect. In morphine overdose, IV dose is 0.4–0.8 mg, which may be repeated as necessary. Alternatively, naloxone may be given by IV infusion [1]. In propoxyphene overdose, IV dose is 0.4–0.8 mg, which may be repeated as necessary [8].

Used as narcotic abuse prophylaxis in methadone maintenance programs (see Methadone, p. 216). Dose is 1 mg of naloxone for every 10 mg of methadone [5, 6].

Special Dosage Situations
Children and neonates: 0.005–0.01 mg/kg. No available information about dosage adjustments in patients with renal or hepatic disease or in the elderly.

Therapeutic Concentrations
Not established.

Adverse Reactions
Ventricular tachyarrhythmias have occurred after IV administration to patients after cardiac surgery [3].

Interactions
Produces acute withdrawal symptoms in narcotic addicts when given by the IV route.

References
1. Evans, J. M., Hogg, M. I. J., et al.   Degree and duration of reversal by naloxone of effects of morphine in conscious subjects. *Br. Med. J.* 2:589–591, 1974.
2. Fishman, J., Roffwarg, H., et al.   Disposition of naloxone-7,8-3 H in normal and narcotic dependent men. *J. Pharmacol. Exp. Ther.* 187:575–580, 1973.
3. Michaelis, L. L., Hickey, P. R., et al.   Ventricular irritability associated with the use of naloxone hydrochloride. Two case reports and laboratory assessment of the effect of the drug on cardiac excitability. *Ann. Thorac. Surg.* 18:608–614, 1974.
4. Ngai, S. H., Berkowitz, B. A., et al.   Pharmacokinetics of naloxone in rats and in man. *Anesthesiology* 44:398–401, 1976.
5. Nutt, J. G., and Jasinski, D. R.   Methadone-naloxone mixtures for use in methadone maintenance programs. 1. An evaluation in man of their pharmacological feasibility. 2. Demonstration of acute physical dependence. *Clin. Pharmacol. Ther.* 15:156–166, 1974.
6. Parwatikar, S. D., and Knowles, R. D.   Methadone-naloxone in combination for the treatment of heroin addicts. *Clin. Pharmacol. Ther.* 14:941–948, 1973.
7. Rumack, B. H., and Temple, A. R.   Lomotil poisoning. *Pediatrics* 53:495–500, 1974.
8. Vlasses, P. M., and Fraker, T.   Naloxone for propoxyphene overdosage. *J.A.M.A.* 229:1167, 1974.
9. Weinstein, S. H., Pfeffer, M., et al.   Metabolites of naloxone in human urine. *J. Pharm. Sci.* 60:1567–1568, 1971.

NITRITES

Agents possessing the nitrite ion or nitrates that are apparently capable of conversion in vitro to the active nitrite by reaction with sulfhydryl groups in smooth muscle. Smooth muscle relaxation is the major action, although the resulting vascular change appears to be modified by local, autonomic, and postural effects. Observations of the factors influencing myocardial oxygen consumption show an increase in heart rate and ejection fraction and a decrease in left ventricular cavity size, left ventricular systolic pressure, and peak systolic tension. Diastolic coronary blood flow and subendocardial perfusion are improved [5]. Indicated in the prophylaxis or acute management of angina pectoris. The effect of nitrites in acute myocardial infarction is under evaluation [3]. A number of short-acting and long-acting preparations are available, although the value of the latter is disputed [4, 7, 11, 12]. Nitroglycerine (NTG, glyceryl trinitrate, GTN), isosorbide dinitrate, and pentaerythritol tetranitrate (PETN) will be discussed.

Absorption

Systemic bioavailability of NTG after oral dosage: unknown. t_{max} of NTG after oral dosage: unknown. There is probably extensive hepatic denitration during first-pass metabolism, since oral doses up to 10 times the size of sublingual doses may be necessary for a similar effect. 60–75% of a sublingual dose is absorbed during 3½ minutes of mucosal contact [1]. t_{max} of NTG: unknown, but maximum effect is seen within 3 minutes [4]. Systemic bioavailability of isosorbide dinitrate: unknown. Systemic bioavailability of PETN: unknown. t_{max} of PETN: unknown.

Distribution

V_d: unknown. Protein binding: unknown.

Elimination

$t_{\frac{1}{2}}$ of NTG: about 30 minutes [1]. Sublingual NTG acts for about 1 hour [4] and NTG ointment for about 3 hours [8]. $t_{\frac{1}{2}}$ of isosorbide dinitrate: 15–30 minutes [9]. $t_{\frac{1}{2}}$ of PETN: unknown. Inactivation by denitration occurs in the liver [7]. Only the trinitrate of PETN appears active [2].

Dosage Schedule

NTG: 0.4 mg sublingually, repeated as necessary for prophylaxis or relief of symptoms. 2.5 mg orally b.i.d. or t.i.d. for prophylaxis. 2% ointment applied 3 times daily to 36 sq in (6-in or 15-cm square area) of skin acts like a sustained-release preparation [8]. Isosorbide dinitrate: 2.5–10 mg sublingually; 10–60 mg orally t.i.d. or q.i.d. PETN: 10–30 mg t.i.d. or q.i.d.

Special Dosage Situations

No available information about use in patients with renal or hepatic disease.

Therapeutic Concentrations

No available information.

Adverse Reactions

Throbbing headache common, although tolerance may develop with repeated use. Burning sensation in the mouth, dizziness, flushing, postural hypotension, palpitations and tachycardia. Withdrawal after heavy exposure (e.g., industrial exposure) may produce nonobstructive ischemic heart disease [6].

Interactions

Cross-tolerance may occur [10, 13]. The beneficial effects of single doses of NTG may be lost after chronic exposure to PETN or isosorbide dinitrate, although this is debated.

Special Note

GTN is volatile, and therefore tablets should be dispensed in small numbers and stored in a small sealed container in a cool place. Loss of sublingual burning sensation indicates deterioration of tablets. Concurrent use of a beta blocker, e.g., propranolol, may be helpful in angina pectoris and may prevent reflex tachycardia and associated symptoms.

References

1. Bogaert, M. G., and Rosseel, M. T.   Plasma levels in man of nitroglycerin after buccal administration. *J. Pharm. Pharmacol.* 24:737–738, 1972.
2. Davidson, I. W. F., Miller, H. S., et al.   Pharmacodynamics and biotransformation of pentaerythritol tetranitrate in man. *J. Pharm. Sci.* 60:274–277, 1971.
3. Epstein, S. E., Kent, K. M., et al.   Reduction of ischemic injury by nitroglycerin during acute myocardial infarction. *N. Engl. J. Med.* 292:29–35, 1975.
4. Goldstein, R. E., Rosing, D. R., et al.   Clinical and circulatory effects of isosorbide dinitrate. *Circulation* 43:629–640, 1971.
5. Greenberg, H., Dwyer, E. M., et al.   Effects of nitroglycerin on the major determinants of myocardial oxygen consumption. An angiographic and hemodynamic assessment. *Am. J. Cardiol.* 36:426–432, 1975.
6. Lange, R. L., Reid, M. S., et al.   Nonatheromatous ischemic heart disease following withdrawal from chronic industrial nitroglycerin exposure. *Circulation* 46:666–678, 1972.
7. Needleman, P., Lang, S., et al.   Organic nitrates: Relationship between biotransformation and rational angina pectoris therapy. *J. Pharmacol. Exp. Ther.* 181:489–497, 1972.
8. Reichek, N., Goldstein, R. E., et al.   Sustained effects of nitroglycerin ointment in patients with angina pectoris. *Circulation* 50:348–352, 1974.
9. Rosseel, M. T., and Bogaert, M. G.   GLC determination of nitroglycerin and isosorbide dinitrate in human plasma. *J. Pharm. Sci.* 62:754–758, 1973.
10. Schelling, J. L., and Lasagna, L.   A study of cross-tolerance to circulatory effects of organic nitrates. *Clin. Pharmacol. Ther.* 8:256–260, 1967.
11. Winsor, T., and Berger, H. J.   Oral nitroglycerin as a prophylactic anti-anginal drug: Clinical, physiologic, and statistical evidence of efficacy based on a three-phase experimental design. *Am. Heart J.* 90:611–626, 1975.

12. Winsor, T., Kaye, H., et al.   Hemodynamic response of oral long-acting nitrates: Evidence of gastrointestinal absorption. *Chest* 62:407–413, 1972.
13. Zelis, R., and Mason, D. T.   Isosorbide dinitrate: Effect on the vasodilator response to nitroglycerin. *J.A.M.A.* 234:166–170, 1975.

NITROPRUSSIDE SODIUM
(Sodium nitroferricyanide)

A hypotensive agent that acts by direct vasodilation of peripheral resistance vessels, causing a slight to moderate tachycardia and a variable influence on cardiac output [3]. Major indication is for the emergency treatment of crises of accelerated hypertension. Other indications include cardiogenic shock, ergot poisoning, hypotensive "dry field" surgery, and, in combination with propranolol, the management of dissecting aneurysm [4].

Absorption
Not relevant, IV use only.

Distribution
V_d: unknown; hypotensive effect is extremely rapid, taking place within minutes.

Elimination
$t_{\frac{1}{2}}$: unknown, probably extremely short because drug's effect disappears within 5 minutes. Combination with red cell and tissue sulfhydryl groups forms cyanide, which is converted to thiocyanate in the liver. $t_{\frac{1}{2}}$ for thiocyanate: 7 days in normal subjects; thiocyanate is excreted almost entirely in urine.

Dosage Schedule
50 mg dissolved in 500 ml 5% dextrose solution (100 μg/ml), administered IV by infusion pump or similar *precise* infusion technique. Starting rate is 0.5 μg/kg/min, increased if necessary to 8 μg/kg/min over a few hours. Institute or increase oral antihypertensive medication and reduce nitroprusside infusion 2–3 hours after each dose of oral drug to check patient's response. Finally, discontinue nitroprusside when control of blood pressure is established. Nitroprusside is photosensitive, and therefore containers, pumps, and tubing should be protected from light. A faint red color is acceptable.

Special Dosage Situations
In patients with known or suspected coronary or cerebrovascular disease, reduce pressure with caution. In renal failure, $t_{\frac{1}{2}}$ of thiocyanate becomes prolonged, with an increasing likelihood of toxicity. No available information about use in women during pregnancy or lactation. Tachyphylaxis and resistance to nitroprusside in children undergoing hypotensive surgery is associated with a greater morbidity and mortality [2]. Contraindicated in

tobacco amblyopia and Leber's hereditary optic atrophy when cyanide levels are high and thiosulfate is reduced [2].

Therapeutic Concentrations

Not known; patient's response to the drug is a useful guide to dosage requirement. If therapy is prolonged, especially in renal failure, thiocyanate level should be monitored (toxicity begins at 50–100 μg/ml and may be fatal above 200 μg/ml).

Adverse Reactions

Too rapid infusion may cause nausea, vomiting, restlessness, apprehension, headache, dizziness, retrosternal discomfort, abdominal pain, and muscle twitching, all of which improve rapidly after slowing or discontinuing the infusion drip. Tetanic spasms, anoxic symptoms, and "smell of almonds" breath indicate that cyanide is responsible. Thiocyanate may cause or aggravate hypothyroidism, produce marked fatigue, nausea, hypotension, and death. Methemoglobinemia has been reported [1]. Thiocyanate may be eliminated by dialysis. Thiosulfate infusion appears beneficial when tachyphylaxis occurs [2]. Hydroxycobalamin may also be used for treatment of toxicity.

Interactions

Patients already receiving oral antihypertensive therapy may be sensitive to the action of nitroprusside.

References

1. Bower, P. J., and Peterson, J. N.   Methemoglobinemia after sodium nitroprusside therapy. *N. Engl. J. Med.* 293:865, 1975.
2. Davies, D. W., Cyreiss, L., et al.   Sodium nitroprusside in children: Observations on metabolism during normal and abnormal responses. *Can. Anaesth. Soc. J.* 22:553–560, 1975.
3. Page, I. H., Corcoran, A. C., et al.   Cardiovascular actions of sodium nitroprusside in animals and hypertensive patients. *Circulation* 11:188–198, 1955.
4. Palmer, R. F., and Lasseter, K. C.   Sodium nitroprusside. *N. Engl. J. Med.* 292:294–297, 1975.

NYSTATIN

A relatively insoluble polyene antibiotic that is fungicidal but devoid of other antimicrobial activity. Adsorption to sterols in cell membranes leads to alteration in membrane function, with leakage of essential metabolites, inhibition of glycolysis, and cell death. Maximum activity at 25–30° C and pH 6–8 [2]. Major clinical indication is for superficial infection with *Candida, Cryptococcus, Histoplasma, Blastomyces, Trichophyton, Epidermophyton,* and *Microsporum audouini.*

Absorption

Significant only if given in oral doses in excess of 8 million units (1 mg = 3500 units). Usually not absorbed after topical application to skin, mucous membranes, or bronchi. A large variety of vehicles for administration of nystatin are available, e.g., aqueous suspensions, aerosols, tablets, pessaries, powders, creams, and ointments.

Distribution
Not relevant.

Elimination
Oral dosage is normally excreted in feces. The very small amount absorbed is excreted in urine. Pharmacokinetics of nystatin are unknown.

Dosage Schedule
Topical application: 3 times daily. Vaginal pessaries: 0.5 million units twice daily. Oral suspension: 0.5–1 million units twice daily.

Continue for 48 hours after clinical improvement (usually total of 8–14 days). Consider management of the possible problems underlying candidiasis, e.g., skin maceration, pregnancy, effects of the birth control pill, diabetes mellitus, lymphoma, leukemia, and effects from topical or systemic steroids, broad-spectrum antibiotics, or immunosuppressive drugs.

Special Dosage Situations
Children: reduce oral dose to 100,000–200,000 units. Cutaneous candidiasis in infants and young children responded to 100,000 units applied topically to the lesions t.i.d. or q.i.d. for 6 days. No side-effects were observed [1].

Renal disease: elimination is reduced, but it is not a problem. Not contraindicated in women during pregnancy or lactation. Nystatin is not recommended for the management of systemic candidiasis, for which amphotericin B should be given by the IV route.

Therapeutic Concentrations
Concentrations of 5000–20,000 units/ml are effective in vitro [3].

Adverse Reactions
Mild gastrointestinal symptoms occur rarely after oral use. Bacterial superinfection is not a problem.

Interactions
Not known.

Review
Whittle, C. H.   Antifungal drugs. *Practitioner* 202:69–78, 1969.

References
1.   Alban, J.   Efficacy of nystatin topical cream in the management of cutaneous candidiasis in infants. *Curr. Ther. Res.* 14:158–161, 1972.
2.   Hamilton-Miller, J. M. T.   The effect of temperature on the

stability and bioactivity of nystatin and amphotericin B. *J. Pharm. Pharmacol.* 25:401–407, 1973.
3. Hazen, E., and Brown, R. Fungicidin, an antibiotic produced by a soil actinomycetin. *Proc. Soc. Exp. Biol. Med.* 76:93–97, 1951.

ORPHENADRINE

o-Methyl analogue of diphenhydramine, possessing more anticholinergic activity and less antihistaminic activity than diphenhydramine, although the anticholinergic action is nevertheless relatively weak. Used in the symptomatic management of muscle spasm and supportive or second-line treatment of Parkinson's disease, in which most benefit is demonstrated by relaxation of muscle stiffness and increased muscle power. Less helpful with akinesia, tremor, and sialorrhea. Also used in the treatment of drug-induced extrapyramidal disorders when the causative agent must be continued, e.g., phenothiazines and butyrophenones in chronic psychosis.

Absorption
Complete as hydrochloride. t_{max}: about 3 hours (total radioactivity of labeled dose) [2]. The citrate is formulated in a slow-release form or with analgesic compounds; no available information about its absorption.

Distribution
V_d: apparently very large. Protein binding: unknown.

Elimination
$t_{\frac{1}{2}}$: 14 hours [2]. Extensive hepatic transformation to 5 major and 2 minor metabolites of no apparent clinical significance. Parent drug (8%) and metabolites excreted in urine, apart from a minimal amount in feces, although 25–30% of both oral and IV doses were not accounted for [2]. Urinary excretion of the basic drug and metabolites is dependent on both urine flow and pH [1].

Dosage Schedule
50 mg orally b.i.d. or t.i.d., increased if necessary to a total daily dose of 400 mg, unless limited by adverse effects. Parenteral forms of both hydrochloride and citrate are available; recommended dosage ranges from 20 to 60 mg.

Special Dosage Situations
No available information about use in women during pregnancy or lactation or in patients with renal or hepatic disease. Children may require similar total doses to adults, but increase the dose cautiously from 25 mg b.i.d. Use carefully in patients with glaucoma and prostatic obstruction.

Therapeutic Concentrations
No available information. A case of severe toxicity in a child was associated with a plasma concentration more than 5 μg/ml [3].

Adverse Reactions

Dry mouth, blurred vision, tachycardia, urinary retention, constipation, and fecal impaction. Mental changes, euphoria, excitement, agitation, confusion, convulsions, and coma may be more
prominent than peripheral anticholinergic effects. Hemodialysis
is of no value in treatment of poisoning. Supportive measures
include the use of anticonvulsants and the administration of the
centrally acting cholinesterase inhibitor physostigmine.

Interactions

Additive effects when used with other anticholinergic and antihistaminic agents.

References

1. Beckett, A. H., and Khan, F.   Metabolism, distribution, and
   excretion of orphenadrine in man. *J. Pharm. Pharmacol.*
   23:222S, 1971.
2. Ellison, T., Synder, A., et al.   Metabolism of orphenadrine
   citrate in man. *J. Pharmacol. Exp. Ther.* 173:284–295, 1971.
3. Gill, D. G., and Sowerby, H. A.   Orphenadrine metabolism
   in childhood. *Practitioner* 214:542–544, 1975.

OXYTOCIN

Naturally occurring neurohypophyseal octapeptide hormone.
Known normal functions are the production of breast milk ejection during lactation and possibly the stimulation of uterine muscle contraction during parturition. Other actions that occur when
pharmacological doses are administered include antidiuresis and
peripheral vasodilation with hypotension and tachycardia. Synthetic oxytocin has only minor pressor activity when compared
with vasopressin.

Indicated in the induction of labor, for which it may be combined with amniotic membrane rupture in the management of
hypocontractile labor, and in the induction of midtrimester
therapeutic abortion, for which it may be used in association with
prostaglandin $F_{2\alpha}$ ($PGF2_{\alpha}$).

The usefulness of the oxytocin challenge test as a means of
predicting the failing fetoplacental unit is also being evaluated.
The consensus of opinion at present is that a negative test result
indicates a viable fetus at the time but that often false positive
results occur (up to 50%), with a possible excess of prematurely
induced deliveries [5, 8].

Absorption

Administered only by IV route by constant infusion, since great
care is required in control of the dose. Buccal preparations are
available, but they have fallen from favor because it is not possible
to monitor the dose accurately.

Distribution

V_d: 0.2 L/kg. Protein binding: 30% [4]. Oxytocin is found in the
umbilical cord blood of about 50% of newborn infants [6], but it is

not clear whether this finding represents maternal or fetal hormone.

Elimination

$t_{\frac{1}{2}}$: 5–10 minutes [3]. Extensively metabolized by hepatic and renal oxytocinase. 0.6–35% excreted unchanged in the urine; this percentage appears to increase with urinary flow [1].

Dosage Schedule

Oxytocin should always be administered by infusion pump in normal saline solution rather than 5% dextrose solution. During this period, the fetal heartbeat must be monitored and the dose decreased or discontinued if fetal distress occurs. The maternal fluid balance must also be carefully observed (see Adverse Reactions). Initial dose for induction of labor is 1 mU/min, with the dose doubled every 15–30 minutes until adequate uterine action is established. Dose may reach 64 mU/min. For hypocontractile labor, 0.5–10 mU/min have been used. For the induction of midtrimester abortion, much higher doses, e.g., 100–200 mU/min, are required.

Special Dosage Situations

Contraindicated when signs of fetal distress exist, in placenta previa, in mothers with previous cesarean section, and when vasoconstrictors have already been administered. Use cautiously in patients with hypertension.

Therapeutic Concentrations

4–120 pg/ml [4]; however, it is more important to adjust dose according to the pharmacological response of the patient than to prescribe a specific amount of the drug.

Adverse Reactions

Maternal: antidiuresis may lead to water intoxication if large volumes of fluid are given as a vehicle for oxytocin [7]. Tachycardia and uterine rupture, which is likely to occur especially in grand multipara who receive high doses of oxytocin. Amniotic fluid embolus is rare. Neonate: hyperbilirubinemia, for which the mechanism is unknown [2]. Fetal distress and low Apgar scores at birth.

Interactions

With cyclopropane, occasional ventricular arrhythmias have been reported, especially in patients with a diseased myocardium. Severe hypertension noted in conjunction with vasopressors, especially pseudoephedrine, ephedrine, methoxamine, and ergot alkaloids.

Review

Pauerstein, C. J. Ecbolic agents. *Clin. Anesth.* 10:299–314, 1973.

References

1. Boyd, N. R. H., Jackson, D. B., et al.   The development of a radioimmunoassay for oxytocin: The extraction of oxytocin from urine and determination of the excretion rate for exogenous and endogenous oxytocin in human urine. *J. Endocrinol.* 52:59–67, 1972.
2. Chalmers, I., Campbell, H., et al.   Use of oxytocin and incidence of neonatal jaundice. *Br. Med. J.* 2:116–118, 1975.
3. Chard, T., Boyd, N. R. H., et al.   The development of a radioimmunoassay for oxytocin: The extraction of oxytocin from plasma and its measurement during parturition in human and goat blood. *J. Endocrinol.* 48:223–234, 1970.
4. Fabian, M., Forsling, M. L., et al.   The clearance and antidiuretic potency of neurohypophysial hormones in man and their plasma binding and stability. *J. Physiol.* 204:653–668, 1969.
5. Freeman, R. K.   The use of the oxytocin challenge test for antepartum clinical evaluation of uteroplacental respiratory function. *Am. J. Obstet. Gynecol.* 121:481–489, 1975.
6. Kumaresan, P., Han, G. S., et al.   Oxytocin in maternal and fetal blood. *Obstet. Gynecol.* 46:272–274, 1975.
7. Silva, P., and Allan, M. S.   Water intoxication due to high doses of synthetic oxytocin. Report of a case. *Obstet. Gynecol.* 27:517–520, 1966.
8. Weingold, A. B., DeJesus, T. P. S., et al.   Oxytocin challenge test. *Am. J. Obstet. Gynecol.* 123:466–472, 1975.

PARA-AMINOSALICYLIC ACID
(PAS)

A salicylic acid derivative with tuberculostatic and hypolipidemic properties. May act in tuberculosis by inhibition of folic acid synthesis by *Mycobacterium tuberculosis*. Para-aminosalicylic acid (PAS) is an effective antituberculosis agent when used in combination drug therapy, but because of the high incidence of side-effects, it has fallen into disuse in many countries. However, in countries in which cost is an important factor, PAS continues to be used. It may also have a place in the management of type II hyperlipoproteinemia in combination with dietary restrictions [2].

Available in the acid form and as sodium, potassium, and calcium salts. All of these preparations deteriorate in water, heat, and sunlight. This deterioration is indicated by a brownish or purple discoloration of the crystals.

Absorption

Bioavailability varies markedly with the formulation of PAS. Bioavailability of PAS in solution form is 100%; in suspension form, 70%; as compressed tablets of salt, 90%; and in acid form, 77%. In the form of enteric-coated tablets PAS is not absorbed at all [4, 5, 7]. t_{max} varies with the preparation of PAS. t_{max} of PAS in sodium salt form: 0.5–1 hour. t_{max} of PAS in potassium salt form:

1 hour. t_{max} of PAS in calcium salt form: 1 hour. t_{max} for PAS in acid form: 3–4 hours [4, 5]. First-pass metabolism by N-acetylation occurs both in the bowel wall and in the liver. This process is saturable, and therefore preparations of PAS that are more rapidly absorbed produce higher plasma concentrations and larger areas *under* the plasma concentration/time curve than the same dose of less rapidly absorbed forms [4, 5, 7].

Distribution
V_d: no available data. Protein binding: 50–60% [9]. No available data about transfer to breast milk or to fetus.

Elimination
$t_{\frac{1}{2}}$: 1 hour [5]. 75% is metabolized; N-acetyl-aminosalicylic acid (N-Ac-PAS) and the glucuronide p-aminosalicyluric acid comprise 90% of the metabolites. These metabolites and the parent drug appear in the urine [8]. $t_{\frac{1}{2}}$ of N-Ac-PAS: 1.5–2 hours [4]. The metabolites have weak antituberculous activity.

Dosage Schedule
PAS should always be administered in combination with other antituberculous chemotherapy. It is most frequently given with streptomycin and isoniazid for 3–6 months and then with isoniazid for 12–24 months. The British Medical Research Council showed that PAS given in a single dose of 12 g daily was as effective as ethambutol 15 mg/kg daily or rifampin 600 mg daily when each of these drugs was given with streptomycin and isoniazid to newly diagnosed patients with tuberculosis caused by a sensitive organism. The sputum culture at 12 months was negative in 95–100% of cases, but patients who had received PAS had a higher incidence of side-effects [1].

The study from the Tuberculosis Chemotherapy Centre in Madras showed that PAS given 0.2 g/kg twice weekly in association with isoniazid was as effective as a daily regimen and produced fewer side-effects [6].

The dose of all the salts should be about 30% lower than the dose of aminosalicylic acid. The urine should be kept alkaline to prevent crystalluria. As a hypolipidemic, PAS may be given in a dose of 4.5–11 g/day [2].

Special Dosage Situations
Children: 200–300 mg/kg/day. Use cautiously in patients with hepatic or renal failure, with hypothyroidism, and with peptic ulcer. Avoid the calcium salt form of PAS in patients with hypercalcemia or nephrocalcinosis and the sodium salt form of PAS in patients in heart failure.

Therapeutic Concentrations
The mean inhibitory concentration of PAS is 0.6 μg/ml; for N-Ac-PAS it is 535 μg/ml; and for salicyluric acid it is 210 μg/ml [3]. In practice, only the parent drug reaches therapeutic concentrations in the plasma during the usual regimens. Cultures are

considered to be resistant if growth occurs at PAS concentrations of 4 μg/ml or more.

Adverse Reactions

Gastrointestinal disturbances, especially watery diarrhea. Crystalluria, hypersensitivity reactions, including hepatitis (a syndrome that resembles infectious mononucleosis), bone marrow depression, hemolytic anemia, Loeffler's syndrome, and vasculitis. Malabsorption with steatorrhea, vitamin B_{12} malabsorption, encephalopathy, hypokalemia, acidosis, and goiter with or without myxedema have been reported.

Interactions

Bentonite excipient in PAS granules impairs systemic bioavailability of rifampin (see Rifampin, p. 271). Renal excretion of PAS is impaired by probenecid. PAS increases the activity of anticoagulants by impairing the synthesis of procoagulant factors. As a potential side-effect, hypokalemia may induce digoxin toxicity. May inhibit acetylation of isoniazid, with an increase in isoniazid plasma concentrations.

References

1. British Medical Research Council Co-operative Study. *Tubercle* 54:99–129, 1973.
2. Kuo, P. T., Fan, W. C., et al.   Combined para-aminosalicylic acid and dietary therapy in long-term control of hypercholesterolemia and hypertriglyceridemia (Types IIa and IIb hyperlipoproteinemia). *Circulation* 53:338–341, 1976.
3. Lauener, H., Hodler, J., et al.   Bildung und Ausscheidung der Stoffwechselselfprodukte von *p*-Aminosalicylsäure. *Klin. Wochenschr.* 35:393–401, 1957.
4. Pentikäinen, P., Wan, S. H., et al.   Bioavailability studies on *p*-aminosalicylic acid and its various salts in man II. Comparison of Parasal and Pascorbic. *Am. Rev. Resp. Dis.* 108:1340–1347, 1973.
5. Pentikäinen, P. J., Wan, S. H., et al.   Bioavailability of aminosalicylic acid and its various salts in humans IV. Comparison of four brands of the sodium salt. *J. Pharm. Sci.* 63:1431–1434, 1974.
6. Tuberculosis Chemotherapy Centre, Madras.   Controlled comparison of oral twice-weekly and oral daily isoniazid plus PAS in newly diagnosed pulmonary tuberculosis. *Br. Med. J.* 2:7–11, 1973.
7. Wagner, J. G., Holmes, P. D., et al.   Importance of the type of dosage form and saturable acetylation in determining the bioactivity of *p*-aminosalicylic acid. *Am. Rev. Resp. Dis.* 108:536–546, 1973.
8. Way, E. L., Peng, C. T., et al.   The metabolism of *p*-aminosalicylic acid (PAS) in man. *J. Am. Pharm. Assoc.* 44:65–69, 1955.
9. Way, E. L., Smith, P. K., et al.   The absorption, distribution, excretion, and fate of para-aminosalicylic acid. *J. Pharmacol. Exp. Ther.* 93:368–382, 1948.

PENICILLINS

Water-soluble, acidic, bactericidal antibiotics derived from 6-aminopenicillanic acid (6-APA). From the natural penicillins (e.g., benzylpenicillin), many semisynthetic penicillins have been produced by chemical reactions with 6-APA isolated from the penicillin mold. The penicillins discussed here can be classified according to their main antibacterial activity as shown in Table 10.

Table 10. *Classification of Penicillins by Antibacterial Activity*

Type of Penicillin	Antibacterial Spectrum
Narrow-spectrum penicillins	
Benzylpenicillin (penicillin G)[a]	Gram-positive
Phenoxymethylpenicillin (penicillin V)	and gram-negative
Phenoxyethylpenicillin (phenethicillin)	cocci, many gram-
Phenoxypropylpenicillin (propicillin)	positive bacilli
Azidocillin	and spirochetes
Penicillinase-resistant penicillins	
Isoxazolylpenicillins	
Oxacillin	*Staphylococcus*
Cloxacillin	*aureus.* Most gram-
Dicloxacillin	negative bacilli
Flucloxacillin	are resistant
Methicillin[a]	
Nafcillin[a]	
Ancillin	
Broad-spectrum penicillins	
Ampicillin	
Pivampicillin[b]	Gram-negative
Hetacillin[b]	bacilli except
Metampicillin[b]	*Pseudomonas* species
Bacampicillin[b]	
Amoxycillin	
Epicillin	
Antipseudomonas penicillins	
Carbenicillin[a]	*Pseudomonas* species and
Ticarcillin[a]	other gram-negative
Suncillin	bacilli except
	Klebsiella species

[a]Unstable in acid.
[b]Transformed rapidly to ampicillin during absorption.

Although compounds of the penicillin-resistant, broad-spectrum, and antipseudomonas penicillins inhibit the growth of many gram-positive and gram-negative cocci, they are less active than the compounds of the narrow-spectrum penicillins against susceptible cocci. Mechanism of action of penicillins is inhibition of muramic acid synthesis on the bacterial wall. All penicillins potentiate the action of other bactericidal antibiotics, but their action is antagonistic to that of chloramphenicol and tetracyclines. Development of resistance during treatment is frequent. Complete cross-allergy among all the penicillins is the rule.

Absorption, Distribution, and Elimination
See Table 11.

t_{max} for oral preparations: about 1 hour. V_d: about 0.25 L/kg. The concentration in CSF is 5–10% of the serum concentration except for ampicillin in meningitis, in which the concentration is 30–40% of the serum concentration.

Two derivatives of ampicillin, pivampicillin and bacampicillin, are 90–100% absorbed, while the other penicillins are not absorbed much better than ampicillin.

Food delays t_{max} and reduces the bioavailability of all penicillins except phenoxymethylpenicillin, pivampicillin, and amoxycillin.

Concentration in bile is 1–5 times the serum concentration except for nafcillin, with which the concentration may be 1–100 times higher than the serum concentration. The concentration in fetal circulation is 30–50% and in breast milk, about 10% of the maternal serum concentration.

Dosage Schedule and Special Dosage Situations
See Table 12.

The total daily dose is usually divided into 2–4 doses. No dosage adjustment required in patients with renal failure unless creatinine clearance is below 10 ml/min; if creatinine clearance is below this figure, the daily dose should be reduced by 25–50%. An exception is carbenicillin; the daily dose is 20 g if creatinine clearance is below 50 ml/min and 5–10 g if creatinine clearance is below 10 ml/min. No dosage adjustment necessary in patients with hepatic failure, in women during pregnancy or lactation, or in the elderly.

Therapeutic Concentrations
Highly variable, depending on species and strain. Examples of minimum inhibitory concentrations (MIC) in micrograms per milliliter are given in Table 13.

Adverse Reactions
Allergic skin reactions are frequent (5–10%); most often scarlatiniform, morbilliform, and urticarial exanthemata, whereas exfoliative dermatitis and Stevens-Johnson syndrome occur rarely. The incidence of allergic skin reactions is highest with ampicillin. Doubt exists about the mechanism, which often seems more toxic than allergic. 90% of patients with mononucleosis develop rash after receiving ampicillin. Anaphylactic reactions are rare (about 0.02%); they include sweating, abdominal pain, vomiting, bronchoconstriction, and hypotensive shock. Therapy is 0.4–0.6 ml of epinephrine in a 1/1000 solution (0.4–0.6 mg) IM or IV combined with corticosteroids and supportive therapy. Other allergic reactions are serum sickness and angioedema. Toxic effects include glossitis, stomatitis, and diarrhea. Convulsions may occur at high doses, particularly in patients with reduced renal function. Other

Table 11. *Absorption, Distribution, and Elimination of Penicillins*

Type of Penicillin	Systemic Bioavailability (%)	Protein Binding (%)	Excreted Unchanged (%)	$t_{\frac{1}{2}}$ (min) in Normal People	$t_{\frac{1}{2}}$ (hr) in Anuria	Removed by Dialysis
Benzylpenicillin [3, 11]	15	60	75 (IV)	30	6–10	Yes
Phenoxymethyl penicillin [7, 11]	50	80	40 (oral)	45	. . .[a]	Yes
Oxacillin [3, 6, 15]	30	90	15 (oral)	40	0.8	No
Cloxacillin [3, 6, 12]	50	93	40 (oral)	30	1.0	No
Flucloxacillin [1, 15]	45	96	40 (oral)	30	. . .[a]	No
Methicillin [3, 5, 13]	0	50	80 (IV)	30	4	No
Nafcillin [8, 17]	0	90	90 (IV)	45	1.2	No
Ampicillin [3, 4, 10]	50	20	80 (IV)	75	12	Yes
Amoxycillin [16]	80	20	70 (oral)	75	. . .[a]	Yes
Carbenicillin [2, 9, 14]	0	50	85 (IV)	60	15	Yes

[a]No available information.

Table 12. *Daily Dosage Schedule of Penicillins*

| Type of Penicillin | Adults | | | Newborn Infants Ages 0–1 Month |
	Oral	Parenteral	Children	
Benzylpenicillin	. . . [a]	2–5 million units[b]	50,000 u[b]/kg	60,000 u[b]/kg
Phenoxymethylpenicillin	1–2 million units	. . . [a]	50,000 u[b]/kg	60,000 u[b]/kg
Oxacillin	2–4 g	2–4 g	50 mg/kg	50 mg/kg
Cloxacillin	2–4 g	2–4 g	50 mg/kg	50 mg/kg
Methicillin	. . . [a]	4–6 g	100 mg/kg	100 mg/kg
Nafcillin	2–4 g	2–4 g	25–50 mg/kg	20–50 mg/kg
Ampicillin	1–4 g	2–6 g	50–100 mg/kg	50–100 mg/kg
Amoxycillin	1–2 g	. . . [a]	20–40 mg/kg	. . . [a]
Carbenicillin	. . . [a]	30–40 g in IV infusion	400–500 mg/kg	200 mg/kg

[a]Not applicable.
[b]1 mg = 1667 units.

Table 13.   *Minimum Inhibitory Concentrations (MIC) of Penicillins ($\mu g/ml$)*

Species of Organism	Benzyl-penicillin	Methi-cillin	Ampi-cillin	Carbeni-cillin
Streptococcus pneumoniae	0.1	2.0	0.2	2.0
Staphylococcus aureus	R[a]	5.0	R[a]	50
Haemophilus influenzae	1.0	5.0	0.5	0.5
E. coli	50	R[a]	5.0	10.0
Klebsiella species	R[a]	R[a]	R[a]	R[a]
Pseudomonas species	R[a]	R[a]	R[a]	50–100

[a]R = resistant.

side-effects are interstitial nephritis (most frequently found with methicillin), bone marrow depression (with methicillin and ampicillin), inhibition of platelet aggregation (with carbenicillin), hyperkalemia (with high doses of potassium benzylpenicillin), hypernatremia (with high doses of carbenicillin), and superinfection (with broad-spectrum antibiotics).

Interactions

Probenecid, sulfinpyrazone, phenylbutazone, sulfafenazole, and indomethacin prolong the half-life of all penicillins by inhibiting renal tubular secretion. Carbenicillin shows a synergistic effect with gentamicin, but it must be given separately because carbenicillin inactivates gentamicin if given in same intravenous drip solution. Compounds of broad-spectrum penicillins may decrease prothrombin formation in patients taking oral anticoagulants by inhibition of the intestinal flora that produce vitamin K.

Reviews

Ball, A. P., Gray, J. A., et al.   Antibacterial drugs today. I. Penicillins. *Drugs* 10:9–28, 1975.

Barza, M., and Weinstein, L.   Pharmacokinetics of the penicillins in man. *Clin. Pharmacokin.* 1:297–308, 1976.

Rolinson, G. N., and Sutherland, R.   Semisynthetic penicillins. *Adv. Pharmacol. Chemother.* 11:151–220, 1973.

References

1.   Bodey, G. P., Vallejos, C., et al.   Flucloxacillin: A new semisynthetic isoxazolylpenicillin. *Clin. Pharmacol. Ther.* 13:512–515, 1972.

2.   Brumfitt, W., and Percival, A.   Clinical and laboratory studies with carbenicillin. *Lancet* 1:1289–1293, 1967.

3.   Dittert, L. W., Griffen, W. O., et al.   Pharmacokinetic interpretation of penicillin levels in serum and urine after intravenous administration. *Antimicrob. Agents Chemother.* 42–48, 1969.

4.   Eickhoff, T. C., and Kislak, J. W.   Sodium ampicillin: Absorption and excretion of intramuscular and intravenous doses in normal young men. *Am. J. Med. Sci.* 249:163–171, 1965.

5. Gilbert, D. M., and Sandford, J. P.   Methicillin: Critical
    appraisal after a decade of experience. *Med. Clin. North Am.*
    54:1113–1125, 1970.
6. Gravekemper, C. F., Bennett, J. V., et al.   Dicloxacillin, *in
    vitro* and pharmacologic comparison with oxacillin and
    cloxacillin. *Arch. Intern. Med.* 116:340–345, 1965.
7. Hellstrom, K., Rosen, A., et al.   Absorption and decomposi-
    tion of potassium ^{35}S-phenoxymethylpenicillin. *Clin. Phar-
    macol. Ther.* 16:825–833, 1974.
8. Klein, J. O., and Finland, M.   Nafcillin. *Am. J. Med. Sci.*
    246:10–26, 1963.
9. Knudsen, E. T., Rolinson, G. N., et al.   Carbenicillin: A new
    semisynthetic penicillin active against *Pseudomonas pyocyanea.*
    Br. Med. J. 3:75–78, 1967.
10. Loo, J. C. K., Foltz, E. L., et al.   Pharmacokinetics of
    pivampicillin and ampicillin in man. *Clin. Pharmacol. Ther.*
    16:35–43, 1974.
11. McCarthy, C. G., and Finland, M.   Absorption and excre-
    tion of four penicillins. *N. Engl. J. Med.* 263:315–326, 1960.
12. Nauta, E. H., and Mattie, H.   Dicloxacillin and cloxacillin:
    Pharmacokinetics in healthy and hemodialysis subjects. *Clin.
    Pharmacol. Ther.* 20:98–108, 1976.
13. Sabath, L. D., Postic, B., et al.   Laboratory studies on
    methicillin. *Am. J. Med. Sci.* 244:484–500, 1962.
14. Smith, C. B., and Finland, M.   Carbenicillin: Activity in
    vitro and absorption and excretion in normal young men.
    Appl. Microbiol. 16:1753–1760, 1968.
15. Sutherland, R., Croydon, E. A. P., et al.   Flucloxacillin, a new
    isoxazolylpenicillin compared with oxacillin, cloxacillin and
    dicloxacillin. *Br. Med. J.* 4:455–460, 1970.
16. Sutherland, R., Croydon, E. A. P., et al.   Amoxycillin: A
    new semi-synthetic penicillin. *Br. Med. J.* 3:13–16, 1972.
17. Whitehouse, A. C., and Morgan, J. G.   Blood levels and
    antistaphylococcal titers produced in human subjects by a
    penicillinase-resistant penicillin, nafcillin, compared with
    similar penicillin. *Antimicrob. Agents Chemother.* 384–392,
    1962.

PENTAZOCINE

A benzomorphan derivative that is usually classified as a nonnar-
cotic analgesic. In addition to its analgesic action, also acts as a
weak narcotic antagonist. In comparison with parenteral
morphine, analgesic potency is 20–30% [3]. Indicated for use in
patients with severe pain.

Absorption

Well absorbed from GI tract, but first-pass metabolism occurs [9].
t_{max}: 1–3 hours orally; 15–60 min (IM) [6]. Plasma and CSF levels
correlate well with the onset, duration, and intensity of analgesia
[1].

Distribution

V_d: about 3 L/kg [1]. Protein binding: 60–70% [1]. Pentazocine passes the blood-brain and placental barriers [1, 4].

Elimination

$t_{\frac{1}{2}}$: 2 hours [1, 6]. Pentazocine is extensively metabolized in liver. Metabolites, glucuronide conjugate, and unchanged drug (about 10%) are excreted by the kidneys.

Dosage Schedule

15–30 mg every 2–4 hours (parenterally). 25–100 mg orally every 3–6 hours as required for relief of pain.

Special Dosage Situations

Pentazocine should be avoided in opiate addicts because of the risk of precipitating the withdrawal syndrome [3]. With frequent and repeated use, tolerance and withdrawal syndromes develop [7]. Gradual dosage reduction is recommended in patients who develop the withdrawal syndrome. Pentazocine should be given with caution to patients with angina and myocardial insufficiency because it increases cardiac work load [2].

Therapeutic Concentrations

0.03–0.1 μg/ml; toxic level is 0.2 μg/ml [6]. Deaths have been reported with plasma levels greater than 0.3 μg/ml.

Adverse Reactions

Sedation, sweating, dizziness, light-headedness, and nausea are the most common adverse reactions. Psychomimetic effects such as anxiety, nightmares, euphoria, and hallucinations have been reported, especially with doses of more than 60 mg [5, 8]. Respiratory depression is observed at high doses and is antagonized by naloxone but not by nalorphine or levellorphan. Subcutaneous atrophy and scarring may occur with prolonged parenteral abuse.

Interactions

Withdrawal syndrome in patients receiving opiates as well as pentazocine.

References

1. Agurell, S. V., Boreus, L. O., et al. Plasma and cerebrospinal fluid concentrations of pentazocine in patients: Assay by mass fragmentography. *J. Pharm. Pharmacol.* 26:1–8, 1974.
2. Alderman, E. L., Barry, W. H., et al. Hemodynamic effects of morphine and pentazocine differ in cardiac patients. *N. Engl. J. Med.* 287:623–627, 1972.
3. Beaver, W. T., Wallenstein, S. L., et al. A comparison of the analgesic effects of pentazocine and morphine in patients with cancer. *Clin. Pharmacol. Ther.* 7:740–751, 1966.
4. Beckett, A. H., and Taylor, J. F. Blood concentrations of pethidine and pentazocine in mother and infant at time of birth. *J. Pharm. Pharmacol.* 19 (Suppl. I):50S–52S, 1967.

5. Bellville, J. W., Forrest, W. H., et al.   Evaluating side effects of analgesics in a cooperative clinical study. *Clin. Pharmacol. Ther.* 9:303–313, 1968.
6. Berkowitz, B. A., Asling, J. H., et al.   Relationship of pentazocine plasma levels to pharmacological activity in man. *Clin. Pharmacol. Ther.* 10:320–328, 1969.
7. Fraser, H. F., and Rosenberg, D. E.   Studies on the human addiction liability of 2'-hydroxy-5,9-dimethyl-2-(3,3-dimethyl-allyl)-6,7-benzomorphan (Win 20228): A weak narcotic antagonist. *J. Pharmacol. Exp. Ther.* 143:149–156, 1964.
8. Paddock, R., Beer, E. G., et al.   Analgesic and side effects of pentazocine and morphine in a large population of postoperative patients. *Clin. Pharmacol. Ther.* 10:355–365, 1969.
9. Rowland, M.   Influence of route of administration on drug availability. *J. Pharm. Sci.* 61:70–74, 1972.

PENTOBARBITAL

An intermediate-acting barbiturate used as a hypnotic. In common with all barbiturates pentobarbital reversibly depresses the activity of both the peripheral nervous system and CNS, probably at the synaptic level. Reduces the time spent in rapid eye movement (REM) sleep.

Absorption

Oral bioavailability: 90–100 [3]. t_{max}: 1 hour in fasting state; in nonfasting state t_{max} is prolonged, but bioavailability is not affected [7].

Distribution

V_d: about 1 L/kg [3, 5]. Protein binding: 60–70% in individuals with normal renal function; 40–70% in patients with severe renal failure [5].

Crosses the placenta. No available data about distribution to breast milk.

Elimination

$t_{\frac{1}{2}}$: 20–35 hours [5]. Inactivated in the liver, the predominant metabolite being an alcohol of barbituric acid [1]. About 20% excreted unchanged in the urine.

Dosage Schedule

100–200 mg as a single dose at bedtime.

Special Dosage Situations

Children: 1–2 mg/kg. Elderly: no available information. Renal disease: protein binding is slightly reduced, but no special precautions are required [5]. Liver disease: in decompensated cirrhosis, $t_{\frac{1}{2}}$ is doubled [4]. $t_{\frac{1}{2}}$ is also increased in extrahepatic biliary obstruction (30%) and cholestatic hepatitis (60%) [2]. This effect has been associated with a decrease in hepatic pentobarbital hydroxylase activity [2], and therefore appropriate dosage adjustments need to be made in patients with these conditions.

Therapeutic Concentrations

Not relevant, since drug is usually administered to achieve sleep that is easily monitored clinically. The levels of about 40 μg/ml have been associated with coma [8], but this relationship of plasma level to clinical effect is influenced by the tolerance of the patient to the drug.

Adverse Reactions

Sedation, occasionally excitement, and hypersensitivity; contrain-dicated in patients with acute intermittent porphyria. Overdosage results in varying degrees of CNS depression, and if sufficient quantity of the drug is ingested, respiratory depression, hypo-thermia, cardiovascular collapse, and death may ensue. In over-dosage, dialysis and forced diuresis are of no value. Meticu-lous supportive care results in mortality of less than 5% [8].

Drug Interactions

Ethanol doubles the $t_{\frac{1}{2}}$ [6].

References

1. Brodie, B. B., Burns, J. J., et al.   The fate of pentobarbital in man and dog and a method for its estimation in biological material. *J. Pharmacol. Exp. Ther.* 109:26–34, 1953.
2. Carulli, N., Manenti, F., et al.   Alteration of drug metabo-lism during cholestasis in man. *Eur. J. Clin. Invest.* 5:455–462, 1975.
3. Ehrnebo, M.   Pharmacokinetics and distribution properties of pentobarbital in humans following oral and intravenous administration. *J. Pharm. Sci.* 63:1114–1118, 1974.
4. Ossenberg, F. W., Denis, P., et al.   Pentobarbital phar-macokinetics in cirrhosis. *Digestion* 8:448–449, 1973.
5. Reidenberg, M. M., Lowenthal, D. T., et al.   Pentobarbital elimination in patients with poor renal function. *Clin. Phar-macol. Ther.* 20:67–71, 1976.
6. Rubin, E., Gang, H., et al.   Inhibition of drug metabolism by acute ethanol intoxication. *Am. J. Med.* 49:801–806, 1970.
7. Smith, R. B., and Dittert, L. W.   Pharmacokinetics of pen-tobarbital after intravenous and oral administration. *J. Phar-macokin. Biopharm.* 1:5–16, 1973.
8. Spear, P. W., and Protass, L. M.   Barbiturate poisoning, an endemic disease. Symposium on acute medicine. *Med. Clin. North Am.* 57:1471–1479, 1973.

PHENFORMIN

Phenethylbiguanide, a member of the biguanide group of oral euglycemic agents. Mechanism of action unclear but appears to inhibit and delay gastrointestinal absorption of glucose, sodium, and water [2] and enhance aerobic glycolysis, with decreased fasting blood glucose levels, improved glucose tolerance, and decreased fasting and postglucose insulinemia [7]. Reduction of serum cholesterol and a decrease in body weight by 2–3 kg may be observed [7]. Possesses antifibrinopathic activity that is manifested by prolonged prothrombin time and increased fibrinolysis [3], which is enhanced by ethylestrenol [5]. Unlike the sulfonylureas does not require residual islet cell activity. Does not stimulate the pancreas or cause hypoglycemia in the normal person. Used in the treatment of patients with nonketotic adult-onset diabetes who have good renal function and in whom reduction of weight and restriction of carbohydrates have not been successful. May be used in combination with insulin in treatment of brittle diabetes. Under evaluation in conditions of excessive vascular thrombosis.

Absorption
Oral bioavailability: about 50–70% [4]. t_{max}: 2–4 hours for both tablets and sustained-release preparation [1, 4, 10].

Distribution
V_d: about 5–10 L/kg. Protein binding: about 20% [10].

Elimination
$t_{\frac{1}{2}}$: 2–4 hours [4]. However, recent work indicates that this figure represents only distribution $t_{\frac{1}{2}}$ and that true elimination $t_{\frac{1}{2}}$ is 13 hours [10]. 33% is parahydroxylated and excreted in urine with the parent drug (about 50% of dose) [4, 10].

Dosage Schedule
Initial dose 25 mg 2–3 times daily before meals. Dosage increased every 2–4 days until diabetic control is established or adverse gastrointestinal effects occur. Total daily dosage is usually 100–200 mg. Sustained-release preparations permit more convenient dosage, either daily or twice daily.

Special Dosage Situations
Contraindicated in renal disease. Use with caution in the elderly because their renal function is usually diminished. If possible, also avoid in patients with heart failure and hepatocellular disease. During crises of the diabetic state, management with soluble insulin is usually necessary and advisable.

Therapeutic Concentrations
Levels of 100–240 ng/ml have been associated with euglycemic response. It is usual to simply monitor blood glucose response to treatment.

Adverse Reactions
A metallic taste in the mouth, gastrointestinal disturbances, lassitude, weakness, and weight loss. Increased cardiovascular mortality is thought to occur in patients treated with phenformin [12], but this finding remains controversial [8]. Lactic acidosis is the

major cause of morbidity and mortality and occurs most frequently in the elderly and those with renal or hepatic impairment. Development of lactic acidosis is a serious crisis that demands urgent treatment to control acidosis, hyperglycemia, and fluid and electrolyte imbalance [6, 11]. IV bicarbonate, insulin, and potassium are indicated [9]. Peritoneal dialysis or hemodialysis may be useful in the most extreme cases.

Interactions

Alcohol inhibits parahydroxylation of phenformin, potentiating its hypoglycemic effect and aggravating lactic acidosis. Phenformin interferes with vitamin B_{12} absorption from the gastrointestinal tract and may invalidate the results of oral glucose tolerance tests.

Review

Danowski, T. S. (Ed.).   Diabetes mellitus and obesity: Phenformin hydrochloride as a research tool. *Ann. N.Y. Acad. Sci.* 148:573–962, 1968.

References

1. Alkalay, D., Khemani, L., et al.   Pharmacokinetics of phenformin in man. *J. Clin. Pharmacol.* 15:446–448, 1975.
2. Arvanitakis, C., Lorenzsonn, V., et al.   Phenformin-induced alterations of small intestinal function and mitochondrial structure in man. *J. Lab. Clin. Med.* 82:195–200, 1973.
3. Banerjee, R. N., Kumar, V., et al.   Antifibrin action of phenformin. *Diabetologia* 11:105–111, 1975.
4. Beckmann, R.   The fate of biguanides in man. *Ann. N.Y. Acad. Sci.* 148:820–832, 1968.
5. Chakrabarti, R., and Fearnley, G. R.   Pharmacological fibrinolysis in diabetes mellitus. *Diabetologia* 10:10–22, 1974.
6. Cleaver, T., and Carretta, R.   Lactic acidosis with phenformin therapy. *Calif. Med.* 117:14–19, 1972.
7. Danowski, T. S., Sunder, J. H., et al.   Phenformin therapy of chemical diabetes. *J. Clin. Pharmacol.* 14:638–650, 1974.
8. Feinstein, A. R.   Clinical biostatistics—VIII. An analytic appraisal of the University Group Diabetes Program (UGDP) study. *Clin. Pharmacol. Ther.* 12:167–191, 1971.
9. Kristensen, O., Andersen, H. H., et al.   Glucose-insulin treatment of lactic acidosis in phenformin-treated diabetics. *Acta Med. Scand.* 197:463–465, 1975.
10. Matin, S. B., Karam, J. H., et al.   Simple electron capture gas chromatographic method for the determination of oral hypoglycemic biguanides in biological fluids. *Anal. Chem.* 47:545–548, 1975.
11. Oliva, T. D.   Lactic acidosis. *Am. J. Med.* 48:209–225, 1970.
12. University Group Diabetes Program.   A study of the effects of hypoglycemic agents on vascular complications in patients with adult-onset diabetes. IV. A preliminary report on phenformin results. *J.A.M.A.* 217:777–784, 1971.

PHENOBARBITAL

An ethylphenyl-substituted long-acting barbiturate available as an acid or as a sodium salt. Used as an anticonvulsant and sedative and in the treatment of chronic cholestasis [2] and neonatal jaundice. Phenobarbital has a nonspecific depressant action on the CNS and is a potent microsomal mixed-function oxidase-inducing agent.

Absorption
At least 80% absorbed after oral administration [14]. t_{max}: 6–18 hours [10] after oral ingestion and 1½ hours after IM injection [3]. The sodium salt is absorbed more rapidly from the gastrointestinal tract than the acid form.

Distribution
V_d: 0.75 L/kg. Protein binding: 46% [15]. CSF and brain levels equilibrate with total plasma levels [15]. Fetal levels equal 95% of maternal levels [12]. 10–30% of maternal plasma levels are found in breast milk [16].

Elimination
$t_{\frac{1}{2}}$: 3–4 days [1]. Inactivated by hepatic p-hydroxylation of the phenyl ring. This inactive metabolite is excreted in the urine conjugated with glucuronic acid and possibly also with sulfuric acid [1]. Up to 25% of the dose may be excreted unchanged in the urine [1]. $t_{\frac{1}{2}}$ in neonates: 59–182 hours [8]. $t_{\frac{1}{2}}$ in children: 37–73 hours [6].

Dosage Schedule
Loading dose: 2–6 mg/kg for 3 days. Maintenance dose: 1–3 mg/kg. Plasma levels bear a constant relationship to the dose in milligrams per kilogram, e.g., 1 mg/kg produces a level of 8 μg/ml, 2 mg/kg a level of 16 μg/ml, etc. [14]. A dose is required only once daily.

Special Dosage Situations
Children: loading dose 4–8 mg/kg for 2 days [11]. Maintenance dose: 2–4 mg/kg [5]. In patients with cirrhosis, $t_{\frac{1}{2}}$ increased to 4–8 days, and conjugation of parahydroxyphenobarbital may be reduced by 50% [1]. There is a strong negative correlation between the serum albumin level and the $t_{\frac{1}{2}}$ of phenobarbital. No dosage adjustment is required in patients with hepatitis [1] or renal failure or in the elderly. Teratogenicity has not been clearly demonstrated, but the usual precautions against prescribing medications for pregnant women should be observed.

Therapeutic Concentrations
15–25 μg/ml in seizure control. Concentrations up to 40 μg/ml may be necessary in some epileptic patients.

Adverse Reactions
Drowsiness; paradoxical excitement, especially in children and the elderly. Tolerance to CNS side-effects may develop. Ma-

crocytosis and occasionally anemia occur [7]. Hemorrhage in a newborn whose mother received phenobarbital in pregnancy is reversed by vitamin K. Contraindicated in acute intermittent porphyria, which may be exacerbated by phenobarbital. Skin rashes occur in 1–2% of patients. Increased serum alkaline phosphatase and hydroxyproline but no overt rickets reported [9].

If coma and cardiopulmonary depression occur in overdose, forced alkaline diuresis and hemodialysis may be of value.

Interactions

At doses that exceed 1.7 mg/kg or at plasma levels that are greater than 7 μg/ml [13], phenobarbital induces the metabolism of warfarin, dicumarol, phenytoin, phenylbutazone, prednisone, hydrocortisone, and possibly digitoxin [4]. The induced state persists for several days after cessation of therapy.

References

1. Alvin, J., McHorse, T., et al.   The effect of liver disease in man on the disposition of phenobarbital. *J. Pharmacol. Exp. Ther.* 192:224–235, 1975.
2. Bloomer, J. R., and Boyer, J. L.   Phenobarbital effects in cholestatic liver disease. *Ann. Intern. Med.* 82:310–317, 1975.
3. Brachet-Liermain, A., Goutieres, F., et al.   Absorption of phenobarbital after the intramuscular administration of single doses in infants. *J. Pediatr.* 87:624–626, 1975.
4. Conney, A. H.   Pharmacological implications of microsomal enzyme induction. *Pharmacol. Rev.* 19:317–366, 1967.
5. Eadie, M. J., and Tyrer, J. H.   *Anticonvulsant Therapy.* London: Churchill/Livingstone, 1974. Pp. 79–99.
6. Garrettson, L. K., and Dayton, P. G.   Disappearance of phenobarbital and diphenylhydantoin from serum of children. *Clin. Pharmacol. Ther.* 11:674–679, 1970.
7. Hawkins, C. F., and Meynell, M. J.   Macrocytosis and macrocytic anemia caused by anticonvulsant drugs. *Q. J. Med.* 27:45–63, 1958.
8. Jalling, B.   Plasma concentrations of phenobarbital in the treatment of seizures in newborns. *Acta Pediatr. Scand.* 64:514–524, 1975.
9. Liakakos, D., Papadopoulos, Z., et al.   Serum alkaline phosphatase and urinary hydroxyproline values in children receiving phenobarbital with and without vitamin D. *J. Pediatr.* 87:291–296, 1975.
10. Lous, P.   Plasma levels and urinary excretion of three barbituric acids after oral administration to man. *Acta Pharmacol. Toxicol.* (Kbh.) 10:147–165, 1954.
11. Maynert, E. W.   Phenobarbital, Mephobarbital, and Metharbital. Absorption, Distribution, and Excretion. In D. M. Woodbury, J. K. Penry, and R. P. Schmidt (Eds.), *Antiepileptic Drugs.* New York: Raven Press, 1972.
12. Melchior, J. C., Svensmark, O., et al.   Placental transfer of phenobarbitone in epileptic women, and elimination in newborns. *Lancet* 2:860–861, 1967.

13. Morselli, P. L., Rizzo, M., et al. Interaction between phenobarbital and diphenylhydantoin in animals and in epileptic patients. *Ann. N.Y. Acad. Sci.* 179:88–107, 1971.
14. Svensmark, O., and Buchthal, F. Accumulation of phenobarbital in man. *Epilepsia* 4:199–206, 1963.
15. Waddell, W. J., and Butler, T. C. The distribution and excretion of phenobarbital. *J. Clin. Invest.* 36:1217–1226, 1957.
16. Westerink, D., and Glerum, J. H. Scheiding en microbepaling van fenobarbital en fenytoine in moedermelk. *Pharm. Weekbl.* 100:577–583, 1965.

PHENYLBUTAZONE

A pyrazolone derivative that has analgesic, antipyretic, anti-inflammatory, and uricosuric effects. Indicated for rheumatoid arthritis, ankylosing spondylitis, osteoarthritis, pseudogout, and acute gout. Actions include inhibition of prostaglandin biosynthesis and stabilization of lysosome membrane [8].

Absorption
Oral bioavailability: 90–100%. t_{max}: 1–2 hours [9].

Distribution
V_d: 0.1–0.35 L/kg [9]. Protein binding: 90–98%. At higher plasma concentrations, the protein binding declines because of saturation of binding sites [11].

Elimination
$t_{\frac{1}{2}}$: 2–5 days [9]. Almost completely metabolized by the hepatic microsomal system; metabolites are excreted by the kidneys [2, 3]. Metabolism is induced by repeated administration. Main active metabolite is oxyphenbutazone, which possesses the same pharmacological potency, toxicity, and pharmacokinetic properties as the parent drug. $t_{\frac{1}{2}}$: 72 hours. The other metabolite, γ-hydroxyphenylbutazone, has only uricosuric action. $t_{\frac{1}{2}}$: 12 hours.

Dosage Schedule
Maintenance dose: 200–400 mg a day in 2–4 divided doses, with meals to lessen gastric distress. Loading dose: 600–800 mg for 1–2 days may be necessary when treatment with phenylbutazone is begun. Should not be given for more than 10 days in any one treatment period because of its toxicity. Patients should be warned that they may develop the symptoms of agranulocytosis and taught to recognize these symptoms should they occur.

Special Dosage Situations
Contraindicated in patients with cardiac, renal, and hepatic dysfunction, especially in patients with edema because of the potential salt and water retention (see Adverse Reactions). Relative contraindication in patients with a history of peptic ulcer. Toxic effects are more common and severe in elderly persons.

Therapeutic Concentrations
50–150 μg/ml [7, 9, 13].

Adverse Reactions
Untoward effects are noted in 10–45% of patients. Gastrointestinal irritation and ulceration. Salt and water retention. Blood dyscrasias, aplastic anemia, leukopenia, agranulocytosis, and thrombocytopenia may occur within a few days of commencing treatment [5, 12]. Blurred vision, vertigo, insomnia, and nervousness. Hypersensitivity reactions such as skin rashes, serum sickness, nephritis, and hepatitis.

Interactions
Phenylbutazone inhibits the metabolism of tolbutamide, which enhances hypoglycemic effects [4, 11]. There is also an increased hypoglycemic effect with chlorpropamide, but the mechanism of this interaction is not yet established [6]. Phenylbutazone potentiates the anticoagulant effects of warfarin by inhibiting the metabolism of the more potent enantiomorph S-warfarin [10] and by displacing it from protein-binding sites [1].

References

1. Aggeler, P. M., O'Reilly, R. A., et al. Potentiation of anticoagulant effect of warfarin by phenylbutazone. *N. Engl. J. Med.* 276:496–501, 1967.
2. Burns, J. J., Rose, R. K., et al. The physiological disposition of phenylbutazone (Butazolidin) in man and a method for its estimation in biological material. *J. Pharmacol. Exp. Ther.* 109:346–357, 1953.
3. Burns, J. J., Rose, R. K., et al. The metabolic fate of phenylbutazone (Butazolidin) in man. *J. Pharmacol. Exp. Ther.* 113:481–489, 1955.
4. Christensen, L. K., Hansen, J. M., et al. Sulphaphenazole-induced hypoglycemic attacks in tolbutamide-treated diabetics. *Lancet* 2:1298–1301, 1963.
5. Clinicopathologic Conference: Agranulocytosis and anuria during phenylbutazone therapy of rheumatoid arthritis. *Am. J. Med.* 30:268–280, 1961.
6. Dalgas, M., Abdel-Maguid, R., et al. Fenylbutazon-inducerat hypoglykaemit ilfaelde hos klorpropamid behandlet diabetikere. *Ugeskr. Laeg.* 127:834–836, 1965.
7. Done, A. K. The toxic emergency. *Emergency Med.* 7: 193–201, 1975.
8. Ferreira, S. H., and Vane, J. R. New aspects of the mode of action of nonsteroid anti-inflammatory drugs. *Annu. Rev. Pharmacol.* 14:57–73, 1974.
9. Hvidberg, E. F., Andreasen, P. B., et al. Plasma half-life of phenylbutazone in patients with impaired liver function. *Clin. Pharmacol. Ther.* 15:171–177, 1974.
10. Lewis, R. L., Trager, W. F., et al. Warfarin. Stereochemical aspects of its metabolism and the interaction with phenylbutazone. *J. Clin. Invest.* 53:1607–1617, 1974.
11. Mahfouz, M., Hansen, J. M., et al. Potentiation of the

hypoglycaemic action of tolbutamide by different drugs. *Arzneim. Forsch.* 20:120–122, 1970.

12. Mauer, E. F. The toxic effect of phenylbutazone (Butazolidin). Review of literature and report of the twenty-third death following its use. *N. Engl. J. Med.* 253:404–410, 1955.

13. Orme, M., Holt, P. J. L., et al. Plasma concentrations of phenylbutazone and its therapeutic effect—studies in patients with rheumatoid arthritis. *Br. J. Clin. Pharmacol.* 3:185–191, 1976.

PHENYTOIN

Diphenylhydantoin, an organic acid that is poorly soluble in water. Inhibits spread of ectopic electrical activity in the brain and the heart. Primary clinical uses are as an anticonvulsant, for all types of epilepsy except petit mal triad, and as an antiarrhythmic; especially useful in digitalis-induced ventricular arrhythmias [21].

Absorption
Oral bioavailability: approximately 90% [6]. t_{max}: 3–10 hours [6]. By IM route absorption is erratic, since the drug crystallizes in muscles, resulting in low plasma levels [20]; it is painful and not recommended.

Distribution
V_d: 0.6 L/kg [6]. Protein binding: approximately 90% [15]; it is reduced in renal failure [19]; in hypoalbuminemia, the usual 10% unbound drug increases by 1% for every 0.1 g reduction of plasma albumin below 3 g/dl [7]. Concentration in fetal plasma equals that of the mother [16]; brain and plasma concentrations are approximately equal [11]. Small amounts are excreted in breast milk [16].

Elimination
"$t_{\frac{1}{2}}$" varies according to plasma level, because elimination changes from apparent first-order process to mainly zero-order process when metabolism becomes saturated [2]. This effect occurs at a plasma concentration of 7–10 μg/ml, after which plasma levels increase disproportionately in relation to an increase in dosage [10]. The dosage required to achieve 7–10 μg/ml varies widely among individuals. Mean elimination "$t_{\frac{1}{2}}$" is 24 hours when plasma levels are in the therapeutic range [2]. "$t_{\frac{1}{2}}$" is increased when plasma levels are in the toxic range. Metabolized by hepatic parahydroxylation, the main metabolite being 5-p-hydroxy 5-phenyl phenylhydantoin (HPPH), which is excreted as glucuronide [4]; no active metabolites are known. 5% is excreted as unchanged drug in stools and 2% in urine [5].

Dosage Schedule
Loading dose: 10–12 mg/kg in 2–3 doses over 12–24 hours. A large single dose may produce gastric irritation. Maintenance dose: 5–6 mg/kg/day given as a single dose will result in therapeu-

tic plasma levels in about 50% of patients [10]. Same IV dose as oral dose; IM route not recommended. By IV route, drug must be given no more rapidly than 50 mg/min. Rapid injection may cause hypotension, cardiovascular collapse, and death. Must be given directly into the vein to prevent crystallization in intravenous drip tubing, preferably by central venous line because parenteral dosage form has pH of 11–12.

Special Dosage Situations

Children: 10 mg/kg/day [9]. Lactation or elderly: no special precautions. Pregnancy: clearance is increased, and therefore dose may need to be increased to maintain therapeutic plasma levels [17]; observe fetus at parturition for evidence of hemorrhagic disease, for which vitamin K is antidote. In acute viral hepatitis, the plasma protein binding is decreased [3]. Dosage may have to be reduced in renal failure, acute hepatitis, and hypoalbuminemia.

Therapeutic Concentrations

10–20 μg/ml [12].

Adverse Reactions

Adverse reactions are related to the plasma level. At 20–30 μg/ml, nystagmus results; at 30–40 μg/ml, ataxia occurs; and over 40 μg/ml, drowsiness and speech disturbance are found [12]. There is a twofold or threefold increase in teratogenic fetal abnormalities. Other effects are gingival hypertrophy, osteomalacia, hirsutism, lymphadenopathy, and folic acid deficiency, but anemia is uncommon. In poisoning, hemodialysis and forced diuresis are of no value [1].

Interactions

Phenytoin metabolism is inhibited and the steady-state plasma levels elevated by isoniazid, *p*-aminosalicylic acid [13], disulfiram [18], sulfamethizole [14], sulthiame [8], chloramphenicol, phenylbutazone, and dicoumarol.

Metabolism is induced by carbamazepine and phenobarbital, with a lowering of phenytoin steady-state plasma levels. Whenever these drugs are to be administered regularly with phenytoin, plasma levels of phenytoin should be checked and the dosage regulated accordingly.

The $t_{\frac{1}{2}}$ of quinidine is decreased by 50% when phenytoin is administered concurrently.

References

1. Adler, D. S., Martin, E., et al. Hemodialysis of phenytoin in a uremic patient. *Clin. Pharmacol. Ther.* 18:65–69, 1975.
2. Arnold, K. and Gerber, N. The rate of decline of diphenylhydantoin in human plasma. *Clin. Pharmacol. Ther.* 11:121–134, 1970.
3. Blaschke, T. F., Meffin, P. J., et al. Influence of acute viral hepatitis on phenytoin kinetics and protein binding. *Clin. Pharmacol. Ther.* 17:685–691, 1975.

4. Butler, T. C. The metabolic conversion of 5,5-diphenyl hydantoin to 5-(*p*-hydroxyphenyl)-5-phenyl hydantoin. *J. Pharmacol. Exp. Ther.* 119:1–11, 1957.

5. Eadie, M. J. and Tyrer, J. H. In *Anticonvulsant Therapy.* London: Churchill/Livingstone. 1974. P. 38.

6. Gugler, R., Manion, C. V., et al. Phenytoin: Pharmacokinetics and bioavailability. *Clin. Pharmacol. Ther.* 19:135–142, 1976.

7. Gugler, R., Shoeman, D. W., et al. Pharmacokinetics of drugs in patients with the nephrotic syndrome. *J. Clin. Invest.* 55:1182–1189, 1975.

8. Hansen, J. M., Kristensen, M., et al. Sulthiame (Ospolot) as inhibitor of diphenylhydantoin metabolism. *Epilepsia* 9:17–22, 1968.

9. Hooper, W. D. Eadie. M. J., et al. Plasma diphenylhydantoin levels in Australian children. *Aust. N.Z. J. Med.* 4:456–461, 1974.

10. Hooper, W. D., Tyrer, J. H., et al. Plasma diphenylhydantoin levels in Australian adults. *Aust. N.Z. J. Med.* 4:449–455, 1974.

11. Houghton, G. W., Richens, A., et al. Brain concentrations of phenytoin, phenobarbitone, and primidone in epileptic patients. *Eur. J. Clin. Pharmacol.* 9:73–78, 1975.

12. Kutt, H. and McDowell, F. Management of epilepsy with diphenylhydantoin sodium. *J.A.M.A.* 203:167–170, 1968.

13. Kutt, H., Winters, W., et al. Depression of parahydroxylation of diphenylhydantoin by antituberculosis chemotherapy. *Neurology* 16:594–602, 1966.

14. Lumholtz, B., Siersbaek-Nielsen, K., et al. Sulfamethizole-induced inhibition of diphenylhydantoin, tolbutamide, and warfarin metabolism. *Clin. Pharmacol. Ther.* 17:731–734, 1975.

15. Lunde, P. K. M., Rane, A., et al. Plasma protein binding of diphenylhydantoin in man. Interaction with other drugs and the effect of temperature and plasma dilution. *Clin. Pharmacol. Ther.* 11:846–855, 1970.

16. Mirkin, B. L. Diphenylhydantoin: Placental transport, fetal localization, neonatal metabolism, and possible teratogenic effects. *J. Pediatr.* 78:329–337, 1971.

17. Mygind, K. I., Dam, M., et al. Phenytoin and phenobarbitone plasma clearance during pregnancy. *Acta Neurol. Scand.* 54:160–166, 1976.

18. Olesen, O. V. Disulfiramum (Antabuse) as inhibitor of phenytoin metabolism. *Acta Pharmacol Toxicol.* 24:317–322, 1966.

19. Reidenberg, M. M., Odar-Cederlöf, I., et al. Protein binding of diphenylhydantoin and desmethylimipramine in plasma from patients with poor renal function. *N. Engl. J. Med.* 285:264–267, 1971.

20. Wilensky, A. J. and Lowden, J. A. Inadequate serum levels after intramuscular administration of diphenylhydantoin. *Neurology* 23:318–324, 1973.

21. Wit, A. L., Rosen, M. R., et al. Appraisal and reappraisal of cardiac therapy. *Am. Heart J.* 90:265–272, 1975.

PREDNISONE AND PREDNISOLONE
Δ^1*PREDNISONE*

Synthetic corticosteroid, Δ^1-cortisone, which is considered inactive as such. Converted within minutes to active prednisolone by 11 β-hydroxydehydrogenase in the liver, probably during the first-pass metabolism. In liver disease this conversion may be delayed and possibly reduced [3]. Prednisolone should be used if liver function is markedly impaired. The dosage requirements, metabolism, and adverse reactions for prednisone are the same as those listed for prednisolone, which follows below.

PREDNISOLONE

Synthetic corticosteroid, Δ^1-cortisol. The glucocorticoid activity of prednisolone is 4 times that of cortisol, but it has approximately 20% less sodium-retaining activity than cortisol [7]. Prednisolone has the same widely diversified physiological effects on many organs as endogenous cortisol, and the pharmacological effects are also similar. Carbohydrate, protein, fat, and purine metabolism and water and electrolyte balance are modified. The mode of action, as for all steroid hormones, is thought to be the control of the rate of protein synthesis.

Used empirically for a wide variety of disorders such as rheumatoid disease and other collagen-vascular diseases, rheumatic carditis, nephrotic syndrome (minimal change), allergic disorders, bronchial asthma, ulcerative colitis, Crohn's disease, chronic active hepatitis, cerebral edema, some demyelinating diseases (e.g., multiple sclerosis), lymphomas, various leukemias, and organ transplantation. The action of steroids in these diseases appears to be related to suppression of inflammation and lymphoid activity.

Absorption

Complete after oral administration. t_{max}: 1 hour [10]. Rectal enemas of prednisolone 21-phosphate result in plasma levels of 20–100% of the equivalent oral dose [11].

Distribution

V_d: 0.5–0.6 L/kg [5, 8]. Protein binding: 54% [9]. Fetal concentration 8–10 times lower than maternal concentration [1]. 0.07–0.23% of a dose is recovered from breast milk [7].

Elimination

$t_{\frac{1}{2}}$: 2.5–3.0 hours [6]. Metabolism is probably similar to that of endogenous cortisol [8], in that 11β-dehydrogenase converts cortisol to cortisone in peripheral tissues [12], the kidneys being an important site [4]. The conversion of prednisone to prednisolone is similarly a reversible process, with the equilibrium markedly in favor of prednisolone [9].

Dosage Schedule

Depends on the nature and the severity of the disease being treated. Doses of prednisone and prednisolone may vary from less than 5 mg daily to more than 100 mg daily. Dosage should be kept as low as possible and still be compatible with disease response; it should be given on alternate mornings if feasible [13]. Duration of treatment should be as short as possible.

Special Dosage Situations

Children and elderly: same dosage as for adults. Pregnancy: caution is advised before 12 weeks of gestation [14] (see Adverse Reactions). Liver disease: protein binding is slightly decreased in patients with chronic active hepatitis and acute hepatitis. This effect is related to the reduced serum albumin concentration in these diseases. Peak prednisolone levels are higher in patients with active or acute liver disease, and the $t_{\frac{1}{2}}$ is prolonged by about 20% in patients with chronic liver disease [10]. Renal disease: no available information.

In preparation for surgery, prednisolone therapy should be substituted with IV hydrocortisone 100–200 mg every 4–6 hours until oral prednisolone therapy can be recommended.

Therapeutic Concentrations

Objective assessment of disease improvement is the usual means of measuring patient's response to the drug. At present, there is no available information that relates plasma concentrations to patients' response in particular disorders.

Adverse Reactions

Adverse reactions are related to dose and time, i.e., the longer the duration of administration and the higher the dose of prednisolone, the greater the incidence of adverse effects. Single large doses, e.g., 100 mg, are devoid of risk, and large doses administered over several days are associated with very little adverse effect. Chronic administration is associated with adrenocortical suppression, with risk of acute adrenocortical insufficiency (addisonian crisis) if prednisolone is withdrawn acutely. Cushingoid features, glucose intolerance, increased susceptibility to infection, possibly increased risk of peptic ulceration with large doses, osteoporosis (especially in postmenopausal females), aseptic necrosis of head of femur, posterior subcapsular cataracts, growth retardation in children, mental changes, myopathy, fluid retention, hypertension, and acne vulgaris may occur. Adverse effects on the fetus remain controversial [14]. A retrospective study revealed a higher incidence of stillbirths to mothers who took prednisolone regularly than to mothers who did not [15].

Interactions

Reduces plasma levels of salicylate [5], potentiates potassium loss when potassium-losing diuretics are given [12], and, if combined with indomethacin, may potentiate gastric ulcer [3]. Phenobarbital may affect asthmatics adversely by increasing the clearance of dexamethasone and prednisone [2].

References

1. Beitins, I. Z., Bayard, F., et al.   The transplacental transfer of prednisone and prednisolone in pregnancy near term. *J. Pediatr.* 81:936–945, 1972.

2. Brooks, S. M., Werk, E. E., et al. Adverse effects of phenobarbital on corticosteroid metabolism in patients with bronchial asthma. *N. Engl. J. Med.* 286:1125–1128, 1972.

3. Emmanuel, J. H., and Montgomery, R. D. Gastric ulcer and the antiarthritic drugs. *Postgrad. Med. J.* 47:227–232, 1971.

4. Jenkins, J. S. The metabolism of cortisol by human extrahepatic tissues. *J. Endocrinol.* 34:51–56, 1966.

5. Klinenberg, J. R., and Miller, F. Effect of corticosteroids on blood salicylate concentration. *J.A.M.A.* 194:601–604, 1965.

6. Kozower, M., Veatch, L., et al. Decreased clearance of prednisolone, a factor in the development of corticosteroid side effects. *J. Clin. Endocrinol. Metab.* 38:407–412, 1974.

7. Liddle, G. W. Clinical pharmacology of the anti-inflammatory steroids. *Clin. Pharmacol. Ther.* 2:615–635, 1961.

8. McKenzie, S. A., Selley, J. A., et al. Secretion of prednisolone into breast milk. *Arch. Dis. Child.* 50:894–896, 1975.

9. Meikle, A. W., Weed, J. A., et al. Kinetics and interconversion of prednisolone and prednisone studied with new radioimmunoassays. *J. Clin. Endocrinol. Metab.* 41:717–721, 1975.

10. Powell, L. W., and Axelsen, E. Corticosteroids in liver disease: Studies on the biological conversion of prednisone to prednisolone and plasma protein binding. *Gut* 13:690–696, 1972.

11. Powell-Tuck, J., Lennard-Jones, J. E., et al. Plasma prednisolone levels after administration of prednisolone-21-phosphate as a retention enema in colitis. *Br. Med. J.* 1:193–195, 1976.

12. Srivastava, L. S., Werk, E. E., et al. Plasma cortisone concentration as measured by radioimmunoassay. *J. Clin. Endocrinol. Metab.* 36:937–943, 1973.

13. Thorn, G. W. Clinical considerations in the use of corticosteroids. *N. Engl. J. Med.* 274:775–781, 1966.

14. Villee, D. B. What risk to fetus from maternal steroid therapy? *J.A.M.A.* 230:1202, 1974.

15. Warrell, D. W., and Taylor, R. Outcome for the fetus of mothers receiving prednisolone during pregnancy. *Lancet* 1:117–118, 1968.

PRIMIDONE

2-Desoxyphenobarbital; biotransformed to phenobarbital and phenylethylmalonylamide (PEMA). Although phenobarbital is a proven anticonvulsant, primidone and PEMA have not definitely been shown to possess anticonvulsant activity in man. Primidone is useful in all types of epilepsy, except petit mal absences.

Absorption

Oral bioavailability: unknown. t_{max} for primidone: 2–4 hours [3]. t_{max} for PEMA: 7–8 hours.

Distribution

V_d: probably about 0.6 L/kg. Protein binding: 19% [4]. The fraction of primidone in the brain equals 87% of the plasma concentration [4], i.e., the unbound fraction. PEMA is negligibly bound to serum proteins. Extent of placental transfer of primidone varies, the maternal to fetal concentration ratio being from 2 : 1 to 1 : 2 [5]. No available information about transfer to breast milk.

Elimination

$t_{\frac{1}{2}}$ for primidone: 3–12 hours [3]. There are two major metabolites—phenobarbital and PEMA. $t_{\frac{1}{2}}$ for PEMA: 29–36 hours [3]. The extent of transformation of primidone to either metabolite varies among individuals, the magnitude of phenobarbital formation being from 15–25% [2, 6].

Dosage Schedule

Initial dose: 250 mg; increased over 2–4 weeks to 750–1500 mg. Probably can be administered once daily, because phenobarbital ($t_{\frac{1}{2}}$: about 120 hours) rather than primidone itself is assumed to be the active principle.

Special Dosage Situations

Children under 8 years: about half of the adult dose (i.e., 125 mg, increasing to 350–750 mg/day). Infants: 100–150 mg daily. Pregnancy: no contraindication known for primidone; vitamin K should be given the last few days before parturition. Elderly: no available information. Hepatic and renal failure: see Phenobarbital, p. 250.

Therapeutic Concentrations

Phenobarbital and primidone levels are usually measured. The therapeutic level for phenobarbital is 15–25 μg/ml. Suggested therapeutic level for primidone is 5–10 μg/ml, but it is not known if primidone is an anticonvulsant in its own right in man [1].

Adverse Reactions

Dizziness, ataxia, nystagmus, diplopia, megaloblastic erythropoiesis, maculopapular rash, and systemic lupus erythematosus syndrome, which rarely occurs. All adverse reactions related to phenobarbital may also occur.

Interactions

See Phenobarbital, p. 250. No interactions have been related to primidone or PEMA specifically.

Review

Hvidberg, E. F., and Dam, M.   Clinical pharmacokinetics of anticonvulsants. *Clin. Pharmacokin.* 1:161–188, 1976.

References

1.   Booker, H. E.   Primidone. Relation of plasma level to clinical control. In D. M. Woodbury, J. K. Penry, and R. P. Schmidt

(Eds.), *Antiepileptic Drugs.* New York: Raven Press, 1972. Pp. 373–376.
2. Butler, T. C., and Waddell, W. J. Metabolic conversion of primidone (Mysoline) to phenobarbital. *Proc. Soc. Exp. Biol. Med.* 93:544–546, 1956.
3. Gallagher, B. B., Baumel, I. P., et al. Primidone. Absorption, distribution, and excretion. In D. M. Woodbury, J. E. Penry, and R. P. Schmidt (Eds.), *Antiepileptic Drugs.* New York: Raven Press, 1972. Pp. 357–359.
4. Houghton, G. W., Richens, A., et al. Brain concentration of phenytoin, phenobarbitone, and primidone in epileptic patients. *Eur. J. Clin. Pharmacol.* 9:73–78, 1975.
5. Martinez, G., and Snyder, R. D. Transplacental passage of primidone. *Neurology* 23:381–383, 1973.
6. Olesen, O. V., and Dam, M. The metabolic conversion of primidone (Mysoline) to phenobarbital in patients under long-term treatment. *Acta Neurol. Scand.* 43:348–356, 1967.

PROBENECID

An inhibitor of renal tubular secretion and reabsorption of organic acids, including uric acid. Main indication for use is as a uricosuric agent in the management of chronic gout but may also be used to prolong penicillin half-life and thus enhance plasma levels of penicillin [1, 8]. Area under the penicillin level–time curve is increased 2–20 times by 2 g of probenecid [1].

Absorption
Oral bioavailability: 100%. t_{max}: 1–5 hours [2].

Distribution
V_d: 0.3 L/kg. Protein binding: 85–95% [2]. No available data about distribution to breast milk and across placenta.

Elimination
Metabolism is dose-dependent. $t_{\frac{1}{2}}$ with usual therapeutic dose: 6–12 hours [2]. Less than 5% is excreted unchanged in the urine. The major metabolic pathways are oxidation of the side chain and glucuronidation to probenecid acyl monoglucuronide. 17–35% is excreted in the urine as the glucuronide and approximately the same amount as hydroxylated metabolites [7]. The hydroxylated metabolites have uricosuric activity in animals.

Dosage Schedule
10–25 mg/kg/day in 2 divided doses. This dosage applies to both adults and children. Commence with low dose to avoid rapid mobilization of urate into joints.

Special Dosage Situations
In patients with diminished renal function, probenecid is less effective because of the inability of the kidneys to clear urate. Contraindicated in patients with a previous history of renal calculi. To avoid the possibility of urate stones, patients should

maintain a urine flow of 3 liters/day and alkalinize the urine with sodium bicarbonate, 10–15 g/day. Contraindicated during an attack of acute gout because probenecid mobilizes additional urate crystals into the synovial fluid, with exacerbation of arthritic pain [3]. Likewise, this mobilization may cause an acute flare-up of gout when therapy is commenced, and this reaction may require treatment with phenylbutazone or colchicine. Use cautiously in patients with a history of peptic ulcer.

Therapeutic Concentrations

100–200 μg/ml [6].

Adverse Reactions

Gastrointestinal irritation (8–18%), hypersensitivity (2–4%), and acute gout (10–20%). In massive overdose, convulsions may occur [5].

Interactions

Decreases the renal clearance of indomethacin, penicillins, dapsone, cephalothin, nitrofurantoin [4], thiazides, salicylic acid, and para-aminohippuric acid, with consequent increases in plasma levels and half-lives of these drugs. Salicylates antagonize the uricosuric effect of probenecid, and concurrent use of salicylates and probenecid should be avoided. Reduces V_d of ampicillin, ancillin, nafcillin, and cephaloridine. Impairs hepatic uptake of bromsulphthalein, rifampin, and indocyanine green.

Review

Kelley, W. N.   Effect of drugs on uric acid in man. *Annu. Rev. Pharmacol.* 15:321–350, 1975.

References

1. Boger, W. P., Beatty, J. P., et al.   The influence of a new benzoic acid derivative on the metabolism of para-aminosalicylic acid (PAS) and penicillin. *Ann. Intern. Med.* 33:18–31, 1950.
2. Dayton, P. G., Yü, T. F., et al.   The physiological disposition of probenecid including renal clearance in man studied by an improved method for its estimation in biological material. *J. Pharmacol. Exp. Ther.* 140:278–286, 1963.
3. Goldfinger, S. E.   Drug therapy. Treatment of gout. *N. Engl. J. Med.* 285:1303–1306, 1971.
4. Jubmann, R., and Bremer, G.   Die Ausscheidung von Furadantin bei manifester Niereninsuffizienz. *Med. Welt* 19:1039–1049, 1965.
5. McKinney, S. E., Peck, H. M., et al.   Benemid, p-(di-n-propyl-sulfamyl)-benzoic acid: Toxicologic properties. *J. Pharmacol. Exp. Ther.* 102:208–214, 1951.
6. Perel, J. M., Dayton, P. G., et al.   Studies of the renal excretion of probenecid acyl glucuronide in man. *Eur. J. Clin. Pharmacol.* 3:106–112, 1971.
7. Skeith, M. D., Simkin, P. A., et al.   The renal excretion of indomethacin and its inhibition by probenecid. *Clin. Pharmacol. Ther.* 9:89–93, 1968.

8. Weiner, I. M., Washington, J. A., et al. On the mechanism of action of probenecid on renal tubular secretion. *Bull. Johns Hopkins Hosp.* 106:333–346, 1960.

PROCAINAMIDE

An antiarrhythmic of the local anesthetic family. Main indication is for use in ventricular arrhythmias. Effect depends on depression of excitability, automaticity, and conduction velocity and on increase in refractoriness of cardiac muscle.

Absorption
Oral bioavailability: 75–95% [9]. t_{max}: 1 hour orally and 30 minutes after IM injection [9].

Distribution
V_d: 1.7–2.2 L/kg [9]. Protein binding: 15% [8].

Elimination
$t_{\frac{1}{2}}$: 2.5–4.5 hours [8, 9]. 50–60% excreted unchanged in the urine [8, 9]. Major metabolite is N-acetyl procainamide (NAPA) [2]. 12% appears as NAPA in slow acetylators and 23% in fast acetylators [6]. 2–10% is excreted as para-aminobenzoic acid and its conjugate [2]. Cleared by both glomerular filtration and by tubular secretion [8]. The renal elimination of procainamide does not seem to be changed by urine flow and pH [5].

NAPA is pharmacologically active and is equipotent with procainamide [4]. Oral bioavailability of NAPA: about 85% [10]. t_{max}: 45–90 minutes [10]. $t_{\frac{1}{2}}$: 6 hours [11]. 80% of NAPA excreted in urine [11]. V_d: 1.4 L/kg [11].

Dosage Schedule
IV loading dose: 8–12 mg/kg at a rate of 25–50 mg/min. Oral maintenance dose: 5–6 mg/kg every 3–4 hours. Oral loading dose: twice that of the maintenance dose.

The following dosage schedule is recommended [7]:

<55 kg body weight	250 mg every 3–4 hr
55 to 90-kg body weight	375 mg every 3–4 hr
>90-kg body weight and greater	500 mg every 3–4 hr

Special Dosage Situations
In patients with renal failure, dose should be adjusted according to Table 1, p. 30. Care should be taken with patients with intraventricular conduction defect (wide QRS complex, prolonged QT interval).

Therapeutic Concentrations
4–8 μg/ml [8, 9].

Adverse Reactions
Adverse reactions occur with drug levels greater than 8 μg/ml. Hypotension, widening of QRS complex, prolongation of QT and

PR intervals, and a syndrome like systemic lupus erythematosus (50–70% of patients develop an asymptomatic positive lupus erythematosus test, antinuclear antibody [ANA], or anti-DNA antibody) [3]. The significance of the development of ANA is not well understood, since many patients with this abnormality remain clinically well. However, clinical SLE develops most frequently in slow acetylators.

Interactions
Increases effect of neuromuscular blockade [1].

References

1. Cuthbert, M. F.   The effect of quinidine and procainamide on the neuromuscular blocking action of suxamethonium. *Br. J. Anaesth.* 38:775–779, 1966.
2. Dreyfuss, J., Bigger, J. T., et al.   Metabolism of procainamide in rhesus monkey and man. *Clin. Pharmacol. Ther.* 13:366–371, 1972.
3. Dubois, E. L.   Procainamide induction of a systemic lupus erythematosus-like syndrome. Presentation of six cases, review of the literature, and analysis and follow-up of reported cases. *Medicine* (Baltimore), 48:217–228, 1969.
4. Elson, J., Strong, J. M., et al.   Antiarrhythmic potency of N-acetyl procainamide. *Clin. Pharmacol. Ther.* 17:134–140, 1975.
5. Galeazzi, R. L., Sheiner, L. B., et al.   The renal elimination of procainamide. *Clin. Pharmacol. Ther.* 19:55–62, 1976.
6. Gibson, T. P., Matusik, J., et al.   Acetylation of procainamide in man and its relationship to isonicotinic acid hydrazide acetylation phenotype. *Clin. Pharmacol. Ther.* 17:395–399, 1975.
7. Koch-Weser, J.   Clinical Application of the Pharmacokinetics of Procainamide. In K. L. Melmon (Ed.), *Cardiovascular Drug Therapy.* Philadelphia: Davis, 1974. P. 71.
8. Koch-Weser, J., and Klein, S. W.   Pharmacokinetics of procainamide in man. *Ann. N.Y. Acad. Sci.* 179:370–382, 1971.
9. Koch-Weser, J., and Klein, S. W.   Procainamide dosage schedules, plasma concentrations, and clinical effects. *J.A.M.A.* 215:1454–1460, 1971.
10. Strong, J. M., Dutcher, J. S., et al.   Procainamide induction of a systemic lupus erythematosus-like syndrome. Presentation of six cases, review of the literature, and analysis and follow-up of reported cases. *Clin. Pharmacol. Ther.* 18:613–622, 1975.
11. Strong, J. M., Dutcher, J. S., et al.   Pharmacokinetics in man of the N-acetylated metabolite of procainamide. *J. Pharmacokin. Biopharm.* 3:223–235, 1975.

PROMETHAZINE

An aliphatic phenothiazine derivative. Potent antihistamine with pronounced sedative, moderate anticholinergic, weak local anesthetic, and very little antipsychotic activity. Acts as a competitive H_1 blocker. The mechanism of its sedative effect is unknown, but it may be related to its anticholinergic effect. Inhibits platelet aggregation in the newborn infant if the mother is treated just before delivery, but clinical significance is uncertain [3]. Indicated in the management of allergic disorders, although antihistamines with less sedative action are usually preferred. Valuable in motion sickness if sedation is not contraindicated [4]. Can also be used as a mild tranquilizer and hypnotic.

Absorption
Systemic bioavailability: unknown. t_{max}: unknown. However, the drug's action starts within 30 minutes after oral administration.

Distribution
V_d: unknown. Protein binding: unknown.

Elimination
$t_{\frac{1}{2}}$: unknown. After a dose of 25 mg orally, the action of promethazine continues for 6–8 hours. The exact fate of the drug is unknown, but most of the promethazine is probably oxidized by side-chain cleavage to the hydroxylamine derivative of phenothiazine [1, 2].

Dosage Schedule
25 mg 2–3 times daily for allergy and sedation. For motion sickness 25 mg 1 hour before travel. Can also be administered by deep IM injection or by IV route after a tenfold dilution in saline. Maximum rate of the injection should be 25 mg/min.

Special Dosage Situations
Children: 0.5–1.0 mg/kg/day. No available information about use in patients with renal or hepatic disease, in the elderly, or in women during pregnancy.

Therapeutic Concentrations
Unknown.

Adverse Reactions
Sedation, fatigue, and incoordination may be pronounced. Nausea, dry mouth, epigastric pain, diarrhea, or constipation are frequent. Palpitations, hypotension, headache, and extrapyramidal symptoms have been reported. Photosensitivity and leucopenia are rare.

Overdose is common, especially in children (from remedies that are sold over the counter). Main symptoms are excitement, ataxia, hallucinations, and convulsions. Dilated pupils, fever, and flushed face are common, particularly in children. The phase of excitation is often preceded by a phase of sedation. Overdose should be treated according to symptoms; the centrally acting cholinesterase inhibitor physostigmine may be useful.

Interactions
The sedative effect is increased by concomitant intake of ethanol and other centrally acting drugs.

References

1. Beckett, A. H. The metabolism of chlorpromazine and promethazine to give new "pink spots." Proposal for the mechanism involved. *Xenobiotica* 5:449–452, 1975.
2. Beckett, A. H., Al-Sarraj, S., et al. The metabolism of chlorpromazine and promethazine to give new "pink spots." *Xenobiotica* 5:325–355, 1975.
3. Corby, D. G., and Schulman, I. The effects of antenatal drug administration on aggregation of platelets in newborn infants. *J. Pediatr.* 79:307–313, 1971.
4. Graybiel, A., Wood, C. D., et al. Human assay of anti-motion sickness drugs. *Aviat. Space Environ. Med.* 46:1107–1118, 1975.

PROPANTHELINE

Synthetic quaternary ammonium compound related to atropine, with antimuscarinic (postganglionic) blocking activity of acetylcholine (ACh) at usual doses. Progressive ganglion blocking action and skeletal muscular blocking activity of ACh occurs at large doses. The polarity of propantheline and related drugs appears to impair their absorption in the gastrointestinal tract and in the blood-brain barrier.

Used as a bromide in the management of chronic duodenal ulcer, but evidence of its benefit is lacking [3, 8] in spite of theoretical considerations of diminished gastric emptying, antacid retention, and diminished acid secretion. In radiology, may be used for the better visualization in hypotonic studies of the duodenum, colon, and urinary tract and to improve detection of esophageal varices [4]. Reduces hyperhidrosis when given systemically or topically by solution and aerosol [5]. Parenteral propantheline is effective in short-bowel syndrome [2]. May relieve spasm associated with opiates in treatment of biliary and renal colic, but theophylline is probably better for this condition.

Absorption

Systemic bioavailability: about 10% [7]. Influenced by intestinal hydrolysis and the relationship to food and the pharmaceutical preparation, with poor availability of the prolonged-acting preparation [1, 6]. t_{max}: about 3–5 hours [1], although this figure represents total radioactivity.

Distribution

Protein binding: unknown. V_d: unknown.

Elimination

$t_{\frac{1}{2}}$: unknown. Exposure of oral drug to the bile and duodenal juices leads to hydrolysis to free xanthene carboxylic acid, which is inactive. In 24 hours about 10% of a single oral dose is excreted unchanged in the urine, with 20% as xanthene carboxylic acid and the remainder as a single unidentified metabolite. 3% to 18% of parent drug is excreted in the feces. After an IV dose about 50% is excreted unchanged in the urine in 24 hours, about 10% as xanthene carboxylic acid and the remainder as the unidentified metabolite. Only 3% is excreted in the feces. Propantheline is excreted in the bile, especially after cholecystokinin is secreted, and is apparently reabsorbed, possibly after hydrolysis [1].

Dosage Schedule

Usual starting dosage 7.5–15 mg 3 times daily before meals and 15–30 mg at night for chronic use. Benefit may be associated in individual patients by increasing the dose until side-effects occur.

15 mg parenterally is usually adequate for radiology procedures.

5% topical solution or aerosol may be used 3 or 4 times daily for troublesome hyperhidrosis or skin maceration in conjunction with mycotic infection [5].

Special Dosage Situations

No available information about use in children, in women during pregnancy, or in patients with renal or hepatic disease. Caution is advised in men with prostatic hyperplasia and in patients with glaucoma.

Therapeutic Concentrations

No available data.

Adverse Reactions

Similar to atropine. Typical anticholinergic effects include dry mouth, iridoplegia and cycloplegia with blurring of vision, acute glaucoma, reduction of secretions of bronchi and GI tract, urinary retention, and tachycardia. CNS effects are fewer than with atropine (possibly because polarity prevents propantheline from crossing the blood-brain barrier), and large doses may produce paralysis by neuromuscular blockade, with little confusion, delirium, or disorientation. Intermediate doses may produce hypotension and impotence due to ganglionic blockade (nicotinic receptors). Treatment includes measures to relieve symptoms and the use of an anticholinesterase such as neostigmine.

Interactions

Additive effects with other drugs that possess anticholinergic effects.

The influence on the absorption of other drugs is of great interest. The absorption of drugs such as digoxin and nitrofurantoin may be enhanced, while peak levels of acetaminophen (paracetamol) may be delayed and diminished.

References

1. Beermann, B., Hellström, K., et al. On the metabolism of propantheline in man. *Clin. Pharmacol. Ther.* 13:212–220, 1972.
2. Cameron, J. L., Gayler, B. W., et al. The use of intramuscular propantheline in the short bowel syndrome. *Johns Hopkins Med. J.* 138:91–95, 1976.

3. Cocking, J. B., Gayler, B. W., et al.   The use of intramuscular propantheline bromide in the long-term treatment of chronic duodenal ulcer. *Gastroenterology* 62:6–10, 1972.
4. Dalinka, M. K., Smith, E. H., et al.   Pharmacologically enhanced visualisation of esophageal varices by Pro-Banthine. *Radiology* 102:281–282, 1972.
5. Frankland, J. C., and Seville, R. H.   The treatment of hyperhidrosis with topical propantheline—a new technique. *Br. J. Dermatol.* 85:577–581, 1971.
6. Gibaldi, M., and Grundhofer, B.   Biopharmaceutical influences on the anticholinergic effects of propantheline. *Clin. Pharmacol. Ther.* 18:457–461, 1975.
7. Möller, J., and Rosén, A.   Comparative studies on intramuscular and oral effective doses of some anticholinergic drugs. *Acta Med. Scand.* 184:201–209, 1968.
8. Sun, D. C. H.   A controlled trial of antacid, propantheline, and amylopectin sulfate in duodenal ulcer. *Am. J. Gastroenterol.* 60:449–458, 1973.

PROPYLTHIOURACIL

A thiocarbamide used in the treatment of hyperthyroidism. Inhibits the synthesis of thyroid hormones but does not interfere with iodine uptake or release of hormones. Inhibits the peripheral conversion of thyroxine to triiodothyronine [1].

Absorption

Oral bioavailability: about 80% [3]. t_{max} orally: about 1 hour.

Distribution

V_d: 0.2–0.4 L/kg [3]. Protein binding: about 75%. Accumulates in the thyroid, usually producing a response in 5–10 days [4]. Passes easily to breast milk and fetal circulation (potentially goitrogenic).

Elimination

$t_{\frac{1}{2}}$: 1–2 hours, unchanged in hyperthyroidism [2, 3, 5]. Transformed to several unknown metabolites and excreted as glucuronides in the urine [2].

Dosage Schedule

Only used orally. Initially 400–800 mg in 2 or 3 daily doses, reduced during first 3–6 weeks to 100–200 mg daily according to laboratory and clinical response. Thyroid activity may be titrated but usually is fully blocked, and replacement thyroxine is given to prevent thyroid enlargement. Maintain treatment 18 months–2 years. Remission is frequent, 20–50%. Patient's response to the drug is diminished with previous iodine treatment and large or nodular goiters.

Special Dosage Situations

Children: relate dose to body weight—5–10 mg/kg/day in 3 doses. Pregnancy: reduce dose, keeping serum thyroxine at the physiologically slightly elevated level. Lactation: contraindicated.

No dose adjustments in renal disease or in the elderly. In severe hepatic disorders a slight dose reduction is advised. A large intrathoracic goiter is a contraindication to use of drug, especially without concurrent thyroxine treatment.

Therapeutic Concentrations
Not known; probably not relevant.

Adverse Reactions
Mainly hypersensitivity effects such as allergic rash, drug fever, joint pains, and jaundice. Agranulocytosis is rare (below 0.5%), but patients should be advised to report sore throats immediately. Severe reactions generally develop during the initial 2 months of treatment. Overdosage results in goiter and eventually in exophthalmos. Teratogenicity and cancerogenicity are not described.

Interactions
Not known.

Review
Mills, L. C.   Drug treatment in thyroid disease. *Semin. Drug Treat.* 3:377–402, 1974.

References
1. Geffner, D. L., Azukizawa, M., et al.   Propylthiouracil blocks extrathyroidal conversion of thyroxine to triiodothyronine and augments thyreotropin secretion in man. *J. Clin. Invest.* 55:224–229, 1976.
2. Kampmann, J. P., and Skovsted, L.   The pharmacokinetics of propylthiouracil. *Acta Pharmacol. Toxicol.* 35:361–369, 1974.
3. Kampmann, J. P., and Skovsted, L.   The kinetics of propylthiouracil in hyperthyroidism. *Acta Pharmacol. Toxicol.* 37:201–210, 1975.
4. Marchant, B., Alexander, W. D., et al.   The accumulation of ^{35}S-antithyroid drugs by the thyroid gland. *J. Clin. Endocrinol. Metab.* 34:847–851, 1972.
5. McMurray, J., Jr., Gilliland, L., et al.   Pharmacodynamics of propylthiouracil in normal and hyperthyroid subjects after a single oral dose. *J. Clin. Endocrinol. Metab.* 41:362–364, 1975.

QUINIDINE

d-Isomer of quinine; weak base. Major indications are for the prevention and treatment of supraventricular arrhythmias, ventricular tachycardia, and ventricular premature contractions. Effect depends on depression of automaticity, excitability, and conduction velocity; refractory period is increased. Also has anticholinergic activity, which may cause an initial paradoxical increase in ventricular rate in atrial fibrillation or flutter.

Absorption
Systemic bioavailability: 40–90% [10]. t_{max}: 1–2 hours for quinidine sulfate and 4–8 hours for quinidine gluconate [9], which is formulated as a slow release preparation. A first-pass effect may exist [10].

Distribution
V_d: 0.5 L/kg [3]. Protein binding: 60–80% [2, 12].

Elimination
$t_{\frac{1}{2}}$: 4–7 hours [3, 6]. 20–50% excreted unchanged in the urine; the remainder is hydroxylated in the liver; and a number of metabolites appear in the urine, most of which are not conjugated [1, 9]. Renal excretion increased by acidification and decreased by alkalinization of the urine [5].

Dosage Schedule
Oral loading dose for quinidine sulfate: a single dose of 5–8 mg/kg. Oral maintenance dose for quinidine sulfate: 10–20 mg/kg/day in 4 or 6 divided doses. Oral maintenance dose for quinidine gluconate: 330–660 mg every 8–12 hours.

Special Dosage Situations
In patients with congestive heart failure V_d is decreased; therefore dosage should be decreased [3]. No alterations appear to be necessary in patients with renal or hepatic failure [6]. Ratio of bound drug to free drug depends on the plasma-protein concentration [12]. Use cautiously in patients with intraventricular conduction defects.

Therapeutic Concentrations
2–6 μg/ml.

Adverse Reactions
Adverse reactions occur at plasma levels greater than 6 μg/ml. Paradoxical tachycardia may occur in patients with atrial fibrillation or flutter; pretreat these patients with digitalis. Nausea, vomiting, diarrhea, anorexia, atrioventricular (A-V) block, widening of QRS complex, prolongation of QT interval, and ventricular premature beats. Treat patients with these side-effects by reducing dose or stopping the drug. In large doses, quinidine can cause cinchonism, which includes tinnitus, blurred vision, photophobia, and altered color perception. Massive overdose may cause hypotension due to direct depression of myocardial contractility or to peripheral vasodilatation. Peritoneal dialysis or hemodialysis may be of value in treating overdosage; the use of hypokalemic dialysis fluid has been suggested [11].

Interactions
Prolongs muscular relaxant properties of curare [8]. Potentiates the action of warfarin by hypoprothrombinemic effect [7]. $t_{\frac{1}{2}}$ of quinidine is reduced 50% by phenobarbital and phenytoin because of increased metabolism in liver [4].

Review

Hoffman, B. F., Rosen, M. R., et al. Electrophysiology and pharmacology of cardiac arrhythmias. VII. Cardiac effects of quinidine and procainamide. *Am. Heart J.* 89:804–808, 1975.

References

1. Brodie, B. B., Baer, J. E., et al. Metabolic products of the cinchona alkaloids in human urine. *J. Biol. Chem.* 188:567–581, 1951.
2. Conn, H. L., Jr., and Luchi, R. J. Ionic influences on quinidine-albumin interaction. *J. Pharmacol. Exp. Ther.* 133:76–83, 1961.
3. Crouthamel, W. G. The effect of congestive heart failure on quinidine pharmacokinetics. *Am. Heart J.* 90:335–339, 1975.
4. Data, J. L., Wilkinson, G. R., et al. Interaction of quinidine with anticonvulsant drugs. *N. Engl. J. Med.* 294:699–702, 1976.
5. Gerhardt, R. E., Knouss, R. F., et al. Quinidine excretion in aciduria and alkaluria. *Ann. Intern. Med.* 71:927–933, 1969.
6. Kessler, K. M., Lowenthal, D. T., et al. Quinidine elimination in patients with congestive heart failure or poor renal function. *N. Engl. J. Med.* 290:706–709, 1974.
7. Koch-Weser, J. Quinidine-induced hypoprothrombinemic hemorrhage in patients on chronic warfarin therapy. *Ann. Intern. Med.* 68:511–517, 1968.
8. Miller, R. D., Way, W. L., et al. The potentiation of neuromuscular blocking agents by quinidine. *Anesthesiology* 28:1036–1041, 1967.
9. Palmer, K. H., Martin, B., et al. The metabolic fate of orally administered quinidine gluconate in humans. *Biochem. Pharmacol.* 18:1845–1860, 1969.
10. Ueda, C. T., Williamson, B. J., et al. Absolute quinidine bioavailability. *Clin. Pharmacol. Ther.* 20:260–265, 1976.
11. Woie, L., and Oyri, A. Quinidine intoxication treated with hemodialysis. *Acta Med. Scand.* 195:237–239, 1974.
12. Wosilait, W. D. A theoretical analysis of the distribution of quinidine in the plasma: The relationship between protein binding and therapeutic drug levels. *Res. Commun. Clin. Pathol. Pharmacol.* 12:147–154, 1975.

RIFAMPIN
(Rifampicin)

Semisynthetic macrocyclic antibiotic with activity against *Mycobacterium tuberculosis,* most gram-positive bacteria, and several gram-negative species such as *Escherichia coli, Pseudomonas, Proteus, Klebsiella,* and *Neisseria meningitidis.* Indicated in the prophylaxis of *N. meningitidis* (meningococcal) meningitis but generally restricted to tuberculous infections. Because resistance to the drug develops easily, rifampin is always used in combination with other antituberculous drugs. Mechanism of action is inhibition of RNA synthesis.

Absorption

Oral bioavailability: 90–95%. t_{max}: 1–2 hours [4]. The bioavailability is reduced by concomitant administration of food.

Distribution

V_d: 0.9 L/kg. Protein binding: 90% [4]. Concentration in CNS is about 50% of the concentration in serum. After a few hours the concentration in pleural fluid is equal to the serum concentration [3]. Crosses the placenta.

Elimination

$t_{\frac{1}{2}}$ at the beginning of therapy: 3–5 hours, decreasing after 2–4 weeks to 2–3 hours, probably as a result of increased biliary elimination [1, 4, 5]. 30% of the drug is excreted in the urine and the remainder in the bile, half as unchanged drug and half as deacetylated metabolite. The deacetylated compound retains full antibacterial activity. The parent compound undergoes extensive enterohepatic circulation, while the deacetylated compound is only slightly reabsorbed.

Dosage Schedule

600 mg daily, 2 hours before or after a meal.

Special Dosage Situations

Children: 10–20 mg/kg daily in 1 dose. Hepatic disease: use cautiously. No dosage adjustments necessary in patients with kidney disease, in the elderly, or in women during lactation. Pregnancy: no available information.

Therapeutic Concentrations

0.1–1.0 μg/ml. Up to 10 μg/ml for some gram-negative species of bacteria.

Adverse Reactions

Nausea, vomiting, diarrhea, drowsiness, headache, dizziness, ataxia, and muscular weakness. The development of severe jaundice and hepatorenal syndrome is a rare but serious effect. Allergy manifested by hemolytic anemia, thrombocytopenia purpura, chills, and myalgia is associated with antibody formation and is more likely to occur with a high dose and intermittent therapy [8].

Interactions

Para-aminosalicylic acid granules (but not the suspension) decrease the bioavailability of rifampin [2]. Rifampin increases the metabolism of warfarin, thus decreasing the efficiency of the latter [7], and it impairs the effectiveness of oral contraceptives, resulting in an increased incidence of pregnancies in women taking the drug [6].

Reviews

Radner, D. B.   Toxicologic and pharmacologic aspects of rifampicin. *Chest* 64:213–216, 1973.

Soffer, A. (Ed.). Rifampicin in the treatment of pulmonary tuberculosis. *Chest* 61:517–598, 1972.

Symposium. Experimental and clinical evaluation of the tuberculostatics. *Antibiot. Chemother.* 16:316–529, 1970.

References

1. Acocella, G., Pagani, V., et al. Kinetic studies on rifampicin. *Chemotherapy* 16:356–370, 1971.
2. Boman, G., Lundgren, P., et al. Mechanism of the inhibitory effect of PAS granules on the absorption of rifampicin: Absorption of rifampicin by an excipient, bentonite. *Eur. J. Clin. Pharmacol.* 8:293–299, 1975.
3. Boman, G., and Malmborg, A. S. Rifampicin in plasma and pleural fluid after single oral doses. *Eur. J. Clin. Pharmacol.* 7:51–58, 1974.
4. Furesz, S., Scott, R., et al. Rifampicin: A new rifamycin. III. Absorption, distribution, and elimination in man. *Arzneim. Forsch.* 17:534–537, 1967.
5. Nitti, V., Veneri, F. D., et al. Rifampicin blood serum levels and half-life during prolonged administration in tuberculous patients. *Chemotherapy* 17:121–129, 1972.
6. Nocke-Finck, L., Breuer, H., et al. Wirkung von Rifampicin auf der Menstruations-zyklus und die Oestrogenausscheidung bei Einnahme oraler Kontrazeptiva. *Dtsch. Med. Wochenschr.* 98:1521–1523, 1973.
7. O'Reilly, R. A. Interaction of chronic daily warfarin therapy and rifampin. *Ann. Intern. Med.* 83:506–508, 1975.
8. Pujet, J.-C., Homberg, J.-C., et al. Sensitivity to rifampicin: Incidence, mechanism, and prevention. *Br. Med. J.* 2:415–418, 1974.

SPIRONOLACTONE

A steroid compound with five-membered lactone ring at C_{17} position of steroid nucleus. Acts as aldosterone antagonist and may also have a weak inotropic effect. Indicated as potassium-sparing diuretic in the management of cardiac failure and ascites associated with cirrhosis and as an antihypertensive agent in patients who have an excess of aldosterone [1]. Should be used only as second-line therapy because of current concern about safety (see Adverse Reactions).

Absorption

Poorly soluble in water. New formulations (e.g., Aldactone A) are finely micronized to enhance dissolution, and absorption of this preparation is about 90% [5]. Older preparations given orally had as little as 5% bioavailability. t_{max} for new preparations: about 3 hours [5].

Distribution

V_d: 0.05 L/kg. Protein binding: 90%. This distribution applies to both spironolactone and to canrenone. No available information about transfer to fetus or to breast milk.

Elimination

$t_{\frac{1}{2}}$ of spironolactone: about 10 minutes. It is dithioacetylated to canrenone, which appears to be the active moiety. Other metabolites of spironolactone are unstable in vitro and convert spontaneously to canrenone [3]. After oral administration of spironolactone, t_{max} for canrenone is the same as that for spironolactone. Canrenone has a long distribution (alpha) phase (12 hours) in which the $t_{\frac{1}{2}}\alpha$ is 2–6 hours, and an elimination (beta) $t_{\frac{1}{2}}$ of 10–22 hours [4]. In addition, canrenone may display dose-dependent kinetics at clinical dosage levels, e.g., $t_{\frac{1}{2}}\beta$ after 25 mg orally is 2–6 hours, while "$t_{\frac{1}{2}}$" after 100 mg is 7–26 hours.

Canrenone exists in plasma in equilibrium with canrenoic acid [3], which is conjugated and excreted in the urine. However, there also appears to be significant biliary excretion [6].

Dosage Schedule

For micronized formulation, 25–200 mg/day. In view of the long $t_{\frac{1}{2}}$ of canrenone, doses once or twice daily should be adequate.

Special Dosage Situations

No special precautions about use in patients with congestive heart failure or hepatic disease [7]. Nothing known about use in pregnant women or in the elderly. Give cautiously to patients with renal failure because of risk of hyperkalemia.

Therapeutic Concentrations

Plasma canrenone levels of 100–500 ng/ml have been observed after 100 mg of spironolactone has been given daily for 4–10 days [7]. No available data about pharmacodynamic relationship with blood levels.

Adverse Reactions

Gynecomastia frequently occurs in men after chronic administration of spironolactone [2]. There is currently concern about tumor production in animals after large doses.

Interactions

Hyperkalemia may occur if spironolactone is given with potassium supplements or with other potassium-sparing diuretics such as triamterene and amiloride. Spironolactone is a weak inducer of the mixed-function oxidase system, but the clinical significance of this effect is uncertain.

References

1. Brown, J. J., Davies, D. L., et al.   Comparison of surgery and prolonged spironolactone therapy in patients with hypertension, aldosterone excess, and low plasma renin. *Br. Med. J.* 1:729–734, 1972.
2. Huffman, D. H., and Azarnoff, D. L.   Effect of spironolactone on metabolic conversion of androgens to estrogens: A preliminary report (abstract). *Clin. Res.* 23:4, 476A, 1975.
3. Karim, A., Hribar, J., et al.   Spironolactone metabolism in

man studied by gas chromatography–mass spectrometry. *Drug Metab. Disp.* 3:467–478, 1975.
4. Karim, A., Zagarella, J., et al. Spironolactone. I. Disposition and metabolism. *Clin. Pharmacol. Ther.* 19:158–169, 1976.
5. Karim, A., Zagarella, J., et al. Spironolactone. II. Bioavailability. *Clin. Pharmacol. Ther.* 19:170–176, 1976.
6. Karim, A., Zagarella, J., et al. Spironolactone. III. Canrenone—maximum and minimum steady state plasma levels. *Clin. Pharmacol. Ther.* 19:177–182, 1976.
7. Sadee, W., Schroder, R., et al. Multiple dose kinetics of spironolactone and canrenoate-potassium in cardiac and hepatic failure. *Eur. J. Clin. Pharmacol.* 7:195–200, 1974.

SULFASALAZINE

A drug produced originally as a result of research in rheumatoid arthritis, combining sulfapyridine and salicylate in one molecule. At present, sole indications for its use are in the prophylaxis and management of exacerbations of ulcerative colitis and the prophylaxis of Crohn's disease. Frequently used in combination with corticosteroids, e.g., prednisolone given orally or by retention enema. Mechanism of action is obscure but may depend on the inhibition of prostaglandin synthesis [1] or on changes in electrolyte transport produced in the bowel wall by sulfasalazine or its metabolites [6].

Absorption
About 30% is absorbed in the upper gastrointestinal tract [4, 11], whereas metabolites are absorbed in the colon [4, 11]. t_{max}: 3–5 hours.

Distribution
V_d: unknown. Protein binding: unknown. Binds to connective tissue [5]; this action is thought to be the mechanism for some of its toxic effects [7] (see Adverse Reactions).

Elimination
$t_{\frac{1}{2}}$: unknown. Sulfasalazine is excreted almost exclusively in the bile as parent drug or as the N-acetyl metabolite and undergoes extensive enterohepatic recirculation; very little drug or metabolite is eliminated in the urine [9]. In the colon, bacteria cleave the molecule into its components, 5-aminosalicylate and sulfapyridine [8, 9]. Sulfapyridine is then absorbed. t_{max}: 8–12 hours [11]. Metabolism is by hydroxylation or N-acetylation and subsequent glucuronidation. These metabolites appear in the urine and the bile [11]. 5-aminosalicylate is not absorbed but may be N-acetylated in the gut and then absorbed; in this case, it appears in the urine and may be secreted in the bile [9]. Therefore, the bowel contains sulfasalazine, sulfapyridine, 5-aminosalicylate, and its acetylated metabolite. It seems likely that 5-aminosalicylate is the therapeutically active compound. Toxicity, however, appears to relate to plasma levels of sulfapyridine [3]. Metabolism in healthy volunteers is not significantly different from that in patients with colitis [10].

Dosage Schedule

1 g 4 times daily in acute exacerbations of colitis. 2–3 g/day during quiescent periods. Doses in excess of 4 g/day produce an unacceptably high incidence of toxicity [3].

Special Dosage Situations

Use cautiously in slow acetylators. Higher serum levels for a given dose tend to occur in slow acetylators [2], but it is not possible to predict what serum level will occur in a given patient.

Therapeutic Concentrations

Serum sulfapyridine level 20–50 μg/ml is associated with clinical improvement.

Adverse Reactions

Cross-allergy with sulfonamides. Hemolytic anemia and methemoglobinemia occur frequently, but agranulocytosis is rare. These reactions occur more frequently when serum levels exceed 50 μg/ml [3]. Therefore, it is wise to check patients' acetylation status and also glucose-6-phosphate dehydrogenase (G-6-PD) status when commencing drug. Minor side-effects are nausea, vomiting, headache, fever and rash, and folate malabsorption. Infrequent but serious reactions are toxic epidermal necrolysis, paresthesiae, fibrosing alveolitis [7], and pancreatitis.

Interactions

Concomitant administration of iron sulfate leads to a lowering of sulfasalazine and sulfapyridine levels in plasma.

Review

Goldman, P., and Peppercorn, M. A. Drug therapy. Sulfasalazine. *N. Engl. J. Med.* 293:20–23, 1975.

References

1. Butt, A. A., Collier, H. O. J., et al. Effects on prostaglandin in biosynthesis of drugs affecting gastrointestinal function (abstract). *Gut* 15:344, 1974.
2. Das, K. M., Eastwood, M. A., et al. The metabolism of salicylazosulphapyridine in ulcerative colitis. 1. The relationship between metabolites and the response to treatment in patients. *Gut* 14:631–641, 1973.
3. Das, K. M., Eastwood, M. A., et al. Adverse reactions during salicylazosulfapyridine therapy and the relation with drug metabolism and acetylator phenotype. *N. Engl. J. Med.* 289:491–495, 1973.
4. Das, K. M., Eastwood, M. A., et al. The role of the colon in the metabolism of salicylazosulphapyridine. *Scand. J. Gastroenterol.* 9:137–141, 1974.
5. Hanngren, Å., Hannsson, E., et al. Distribution and metabolism of salicyl-azo-sulfapyridine. II. A study with S35-

salicyl-azo-sulfapyridine and S35-sulfapyridine. *Acta Med. Scand.* 173:391–399, 1963.

6. Harris, J., Archampong, E. Q., et al. The effect of salazopyrin on water and electrolyte transport in the human colon measured in vivo and in vitro (abstract). *Gut* 13:855, 1972.

7. Editorial. Sulphasalazine-induced lung disease. *Lancet* 2:504–505, 1974.

8. Peppercorn, M. A, and Goldman, P. The role of intestinal bacteria in the metabolism of salicylazosulfapyridine. *J. Pharmacol. Exp. Ther.* 181:555–562, 1972.

9. Peppercorn, M. A., and Goldman, P. Distribution studies of salicylazosulfapyridine and its metabolites. *Gastroenterology* 64:240–245, 1973.

10. Schroder, H., Lewkonia, R. M., et al. Metabolism of salicylazosulfapyridine in healthy subjects and in patients with ulcerative colitis. Effect of colectomy and of phenobarbital. *Clin. Pharmacol. Ther.* 14:802–809, 1973.

11. Schroder, H., and Campbell, D. E. S. Absorption, metabolism, and excretion of salicylazosulfapyridine in man. *Clin. Pharmacol. Ther.* 13:539–551, 1972.

SULFINPYRAZONE

A strongly acidic compound that is closely related chemically to phenylbutazone. Main action is inhibition of the tubular transport of organic acids, including uric acid. As with other uricosuric agents, small doses selectively inhibit the tubular secretion of uric acid, resulting in a decrease in uric acid excretion. Clinical doses, however, also block uric acid reabsorption, resulting in increased uric acid excretion and decreased serum uric acid concentrations. The uricosuric action is additive to that of probenecid and phenylbutazone but mutually antagonistic to high doses of salicylates [9]. No anti-inflammatory, analgesic, or antipyretic effects. Only established indication is for the treatment of chronic gout. Sulfinpyrazone prolongs platelet survival and inhibits platelet aggregation in response to collagen [1, 7]. Appears to be of value in prevention of arteriovenous shunt thrombosis [4]. Other clinical benefits in thrombotic diseases are under investigation [8].

Absorption

Oral bioavailability: 90–100% [1]. t_{max}: about 1 hour.

Distribution

V_d: about 0.15 L/kg [5]. Protein binding: 98–99% [2]. No available information about distribution in breast milk, CNS, or across placenta.

Elimination

$t_{\frac{1}{2}}$: 3–5 hours [1, 3]. 30–50% is excreted unchanged [3]. About 50% is transformed to the para-hydroxy metabolite, which is also a potent uricosuric agent with a $t_{\frac{1}{2}}$ of about 1 hour [2].

Dosage Schedule

Initial dose: 100–200 mg daily in 3 divided doses given without meals. Increase dose gradually up to 400 mg daily. To avoid acute attacks of gout, treatment with sulfinpyrazone can be supplemented with colchicine (0.5–2 mg daily for 1–2 months) or phenylbutazone. Large alkaline urine output decreases the risk of the formation of urate renal calculi. Therapy with uricosuric agents should not be initiated during an acute attack of gout but may well be continued if therapy has already been started. Sulfinpyrazone can also be used in secondary gout induced by diseases or drugs, e.g., cytotoxics, diuretics, levodopa, etham-butol, and pyrazinamide.

Special Dosage Situations

No available data about dosage in children, in the elderly, in women during pregnancy or lactation, or in patients with hepatic disease. Of no use in patients with severe renal failure (al-lopurinol is the drug of choice for this condition).

Therapeutic Concentrations

Not established. Relate dose to serum uric acid concentration.

Adverse Reactions

Gastrointestinal irritation and occasionally ulceration. Rarely, hypersensitivity, with fever and skin rashes. Hematopoiesis can be reversibly depressed, but severe hematological reactions have not been described. No salt or water retention.

Interactions

Salicylates even in small doses block the effect of sulfinpyrazone [1]. Probenecid increases the plasma concentration of sulfinpyrazone and its hydroxy metabolite [6].

Review

Gutman, A. B.   Uricosuric drugs, with special reference to pro-benecid and sulfinpyrazone. *Adv. Pharmacol. Chemother.* 4:91–142, 1966.

References

1. Burns, J. J., Yü, T. F., et al.   A potent new uricosuric agent, the sulfoxide metabolite of the phenylbutazone analogue, G-25671. *J. Pharmacol. Exp. Ther.* 119:418–426, 1957.
2. Dayton, P. G., Sicam, L. E., et al.   Metabolism of sulfinpyrazone (Anturan) and other thio analogues of phenylbutazone in man. *J. Pharmacol. Exp. Ther.* 132:287–290, 1961.
3. Kadar, D., Inaba, T., et al.   Comparative drug elimination capacity in man—glutethimide, amobarbital, antipyrine, and sulfinpyrazone. *J. Clin. Pharmacol. Ther.* 14:552–560, 1973.
4. Kaegi, A., Pineo, G. F., et al.   The role of sulfinpyrazone in the prevention of arteriovenous shunt thrombosis. *Circulation* 52:497–499, 1975.

5. Packam, M. A., Warrior, E. S., et al. Alteration of the response of platelets to surface stimuli by pyrazole compounds. *J. Exp. Med.* 126:171–188, 1967.
6. Perel, J. M., Dayton, P. G., et al. Studies of interactions among drugs in man at the renal level: Probenecid and sulfinpyrazone. *Clin. Pharmacol. Ther.* 10:834–840, 1969.
7. Smythe, H. A., Ogryzlo, M. A., et al. The effects of sulfinpyrazone (Anturan) on platelet economy and blood coagulation in man. *Can. Med. Assoc. J.* 92:818–821, 1965.
8. Steele, P., Battock, D., et al. Effects of clofibrate and sulfinpyrazone on platelet survival time in coronary heart disease. *Circulation* 52:473–476, 1975.
9. Yü, T. F., Dayton, P. G., et al. Mutual suppression of the uricosuric effects of sulfinpyrazone and salicylate. A study in interaction between drugs. *J. Clin. Invest.* 42:1330–1339, 1963.

SULFONAMIDES

Acidic, bacteriostatic, synthetic antimicrobial agents derived from para-aminobenzenesulfonamide (sulfanilamide). A free para-amino group is essential for the sulfonamides to be effective, and acetylation abolishes all of their activity. Mechanism of action is inhibition of bacterial growth by preventing the conversion of para-aminobenzoic acid (PABA) to folic acid. The bacteriostatic effect is counteracted competitively by PABA. Therefore, folic acid is contraindicated during sulfonamide therapy.

All sulfonamides have the same antibacterial spectrum, with activity against most strains of *Streptococcus, Pneumococcus, Bacillus anthracis, Corynebacterium diphtheriae,* and *Chlamydia trachomatis* and some strains of *Hemophilus influenzae, Yersinia, Nocardia,* and *Actinomycetes.* Many *Neisseria meningitidis* strains are now insensitive to the sulfonamides, and many strains of *Proteus, Escherichia coli, Klebsiella, Salmonella,* and *Shigella* have also acquired resistance to the sulfonamides. *Enterococci* have always been resistant.

Indications for the sulfonamides have been narrowed because of increasing resistance of many common pathogens and the discovery of antibiotics. Main indications are for urinary tract infections that are caused by susceptible organisms, for yersiniosis, for nocardiosis, and for the treatment of trachoma and lymphogranuloma venereum when combined with tetracyclines. Used as a prophylactic for meningococcal infections, but increasing resistance of meningococcus to the sulfonamides has made rifampin the drug of choice. Special indications are toxoplasmosis (sulfisoxazole) and dermatitis herpetiformis (sulfadiazine).

The long-acting sulfonamides ($t_{\frac{1}{2}}$: 1–2 days), sulfadimethoxine and sulfamethoxypyridazine, are not recommended because adverse reactions persist for a longer time if toxicity develops.

Absorption

Oral bioavailability: 85–100%. t $_{max}$: 2–4 hours [4, 8].

Distribution and Elimination

Sulfonamide	V_d (L/kg)	Protein Binding (%)	$t_{\frac{1}{2}}$ (hr)	Excreted Unchanged (%)
Sulfamerazine [2]	0.35	75	15–30	Unknown
Sulfisoxazole [2, 4] (sulphafurazole)	0.15	85	5–8	40–70
Sulfamethoxazole [2, 3, 5]	0.30	65	8–12	30–50
Sulfamethizole [6]	0.35	90	1–2	40–70
Sulfamethazine [8, 9] (sulphadimidine)	0.50	80	8–10	20–40[a]
Sulfadiazine [1, 2, 7]	0.60	40	10–24	60–80

[a]Slow acetylators; rapid acetylators excrete 70–80% of the drug acetylated.

The concentration in CSF is 30–60% of the serum concentration. The concentration in fetal circulation is 50–90% of the maternal serum concentration. Concentrations in breast milk and plasma are similar. The major metabolites of all sulfonamides are inactive, amino-acetylated compounds. The acetylated metabolites seem to be responsible for several of the side-effects of the sulfonamides, in particular crystalluria. Free and acetylated sulfonamides are excreted by glomerular filtration and to a lesser degree by tubular secretion.

Dosage Schedule

Sulfamethizole, sulfamerazine, sulfamethazine, sulfisoxazole, or sulfadiazine: 2–4 g initially, followed by 0.5–1 g 4–6 hourly. Sulfamethoxazole: 2 g initially, followed by 1 g 8–12 hourly.

The IM dose of sulfisoxazole is 100 mg/kg daily in 3–4 divided doses. In all cases urine volume should be above 1200 ml and urine pH above 6.

Topical use of all sulfonamides is not recommended.

Special Dosage Situations

Children: sulfisoxazole, sulfamethizole, or sulfadiazine—150 mg/kg daily in 4–6 divided doses after a loading dose of 75 mg/kg. Sulfamethoxazole: 60 mg/kg daily in 3 divided doses after a loading dose of 30 mg/kg.

In patients with uremia $t_{\frac{1}{2}}$ is prolonged according to the fraction of drug that is excreted unchanged. Excretion of the acetylated compounds is also inhibited, increasing the likelihood of some of the side-effects. Decreased acetylation of sulfisoxazole has been demonstrated in patients with uremia. Decreased protein binding has been described for many sulfonamides in uremic patients. As a result of these actions, all sulfonamides have to be used cautiously in patients with uremia; the dose should be reduced according to Table 1, p. 30.

Avoid giving drug to pregnant women in the last trimester because of bilirubin displacement from serum albumin in the fetus. Elderly: reduce dose according to the decrease in renal function. No dose adjustment necessary in women during lactation. No available information about use of the sulfonamides in patients with hepatic disease.

Therapeutic Concentrations

Minimum inhibitory concentration (MIC) varies with the bacterial species; for many gram-negative organisms it is 50–200 μg/ml.

Adverse Reactions

Drug fever and skin rashes, including the Stevens-Johnson syndrome. Hemolytic anemia, agranulocytosis, and thrombocytopenia, which are all probably allergic reactions, are rare but serious. Toxic aplastic anemia is extremely rare. Renal failure may be caused by hypersensitivity. Diffuse necrosis of the liver, arthritis, pulmonary eosinophilic alveolitis, photosensitivity, peripheral neuritis, and a syndrome similar to systemic lupus erythematosus are all rare. There is cross-allergy between all sulfonamides.

All sulfonamides are eliminated by hemodialysis.

Interactions

The use of sulfonamides in the newborn and in the last trimester of pregnancy may result in kernicterus, caused by displacement of bilirubin from plasma proteins. Sulfamethizole and sulfaphenazole prolong the half-life of phenytoin and warfarin, probably by inhibition of hepatic metabolism. Sulfadiazine prolongs the half-life of tolbutamide. In addition, the sulfonamides may increase the effect of coumarin anticoagulants by depression of the intestinal bacterial flora that produce vitamin K.

Review

Weinstein, L., Madoff, M. A., et al. The sulfonamides. *N. Engl. J. Med.* 263:793–799, 842–849, and 900–907, 1960.

References

1. Andreasen, F. Protein binding of drugs in plasma from patients with acute renal failure. *Acta Pharmacol. Toxicol.* 32:417–429, 1973.
2. Bünger, P., Diller, W., et al. Vergleichende Untersuchungen an neueren Sulfanilamiden. *Arzneim. Forsch.* 11:247–255, 1961.
3. Craig, W. A., and Kunin, C. M. Trimethoprim-sulfamethoxazole: pharmacodynamic effects of urinary pH and impaired renal function. *Ann. Intern. Med.* 78:491–497, 1973.
4. Kaplan, S. A., Weinfeld, R. E., et al. Pharmacokinetic profile of sulfisoxazole following intravenous, intramuscular, and oral administration to man. *J. Pharm. Sci.* 61:773–778, 1972.
5. Kremers, P., Duvivier, J., et al. Pharmacokinetic studies of

cotrimoxazole in man after single and repeated doses. *J. Clin. Pharmacol.* 14:112–117, 1974.

6. Nelson, E., and O'Reilly, I.   Kinetics of sulfamethyl-thiadiazole acetylation and excretion in humans. *J. Pharm. Sci.* 50:417–420, 1961.

7. Ohnhaus, E. E., and Spring, P.   Elimination kinetics of sul-fadiazine in patients with normal and impaired renal func-tion. *J. Pharmacokin. Biopharm.* 3:171–179, 1975.

8. Taraszka, M. J., and Delor, R. A.   Effect of dissolution rate of sulfamethazine from tablets on absorption and excretion of sulfamethazine. *J. Pharm. Sci.* 58:207–210, 1969.

9. White, T. A., and Evans, D. A. P.   The acetylation of sul-famethazine and sulfamethoxypyridazine by human subjects. *Clin. Pharmacol. Ther.* 9:80–88, 1968.

TERBUTALINE

A noncatechol, highly selective beta-2-adrenergic stimulant used as a bronchodilator in the treatment of reversible airway obstruc-tion [6], including obstruction induced by exercise [5]. Stimulates adenylcyclase activity, increasing $3' : 5'$-cAMP in the bronchial wall. Prevents uterine contractions at full-term [1] and also over-comes midtrimester uterine contractions produced by prosta-glandin $F_{2\alpha}$ and intrauterine hypertonic saline [2].

Absorption

Oral bioavailabilities of tablet and elixir are comparable, i.e., about 45% [7]. The use of a pro-drug, ibuterol, appears to en-hance substantially the amount of terbutaline absorbed [3]. t_{max}: unknown, but maximum effect occurs 2 hours after an oral dose [4]. First-pass metabolism of terbutaline appears to be significant.

Distribution

V_d: unknown. Protein binding: unknown.

Elimination

$t_{\frac{1}{2}}$: unknown. Exact metabolism: unknown. Catechol-0-methyltransferase is not involved in metabolism, which appears responsible for the prolonged duration of action of 4–8 hours.

Dosage Schedule

Inhalations: 1–2 puffs (0.25–0.5 mg) as required, or every 6 or 8 hours for regular prophylaxis. No more than 12 puffs in 24 hours.
    Oral: 2.5–5.0 mg every 8 hours as tablets or elixir.
    Injection: 0.25–0.5 mg subcutaneously as required.

Special Dosage Situations

Use cautiously in the elderly and in patients with known ischemic heart disease. No available special information about use in women during pregnancy or lactation or in patients with renal or hepatic disease. Children: 25–50 μg/kg as elixir every 8 hours.

Therapeutic Concentrations

No available information. For chronic management of reversible airway obstruction, it is advisable to assess changes in respiratory function by objective tests.

Adverse Reactions

Tremulousness, apprehension, occasional palpitations, flushing, and headache. Excessive doses produce tachycardia, which may be detrimental to patients with angina pectoris. Blood glucose level may rise slightly [4].

Interactions

Adverse effects are likely to be aggravated by concurrent use of other sympathomimetic drugs and theophylline.

References

1. Andersson, K.-E., Bengtsson, L. P., et al. The relaxing effect of terbutaline on the human uterus during term labor. *Am. J. Obstet. Gynecol.* 121:602–609, 1975.
2. Andersson, K.-E., and Bengtsson, L. P. Terbutaline inhibition of midtrimester uterine activity induced by prostaglandin F_2 alpha and hypertonic saline. *Br. J. Obstet. Gynaecol.* 82:745–749, 1975.
3. Arner, B., and Magnusson, P. O. Comparison between ibuterol hydrochloride and terbutaline in asthma. *Br. Med. J.* 1:72–74, 1976.
4. Geumei, A., Miller, W. F., et al. Evaluation of a new oral beta-2-adrenoceptor stimulant bronchodilator, terbutaline. *Pharmacology* 13:201–211, 1975.
5. Morse, J. L., Jones, W. L., et al. The effect of terbutaline on exercise-induced asthma. *Am. Rev. Respir. Dis.* 113:89–92, 1976.
6. Sackner, M. A., Greeneltch, M., et al. Bronchodilator effects of terbutaline and epinephrine in obstructive lung disease. *Clin. Pharmacol. Ther.* 16:499–506, 1974.
7. Sitar, D. S., Piafsky, K. M., et al. The relative bioavailability of terbutaline (Bricanyl®) elixir and tablet formulations. *Curr. Ther. Res.* 19:266–273, 1976.

TETRACYCLINES

Water-insoluble, basic, unstable, bacteriostatic polycyclic naphthacene-carboxamide antibiotics. The salts are water-soluble, and the dry powder is stable. The antibacterial spectra of all tetracyclines are the same, with activity against most gram-positive and gram-negative organisms except *Proteus vulgaris* and *Pseudomonas*. Ineffective against viruses, yeasts, and fungi. Mechanism of action is inhibition of protein synthesis by binding to 30 S ribosomal units. Negligible tendency to development of resistance during treatment, but an increasing number of gram-positive cocci have become insensitive to the tetracyclines. Because of toxicity, the tetracyclines should not be used if other less toxic antibiotics are available. Primarily indicated in rickettsial diseases such as Rocky Mountain spotted fever and Q fever and for diseases caused by *Chlamydia* such as lymphogranuloma inguinale, psittacosis, and trachoma. Anaerobic infections are better treated with lincomycin than with the tetracyclines. Erythromycin is preferable for infections caused by *Mycoplasma*. A low dose of 250 mg tetracycline daily has been used for acne vulgaris.

Absorption

Oral bioavailability: 60–80% for tetracycline, chlortetracycline, oxytetracycline, demeclocycline, and methacycline [3, 5], and about 90% for minocycline and doxycycline. Oral t_{max}: 1–3 hours.

Distribution and Elimination

Drug	Protein Binding (%)	$t_{\frac{1}{2}}$ (hr)	% Excreted Unchanged in Urine
Tetracycline [1, 4, 11]	20	6–10	60
Chlortetracycline [4, 11]	60	6–9	15
Oxytetracycline [4, 11]	25	6–9	40
Demeclocycline [1, 4, 6]	50	10–16	40
Methacycline [1, 6]	80	10–16	40
Minocycline [6, 12]	70	15–20	10
Doxycycline [2, 6, 7, 12]	30	14–20[a]	30

[a]Unchanged in renal failure.

V_d: 1–2 L/kg.

The concentration in CSF is 15–30% of the serum concentration [6], even in meningitis. Drug diffuses to joints, pleura, and other tissues. The concentration in fetal circulation is 50–75% and in breast milk, about 75% of the maternal plasma concentration. The biliary concentration is 5–10 times higher than the serum concentration. The renal excretion is by glomerular filtration. The fraction not excreted is metabolized, but details are unknown.

Dosage Schedule

Drug	Daily Dose for Adults (mg)		Daily Dose for Children (mg)[a] (oral only)
	Oral	IV	
Tetracycline	250–500 q6h	500 q12h	6–12/kg q6h
Oxytetracycline	250–500 q6h	500 q12h	6–12/kg q6h
Chlortetracycline	250–500 q6h	500 q12h	6–12/kg q6h
Demeclocycline	300 q12h	. . .	6/kg q12h
Methacycline	300 q12h	. . .	6/kg q12h
Minocycline	100 q12h	100–200	2/kg q12h
Doxycycline	100 q12–24 h	100–200	2/kg q12h

[a]Not recommended in children below the age of 8.

Gastrointestinal irritation during oral treatment; can be minimized by concomitant administration of food, without milk. IM administration is not recommended because of pain and erratic absorption. The tetracyclines should not be used topically except for ophthalmological purposes.

Special Dosage Situations

The tetracyclines should be avoided if possible in patients with renal failure. Contraindicated in women during pregnancy because of increased risk of maternal hepatotoxicity and of damage to the fetus' teeth. If used in the elderly, dosage should be reduced according to the decreased renal function, see Table 1, p. 30. The tetracyclines should never be used intrathecally.

Therapeutic Concentrations

Depends on bacterial strain; usually 1–10 μg/ml.

Adverse Reactions

Skin rashes, urticaria, angioedema, eosinophilia, fever, and serum sickness. Burning of the eyes, black-coated tongue, epigastric pain, nausea, vomiting, diarrhea, and pruritus ani. Liver damage, particularly during pregnancy. Old tablets may result in a Fanconi-like syndrome. Negative nitrogen balance with an increase in blood urea nitrogen is frequent. Phototoxicity has been reported, especially after demeclocycline. Brown discoloration of the teeth and hypoplasia of the enamel may develop in children to 8 years old. Deposits in bones may cause growth retardation. A serious side-effect is superinfection with resistant staphylococci (staphylcoccal enteritis). Tetracyclines are not eliminated by dialysis.

Interactions

Barbiturates and phenytoin shorten the half-life of doxycycline more than 50% [9, 10]. Fe^{++}, Al^{+++}, Ca^{++} and Mg^{++} (iron, milk, and antacids) reduce the bioavailability of the tetracyclines, and the tetracyclines reduce the absorption of Fe^{++} [8]. The use of a tetracycline in combination with methoxyflurane seems to be especially nephrotoxic [5]. The tetracyclines may decrease plasma prothrombin activity in patients who are taking oral anticoagulants by decreasing the intestinal flora that produce vitamin K.

References

1. Doluisio, J. T., and Dittert, L. W.   Influence of repetitive dosing of tetracyclines on biological half-life in serum. *Clin. Pharmacol. Ther.* 10:690–701, 1969.
2. Fabre, J., Pitton, J. S., et al.   Distribution and excretion of doxycycline in man. *Chemotherapy* 11:73–85, 1966.
3. Kunin, C. M.   Comparative serum binding, distribution, and excretion of tetracycline and a new analogue, methacycline. *Proc. Soc.* 110:311–315, 1962.
4. Kunin, C. M., and Finland, M.   Clinical pharmacology of the tetracycline antibiotics. *Clin. Pharmacol. Ther.* 2:51–109, 1961.

5. Kuzucu, E. Y. Methoxyflurane, tetracycline, and renal failure. *J.A.M.A.* 211:1162–1164, 1970.
6. MacDonald, H., Kelly, R., et al. Pharmacokinetic studies on minocycline in man. *Clin. Pharmacol. Ther.* 14:852–861, 1973.
7. Mahon, W. A., Wittenberg, J.-V. P., et al. Studies on the absorption and distribution of doxycycline in normal patients and in patients with severely impaired renal function. *Can. Med. Assoc. J.* 103:1031–1034, 1970.
8. Neuvonen, P. J., Gothoni, G., et al. Interference of iron with the absorption of tetracyclines in man. *Br. Med. J.* 4:532–536, 1970.
9. Neuvonen, P. H., and Pentillä, O. Interaction between doxycycline and barbiturates. *Br. Med. J.* 1:535–536, 1974.
10. Pentillä, O., Neuvonen, P. H., et al. Interaction between doxycycline and some antiepileptic drugs. *Br. Med. J.* 2:470–474, 1974.
11. Spitzy, K. H., and Hitzenberger, G. The distribution volume of some antibiotics. *Antibiotics Annual* 1957–58, 996–1003.
12. Steigbigel, N. H., Reed, C. W., et al. Absorption and excretion of five tetracycline analogues in normal young men. *Am. J. Med. Sci.* 255:296–312, 1968.

THEOPHYLLINE

1, 3-Dimethylxanthine, a relative of caffeine, thought to promote diuresis, cardiac and gastric stimulation, and smooth muscle relaxation by increasing adenosine $3':5'$-cyclic monophosphate (cAMP) by inhibition of phosphodiesterase. Major indications are for reversible airway obstruction and for acute left ventricular failure. May be used in the treatment of biliary and urinary tract colic.

Absorption

Ethanol solution, salt formation (choline theophyllinate), and chemical combination (aminophylline or theophylline ethylenediamine) enhance solubility but do not greatly influence the extent of absorption. Absorption is nearly complete after oral dosage. t_{max}: 1–3 hours; 3–6 hours for slow-release preparations. Rectal absorption is variable, and local irritation is troublesome. Administration of theophylline by the IM route is very painful, and therefore this route is not used.

Distribution

V_d: 0.3–0.6 L/kg [4, 5]. Protein binding: about 15%.

Elimination

$t_{\frac{1}{2}}$: 3–9 hours [3, 5]. Theophylline is partly demethylated and oxidized, although xanthinoxidase is apparently not involved. 1-methyluric acid (16%) and 1,3-dimethyluric acid, which are very soluble (unlike uric acid), methylxanthines (36%), which are probably inactive, and unchanged drug (8%) are excreted, mainly in urine [2]. Cigarette-smoking reduces $t_{\frac{1}{2}}$, probably by enzyme induction [3].

Dosage Schedule

The theophylline content of individual compounds is important [1]. Aminophylline (80% theophylline): a loading dose of 5–6 mg/kg IV over 20 minutes that is followed by a maintenance dose 0.9 mg/kg/hr by IV infusion should produce a plasma theophylline concentration 5–15 μg/ml in 95% of individuals [6] (see Special Dosage Situations). Oral dosage: 10–15 mg/kg/day theophylline equivalent in 3 or 4 doses.

Special Dosage Situations

Young children are considered susceptible to CNS effects such as excitement. Diuresis and vomiting may produce dehydration, which is especially dangerous in this age group. In children, only half the adult dose per kilogram of body weight is recommended, with cautious adjustment according to patient's response. Use requires care in patients with advanced liver disease or heart failure, since unusually high plasma levels are reported under these circumstances [8]. No specific precautions for use in the elderly, in women during pregnancy, or in patients with renal disease.

Therapeutic Concentrations

5–20 μg/ml plasma [6]. It is usual to monitor clinical response objectively by respiratory function tests.

Adverse Reactions

Mainly excessive pharmacological effects such as nausea, dyspepsia, tachycardia, vomiting, dehydration, cardiac arrhythmias, convulsions [7, 8], and coma. Anoxia and acidosis are said to aggravate toxicity.

Toxicity is treated according to symptoms. Acidosis and anoxia should be relieved. Any measure that may make a basic cardiopulmonary disorder worse, e.g., sodium and fluid load, oxygen therapy, sedative tranquilizers, antihistamine antiemetics, and antiarrhythmic agents with beta-blocking activity, should be carefully monitored.

Interactions

Care must be exercised if theophylline is used with catecholamines and other sympathomimetic amines that potentiate tachyarrhythmias.

Review

Salem, H., and Jackson, R. H. Oral theophylline preparations. A review of their clinical efficacy in the treatment of bronchial asthma. *Ann. Allergy* 32:189–199, 1974.

References

1. Eddy, E. F., and Eddy, E. D. Anhydrous theophylline equivalence of commercial theophylline formulations. *J. Allergy Clin. Immunol.* 53:116–119, 1974.
2. Jenne, J. W., Nagasawa, H. T., et al. Relationship of urinary metabolites of theophylline to serum theophylline levels. *Clin. Pharmacol. Ther.* 19:375–381, 1972.

3. Jenne, J. W., Nagasawa, H. T., et al.   Decreased theophylline half-life in cigarette smokers. *Life Sci.* 17:195–198, 1975.
4. Mitenko, P. A., and Ogilvie, R. I.   Rapidly achieved plasma concentration plateaus, with observations on theophylline kinetics. *Clin. Pharmacol. Ther.* 13:329–335, 1972.
5. Mitenko, P. A., and Ogilvie, R. I.   Pharmacokinetics of intravenous theophylline. *Clin. Pharmacol. Ther.* 14:509–513, 1973.
6. Mitenko, P. A., and Ogilvie, R. I.   Rational intravenous doses of theophylline. *N. Engl. J. Med.* 289:600–603, 1973.
7. Yarnell, P. R., and Nai-Shin Chu: Focal seizures and aminophylline. *Neurology* 25:819–822, 1975.
8. Zwillich, C. W., Sutton, F. D., Jr., et al.   Theophylline-induced seizures in adults. Correlation with serum concentrations. *Ann. Intern. Med.* 82:784–787, 1975.

THIAZIDE DIURETICS

Sulfanilamide derivatives that exert their diuretic action by the inhibition of sodium and chloride reabsorption at the distal convoluted tubule of the kidneys. In high dosages these drugs are carbonic anhydrase inhibitors, but this action is insignificant at usual dosage levels. Administration of the thiazide diuretics results in increased excretion of sodium, potassium, chloride, and bicarbonate. Sodium and free-water clearance increase equally. Renal blood flow and glomerular filtration rate are not increased, but plasma volume is decreased acutely. Although not as effective as diuretics as furosemide, the thiazide diuretics are indicated for use in all forms of edema, in ascites, and as hypotensives. Also specifically indicated for the management of nephrogenic and partial pituitary diabetes insipidus and in the treatment of calcium nephrolithiasis (but not hypercalcemia; see Furosemide, p. 177).

Although the potencies of the various thiazide diuretics vary, the maximal response obtainable is the same for each drug. The mechanisms of action and side-effects are also identical, and therefore the thiazides will be dealt with as a group.

Absorption

Oral bioavailability: 60–90%. t_{max}: 1–3 hours. Onset of action: 1 hour after oral dose [1, 3].

Distribution

V_d: unknown. Protein binding: about 99% [8]. All cross placenta in humans [9].

Elimination

$t_{\frac{1}{2}}$ of the short-acting diuretics appears to be 1–4 hours [3, 4, 9]. All thiazide diuretics are believed to be excreted unchanged by the proximal convoluted tubule of the kidneys. They compete for transport sites with para-aminohippuric acid and the penicillins, and their secretion is in turn inhibited by probenecid. $t_{\frac{1}{2}}$ of chlorothiazide: 13 hours [3].

The duration of action of most of the thiazides is about 12

hours, with the exception of quinethazone[a] (18
methylclothiazide (24 hours), polythiazide (24 hours
thalidone[a] (48 hours).

Dosage Schedule

Type of Thiazide Diuretic	Daily Dose
Chlorothiazide	500–1500 mg/day
Hydrochlorothiazide	50–150 mg/day
Hydroflumethiazide	50–150 mg/day
Bendrofluazide	5–10 mg/day
Cyclopenthiazide	2–4 mg/day
Methylclothiazide	5–10 mg/day
Polythiazide	2–8 mg/day
Quinethazone[a]	50–150 mg/day
Chlorthalidone[a]	50–100 mg/day or every second day

[a]Although they are structurally not true thiazides, quinethazone and chlorthalidone are conveniently included here.

Special Dosage Situations

Use cautiously in patients with hepatic failure and those undergoing digitalis therapy; in these circumstances hypokalemia may become a problem. Patients with hepatic failure or patients who are receiving digitalis therapy should be given potassium supplements of 40 mEq potassium daily. Use carefully in patients with gout or with renal insufficiency, in whom exacerbations of the illness may be provoked, and in women during pregnancy, in whom hyponatremia occurs frequently in both the mother and the neonate [7]. The thiazides are contraindicated as diuretics in patients with severe renal failure, since these drugs are unlikely to be effective in this situation.

Therapeutic Concentrations

No available data.

Adverse Reactions

Metabolic side-effects include hypochloremic alkalosis, hypokalemia, hypomagnesemia, and hyponatremia. Hypokalemia may occasionally be severe enough to provoke flaccid paresis or hypokalemic nephropathy. Hyperglycemia and hyperuricemia, which are generally thought to be clinically insignificant, azotemia, and hyperammonemia are other side-effects.

Systemic side-effects, although rare, include skin rashes, photosensitivity, pancreatitis, intrahepatic cholestasis, bone marrow depression, especially thrombocytopenia, neonatal hemolytic anemia (caused by maternal ingestion of the drug), acute pulmonary edema [2], the development of serum antinuclear factor [5], and increased serum triglyceride and pre-beta-lipoprotein concentrations [6].

Interactions

Hypokalemia may potentiate digitalis toxicity and skeletal muscle relaxants. Action of oral hypoglycemics is counteracted by the thiazides, and the dose of these drugs may have to be increased.

Reviews

Beyer, K. H., and Baer, J. E.   Physiological basis for the action of newer diuretic agents. *Pharmacol. Rev.* 13:571–562, 1961.
Lant, A. F., and Wilson, C. M.   Diuretics. In D. A. K. Black (Ed.), *Renal Disease.* Oxford, Eng.: Blackwell, 1973. Pp.655–704.

References

1. Anderson, K. V., Brettell, H. R., et al. C^{14}-labeled hydrochlorothiazide in human beings. *Arch. Int. Med.* 107:736–742, 1961.
2. Beaudry, C., and Laplante, L.   Severe allergic pneumonitis from hydrochlorothiazide. *Ann. Int. Med.* 78:251–253, 1973.
3. Beermann, B.   Absorption, metabolism, and excretion of hydrochlorothiazide. *Clin. Pharmacol. Ther.* 19:531–537, 1976.
4. Brettell, H. R., Smith, J. G., et al. S^{35}-labeled bendroflumethiazide in human beings. *Arch. Int. Med.* 113:373–377, 1964.
5. Feltkamp, T. E. W., Mees, E. J. D., et al.   Autoantibodies related to treatment with chlorthalidone and alpha-methyldopa. *Acta Med. Scand.* 187:219–223, 1970.
6. Johnson, B., Bye, C., et al.   The relation of antihypertensive treatment to plasma lipids and other vascular risk factors in hypertensives (abstract). *Clin. Sci. Mol. Med.* 47:9, 1974.
7. Lindheimer, M. D., and Katz, A. I.   Sodium and diuretics in pregnancy. *N. Engl. J. Med.* 288:891–894, 1973.
8. Sellers, E. M., and Koch-Weser, J.   Binding of diazoxide and other benzothiadiazines to human albumin. *Biochem. Pharmacol.* 23:553–894, 1974.
9. Vandenheuvel, W. J. A., Gruber, V. F., et al.   GLC analysis of hydrochlorothiazide in blood and plasma. *J. Pharm. Sci.* 64:1309–1312, 1975.

THYROXINE (T₄) AND TRIIODOTHYRONINE (T₃)

Hormones produced by the thyroid gland. These hormones increase cellular oxygen uptake, elevating basal metabolic rate, and increase the uptake of adenosine diphosphate (ADP) by mitochondria, but biochemical mechanism of the calorigenic action is unknown. Used in replacement therapy for hypothyroidism (myxedema) and in suppression of nontoxic goiter. Only the L-isomers are used. Daily production is about 75 μg thyroxine and 25–50 μg triiodothyronine. Triiodothyronine (T₃) is about 5 times more potent than thyroxine (T₄).

Absorption

Oral bioavailability of T_4: 50–75%. Oral bioavailability of T_3: 90–95% [2, 3]. Unchanged by hypothyroidism [7]. T_3 can be given by IV route.

Distribution

	T_4	T_3
V_d [4]	0.1–0.2 L/kg	0.6 L/kg
Protein binding [1]	99.95%	99.5%

Thyroxine achieves equal concentrations in mother and fetus.

Elimination

$t_{\frac{1}{2}}$ of T_4: 6–7 days, decreased to 3–4 days in hyperthyroidism and increased to 9–10 days in hypothyroidism [8]. $t_{\frac{1}{2}}$ of T_3: 1–1.5 days, decreased to about 0.8 day in hyperthyroidism [9]. The liver conjugates about 30% of T_4 (and possibly T_3) to glucuronide and sulfate and excretes the conjugates into the bile. Some T_4 is converted to T_3 in peripheral tissues [6]. A major fraction of both hormones is deiodinated and deaminated to thyroacetic and thyropropionic acid derivatives and thyronine [5].

Dosage Schedule

Main indication for T_3 is myxedematous coma. Combined treatment with both hormones has not been shown to be superior to treatment with thyroxine alone in patients with hypothyroidism. 100 μg synthetic T_4 is equivalent to 60 mg thyroid extract (crude extract from powdered thyroid glands obtained from pigs).

Hypothyroidism

0.05–0.1 mg daily initially. Increase dose every 3–6 weeks up to maintenance dose of 0.15–0.30 mg daily. Treatment is lifelong and is controlled by clinical assessment and measurement of serum thyroxine and thyroid-stimulating hormone (TSH).

Nontoxic (Diffuse) Goiter

0.2–0.3 mg daily. Maximal response usually within 3 months. After discontinuation of therapy (1–2 years), there is often a return to pretreatment size of the gland. The treatment is of little value in nodular goiter.

Triiodothyronine in Myxedema Coma

25–100 μg IV daily, depending on cardiac status.

Thyrotoxicosis

0.1–0.3 mg daily in conjunction with fully suppressing doses of propylthiouracil, carbimazole, or methimazole.

Special Dosage Situations

Children: daily dose of thyroxine is reduced. Below 1 year of age: 25–50 μg. From 2–5 years of age: 50–100 μg. Above 5 years of age: 100–200 μg.

Pregnancy and lactation: no dosage adjustments. Elderly and patients with ischemic heart disease: start with 0.025 mg on alternate days and increase dose very slowly. Renal or hepatic failure: no available information about dosage adjustments.

Therapeutic Concentrations

Normal values of T_4: 4–13 μg/100 ml. Normal values of T_3: 70–160 ng/100 ml. Goal of therapy is to reduce TSH to normal level and restore euthyroid clinical state.

Adverse Reactions

Clinical signs of hyperthyroidism. Angina pectoris and myocardial infarction in the elderly and in patients with heart disease if initial dose is increased too rapidly. Overdose can be treated with beta blockers.

Interactions

Phenytoin, androgens, and salicylates result in low values of total thyroxine and estrogens in elevated values. In all cases, unbound thyroxine is unchanged, and no dose adjustments are required.

Reviews

Pappenheimer, J. R. (Ed.). *Handbook of Physiology.* Section F, Endocrinology. Vol. III, Thyroid. Washington, D.C.: American Physiological Society, 1974. Pp. 1–491.

Larsen, P. R.   Triiodothyronine: Review of recent studies of its physiology and pathophysiology in man. *Metabolism* 21:1073–1092, 1972.

Oddie, T. H., Meade, J. H., et al.   An analysis of published data on thyroxine turnover in human subjects. *J. Clin. Endocrinol. Metab.* 26:425–436, 1966.

References

1.   Brown-Grant, K., Brennan, R. D., et al.   Simulation of thyroid hormone-binding protein interactions in human plasma. *J. Clin. Endocrinol.* 30:733–751, 1970.

2.   Hays, M. T.   Absorption of oral thyroxine in man. *J. Clin. Endocrinol.* 28:749–756, 1968.

3.   Hays, M. T.   Absorption of triiodothyronine in man. *J. Clin. Endocrinol.* 30:675–677, 1970.

4.   Nicoloff, J. T., Low, J. C., et al.   Simultaneous measurements of thyroxine and triiodothyronine peripheral turnover kinetics in man. *J. Clin. Invest.* 51:473–483, 1971.

5.   Pittman, C. S., Buck, M. W., et al.   Urinary metabolites of ¹⁴C-labeled thyroxine in man. *J. Clin. Invest.* 51:1759–1766, 1972.

6.   Pittman, C. S., Chambers, J. B., et al.   The extra thyroidal conversion rate of thyroxine to triiodothyronine in normal man. *J. Clin. Invest.* 50:1187–1196, 1971.

7. Read, D. G., Hays, M. T., et al. Absorption of oral thyroxine in hypothyroid and normal man. *J. Clin. Endocrinol.* 30:798–799, 1970.
8. Sterling, K., and Chodos, R. B. Radiothyroxine turnover studies in myxedema, thyrotoxicosis, and hypermetabolism without endocrine disease. *J. Clin. Invest.* 35:806–813, 1956.
9. Woeber, K. A., Sobel, R. J., et al. The peripheral metabolism of triiodothyronine in normal subjects and in patients with hypothyroidism. *J. Clin. Invest.* 49:643–649, 1970.

TOLBUTAMIDE

A short-acting sulfonylurea with hypoglycemic action mediated, at least initially, by stimulation of pancreatic insulin release. Indicated in the treatment of patients with nonketotic adult-onset diabetes, with functioning islet tissue, and in whom reduction of weight and restriction of carbohydrates have been unsuccessful in controlling hyperglycemia. The IV tolbutamide stimulation test has been used as a test of diabetic status [9] and in the diagnosis of insulinoma.

Absorption
Oral bioavailability: 85–100% [1, 7]. t_{max}: 2–3 hours [6].

Distribution
V_d: 0.1–0.15 L/kg [1, 4]. Protein binding: 88% [4]. Salivary concentrations bear a direct relationship to plasma concentrations, equal to the fraction of unbound drug (12%) [4].

Elimination
$t_{\frac{1}{2}}$: 4–8 hours [1, 3, 4]. A small amount of unidentified drug or metabolite is excreted in the feces, but the remainder is completely metabolized and excreted in the urine as carboxy derivative (67%) and hydroxymethyl derivative (33%). Both metabolites are apparently inactive [7].

Dosage Schedule
500 mg once or twice daily initially, increased to a maximum of 2 g in 2–4 divided doses.

Special Dosage Situations
Like all sulfonylurea hypoglycemic agents, tolbutamide is *not* indicated in juvenile diabetes mellitus, in patients with ketoacidosis, or in patients who have undergone pancreatectomy. Hepatocellular disease predisposes patients to hypoglycemic reactions. Congestive heart failure, malignant disease, or other severe intercurrent illnesses tend to prolong elimination half-life, while a history of heavy alcohol consumption may be associated with a reduction in elimination half-life [5]. No dosage adjustment necessary in patients with renal disease. Diabetic control may require insulin during acute intercurrent illness. Occasionally, sulfonylureas are used in conjunction with insulin in the chronic management of labile diabetics.

294   11: Drug Profiles   Tolbutamide

Therapeutic Concentrations

It is usual to monitor the blood glucose response. This control is especially important during acute illness and following dosage adjustments.

Adverse Reactions

Gastrointestinal disturbance and skin rash are fairly common. Cholestatic jaundice and depression of bone marrow are rare. Hypoglycemic reactions are generally less prolonged than with chlorpropamide, but nevertheless they require careful observation.

Cardiovascular mortality may be higher in patients treated with sulfonylureas and dietary control than with diet alone or diet and insulin [8], although these findings remain controversial [2].

Interactions

If alcohol is consumed by the patient while taking tolbutamide the "disulfiram reaction" may occur, but this reaction appears to be less frequent than when chlorpropamide is taken for diabetes. Elimination half-life prolonged 50% by sulfamethizole [3]. A number of other interactions are described, but their significance is uncertain. Chloramphenicol, dicumarol, phenylbutazone, propranolol, and salicylates may enhance the hypoglycemic effect of the sulfonylureas, while corticosteroids, thiazides, and hydantoins may antagonize this effect.

References

1. Andreasen, P. B., and Vesell, E. S.   Comparison of plasma levels of antipurine, tolbutamide, and warfarin after oral and intravenous administration. *Clin. Pharmacol. Ther.* 16:1059–1065, 1974.
2. Feinstein, A. R.   Clinical biostatistics *XXXV*. The persistent clinical failures and fallacies of the UGDP study. *Clin. Pharmacol. Ther.* 19:78–93, 472–485, 1976.
3. Lumholtz, B., Siersbaek-Nielsen, K., et al.   Sulfamethizole-induced inhibition of diphenylhydantoin, tolbutamide, and warfarin metabolism. *Clin. Pharmacol. Ther.* 17:731–734, 1975.
4. Matin, S. G., Suk, H. W., et al.   Pharmacokinetics of tolbutamide: Prediction by concentration in saliva. *Clin. Pharmacol. Ther.* 16:1052–1058, 1974.
5. Sotaniemi, E. A., and Huhti, E.   Half-life of intravenous tolbutamide in the serum of patients in medical wards. *Ann. Clin. Res.* 6:146–154, 1974.
6. Stowers, J. M., Constable, L. W., et al.   A clinical and pharmacological comparison of chlorpropamide and other sulfonylureas. *Ann. N.Y. Acad. Sci.* 74:689–695, 1959.
7. Thomas, R. C., and Ikeda, G. J.   The metabolic fate of tolbutamide in man and in the rat. *J. Med. Chem.* 9:507–510, 1966.
8. University Group Diabetes Program.   A study of the effects of hypoglycemic agents on vascular complications in patients

with adult-onset diabetes. *Diabetes* 19(Suppl. 2):747–830, 1970.

9. Zarowitz, H., and Eis, B.   The role of a tolbutamide tolerance test in the detection of the mild diabetic state: A preliminary report. *Ann. N.Y. Acad. Sci.* 74:662–666, 1959.

TRIMETHOPRIM AND SULFAMETHOXAZOLE
(Co-trimoxazole)

Antimicrobial combination that interferes with bacterial folic acid metabolism significantly better than either agent given alone. Sulfamethoxazole, a sulfonamide, competes with para-aminobenzoic acid (PABA), inhibiting dihydrofolate synthesis. Trimethoprim, a basic diaminopyrimidine, directly inhibits dihydrofolate reductase, preventing the production of tetrahydrofolic acid from dihydrofolic acid. Two consecutive essential steps are blocked, and bacteria are deprived of materials required for nucleoprotein and amino acid production.

Bacteriostatic or bactericidal, depending on tissue level of drug and on infecting organism. Essentially broad-spectrum; major indications include the treatment of gram-negative infections of respiratory and urinary tract. Usually sensitive species include *Hemophilus influenzae, Escherichia coli, Proteus mirabilis,* indole-positive *Proteus, Klebsiella, Neisseria gonorrhea,* some *Streptococci* and *Staphylococci, Nocardia, Actinomycetes,* and *Pneumocystis.* Little activity against *Pseudomonas, Mycobacterium,* or *Treponema pallidum.*

Absorption

Oral bioavailability: 100%. t_{max}: 1–4 hours for each component [3].

Distribution

V_d: not well defined. Protein binding for sulfamethoxazole: 64%. Protein binding for trimethoprim: 44% [5]. At equilibrium the trimethoprim sulfamethoxazole ratio in blood is 1:20.

Elimination

Sulfamethoxazole ($t_{\frac{1}{2}}$: 10 hours) [2] is metabolized in the liver by acetylation and glucuronidation. Parent drug (30–50%) and metabolites excreted in the urine by both filtration and tubular secretion. Trimethoprim ($t_{\frac{1}{2}}$: 10 hours) [5] has 4 metabolites; apparently none is active. Parent drug (65–70%) and metabolites are excreted in the urine, also by filtration and tubular secretion. Urine volume and pH changes may produce changes in the urinary ratio of the two drugs [6].

Dosage Schedule

Preparations contain a 5:1 ratio of sulfamethoxazole and trimethoprim. Most susceptible infections respond to 800 mg sulfamethoxazole and 160 mg trimethoprim (e.g., 2 tablets) given at 12-hour intervals for 8–14 days.

Special Dosage Situations

In patients with renal failure reduce dosage: if creatinine clearance is less than 10 ml/min, give a loading dose of 2 tablets and a maintenance dose of 1 tablet daily; if creatinine clearance is 10–30 ml/min, give 1 tablet every 12 hours. Uremic patients, even patients with normal concentrations of plasma proteins, have reduced protein binding of sulfonamides [1], but trimethoprim (a basic drug) is probably not affected. Little available information about dosage in children and in women during pregnancy or lactation.

Therapeutic Concentrations

Depends on microorganism. In vitro individual minimum inhibitory concentrations (MIC) are 0.25–4 μg/ml (trimethoprim) and 50–200 μg/ml sulfamethoxazole. Synergistic activity of the agents complicates the assessment of therapeutic concentrations in vivo.

Adverse Reactions

Allergic reactions (particularly to sulfonamide component) include urticaria, pruritus, periorbital edema, erythema multiforme, exfoliative dermatitis, Stevens-Johnson syndrome, serum sickness, and anaphylaxis. Blood dyscrasias include depression of all formed elements (important to note sore throats early), megaloblastic anemia, methemoglobinemia, and hypoprothrombinemia. Other adverse effects include glossitis, stomatitis, and gastrointestinal disturbances; and peripheral neuropathy, convulsions, ataxia, tinnitus, vertigo, and other nonspecific neurological complaints. Renal damage, periarteritis nodosa, and lupus erythematosus phenomenon may occur.

Interactions

Prolongation of phenytoin $t_{\frac{1}{2}}$ and possible enhancement of warfarin activity suggest that co-trimoxazole may be an inhibitor of drug metabolism [4]. Destruction of organisms in the gut that produce vitamin K is another possible mechanism for increasing anticoagulant action. Clinical relevance uncertain at present.

Review

Garrod, L. P., James, D. G., et al. (Eds.). The synergy of trimethoprim and sulphonamides. *Postgrad. Med. J.* 45(Nov. Suppl.):1–104, 1969.

References

1. Anton, A. H., and Corey, W. T.   Plasma protein binding of sulfonamides in anephric patients. *Fed. Proc.* 30:629, 1971.
2. Bünger, P., Diller, W., et al. Vergleichende Untersuchungen an neueren Sulfanilamiden. *Arzneim. Forsch.* 11:247–255, 1961.
3. Craig, W. A., and Kunin, C. M.   Trimethoprim/sulfamethoxazole: Pharmacodynamic effects of urinary pH and impaired renal function. *Ann. Intern. Med.* 78:491–498, 1973.

4. Mølholm Hansen, J., Siersbaek-Nielsen, K., et al. Potentiation of warfarin by co-trimoxazole. *Br. Med. J.* 2:684, 1975.
5. Schwartz, D. E., and Ziegler, W. H. Assay and pharmacokinetics of trimethoprim in man and animals. *Postgrad. Med. J.* 45(Nov. Suppl.):32–37, 1969.
6. Sharpstone, P. The renal handling of trimethoprim and sulphamethoxazole in man. *Postgrad. Med. J.* 45(Nov. Suppl.):38–42, 1969.

VALPROATE SODIUM
(Dipropylacetate sodium)

Sodium salt of N-dipropylacetic acid. Anticonvulsant, which is most effective in the treatment of absence seizures and also shows promise in the management of partial and tonic-clonic seizures. Usually administered as the sodium salt but magnesium salt and amide are also available. It is known to cause small elevations of brain levels of the synaptic inhibitor gamma-aminobutyric acid (GABA), by inhibiting GABA transaminase [7], but whether this represents its mechanism of action remains unclear.

Absorption
Oral bioavailability: unknown. t_{max}: 1–4 hours for sodium valproate and 3–6 hours for the amide.

Distribution
V_d: 0.15–0.40 L/kg [6]. Protein binding: 90% [2, 3]. Breast milk concentration is about 10% of plasma concentration [3].

Elimination
$t_{\frac{1}{2}}$: 8–15 hours [4]. No available information about metabolism in human beings.

Dosage Schedule
3–30 mg/kg/day. Average adult dosage is about 1200 mg/day.

Special Dosage Situations
Children: 15–60 mg/kg/day. No available information about dosage adjustment in patients with renal or hepatic disease, in the elderly, and in women during pregnancy or lactation.

Therapeutic Concentrations
No clear relationship has yet been established between plasma levels, dosage, and optimal efficacy. A level of 60–100 μg/ml is associated with suppression of seizures [6].

Adverse Reactions
Transient anorexia, nausea, and vomiting in about 15% of patients but generally not severe enough to require cessation of treatment.

Interactions

Increases phenobarbital levels by 35–200% [5, 6] and lowers serum phenytoin levels [1].

Review

Simon, D., and Penry, J. K.   Sodium di-N-propylacetate (DPA) in the treatment of epilepsy. A review. *Epilepsia* 16:549–573, 1975.

References

1. Bardy, A., Hari, R., et al.   Valproate may lower serum-phenytoin. *Lancet* 2:1297–1298, 1976.
2. Espir, M. L. E., Benton, P., et al.   Sodium valproate (Epilim)—some clinical and pharmacological aspects. In N. J. Legg (Ed.), *Clinical and Pharmacological Aspects of Sodium Valproate (Epilim) in the Treatment of Epilepsy*. London: MCS Consultants, 1976. Pp. 146–151.
3. Jordan, B. J., Shillingford, J. S., et al.   Preliminary observations on the protein binding and enzyme inducing properties of sodium valproate (Epilim). In N. J. Legg (Ed.), *Clinical and Pharmacological Aspects of Sodium Valproate (Epilim) in the Treatment of Epilepsy*. London: MCS Consultants, 1976. Pp. 112–118.
4. Loiseau, P., Brachet, A., et al.   Concentration of dipropylacetate in plasma. *Epilepsia* 16:609–615, 1975.
5. Richens, A., and Ahmad, S.   Controlled trial of sodium valproate in severe epilepsy. *Br. Med. J.* 4:255–256, 1975.
6. Schobben, F., van der Kleijn, E., et al.   Pharmacokinetics of dipropylacetate in epileptic patients. *Eur. J. Clin. Pharmacol.* 8:97–105, 1975.
7. Simler, S., Ciesielski, L., et al.   Effect of sodium N-dipropylacetate on audiogenic seizures and brain gamma-aminobutyric acid level. *Biochem. Pharmacol.* 22:1701–1708, 1973.

WARFARIN

A coumarin anticoagulant, antagonizes vitamin K, which is a cofactor in the synthesis of Factors II, VII, IX, and X [6]. Indicated for the management of pulmonary thromboembolic disease, deep venous thrombosis, and prophylactic anticoagulation of cardiac valve prostheses. May also be of value in prevention of systemic embolus (in association with atrial fibrillation in mitral valve disease), vertebrobasilar insufficiency, transient ischemic attacks, and the thrombotic crises of paroxysmal nocturnal hemoglobinuria. No evidence of value in prophylaxis of myocardial infarction [1, 5].

Absorption

Oral bioavailability: 100%.

Distribution

V_d: 0.1 L/kg. Protein binding: 99.5%. Crosses placenta.

Elimination

Warfarin exists as two optical enantiomorphs, (R+) and (S−), which are metabolized differently and have differing anticoagulant potency [6]. Administered clinically as the racemate:

	S−	R+	Racemic
$t_{\frac{1}{2}}$	29–37 hr	48–68 hr	40–44 hr
Metabolites	7-OH warfarin	(+) (−)	
	(−) (−)	Warfarin alcohol	
	Warfarin alcohol	6-OH warfarin	
Potency	+ + + + +	+	

Completely metabolized with first-order kinetics. Metabolites appear in urine for 4 weeks after a single dose. Hydroxy-metabolites have some anticoagulant activity.

Dosage Schedule

Effect of warfarin generally monitored by one-stage prothrombin time [3]. Effect of anticoagulant is dependent on $t_{\frac{1}{2}}$ of clotting factors:

Factor VII	1.5–6 hr
Factor II	60–123 hr
Factors IX, X	20–40 hr

Protime is diminished at 48 hours, but this effect mainly reflects decrease in Factor VII. Full antithrombotic effect may not be achieved for about a week. For this reason, loading doses are not recommended, since they do not speed the onset of complete anticoagulation. Initial dosage should be 5–10 mg/day, and the dosage should be adjusted after 1 week if protime is not satisfactory. Further monitoring of protime is always necessary.

Special Dosage Situations

Patients with severe congestive heart failure or liver failure and the elderly, malnourished, and thyrotoxic are especially sensitive to warfarin. Occasionally resistance to the drug may require high dosage and may indicate either a faster rate of metabolism, which may be congenital or acquired, or congenital resistance to plasma warfarin levels. Warfarin will cause fetal hemorrhage if it is taken up to term during pregnancy. This reaction may be avoided by stopping warfarin 3–4 weeks before term, substituting heparin, and closely controlling clotting time during pregnancy [2].

Therapeutic Concentrations

Prothrombin time twice that of normal.

Adverse Reactions

For hemorrhage, antidote is vitamin K_1 (mephyton) and discontinuation of drug. Necrosis of subcutaneous tissue, alopecia, and osteoporosis may also occur. Absolute contraindication to use of drug is bleeding diathesis; relative contraindications are peptic ulcer and uncontrolled hypertension.

Interactions

Diminished absorption of vitamin K from bowel is caused by antibiotics, which alter bowel flora and increase effectiveness of warfarin. Warfarin is bound in the gut lumen by cholestyramine, which may inhibit its absorption.

Displaced from albumin-binding sites by phenytoin, phenylbutazone, mefenamic acid, oxyphenbutazone, salicylates, and trichloroacetic acid. In all cases, anticoagulation is increased.

Metabolism increased by barbiturates, meprobamate, ethanol, griseofulvin, ethchlorvynol, haloperidol, chloral hydrate, glutethimide, and carbamazepine.

Metabolism inhibited by chloramphenicol, disulfiram, indomethacin, and metronidazole.

Phenylbutazone and metronidazole induce metabolism of (R+) warfarin and inhibits metabolism of (S−) warfarin. Net effect is increase of anticoagulant effect [4].

In all cases, the degree of inhibition or induction is not predictable, and if any of these drugs is to be administered at the same time as warfarin, the protime must be checked frequently.

Obviously care should also be exercised when any of these drugs is discontinued.

References

1. Gifford, R. H., and Feinstein, A. R.   A critique of methodology in studies of anticoagulant therapy for acute myocardial infarction. *N. Engl. J. Med.* 280:351–357, 1969.
2. Hirsh, J., and Cade, J. F.   Anticoagulants in pregnancy: A review of indications and complications. *Am. Heart. J.* 83:301–305, 1972.
3. Ingram, G. I. C.   Symposium standardizing the control of oral anticoagulant treatment. *Thrombos. Diathes. Haemorrh.* 33:142–147, 1975.
4. Lewis, R. L., Trager, W. F., et al.   Warfarin. Stereochemical aspects of its metabolism and the interaction with phenylbutazone. *J. Clin. Invest.* 53:1607–1617, 1974.
5. O'Reilly, R. A.   Vitamin K and oral anticoagulant drugs as competitive antagonists in man. *Pharmacology* 7:149–158, 1972.
6. O'Reilly, R. A.   Studies on the optical enantiomorphs of warfarin in man. *Clin. Pharmacol. Ther.* 16:348–354, 1974.

Index

Boldface type indicates a drug or group of drugs as they are shown in the drug profiles (Chapter 11).